Methods in Narcotics Research

MODERN PHARMACOLOGY-TOXICOLOGY

A Series of Monographs and Textbooks

Additional Volumes in Preparation

Methods in Narcotics Research

Edited by

Seymour Ehrenpreis and Amos Neidle

NEW YORK STATE RESEARCH INSTITUTE
FOR NEUROCHEMISTRY AND DRUG ADDICTION
WARD'S ISLAND, NEW YORK

MARCEL DEKKER, INC. New York

MARCEL DEKKER, INC.
270 Madison Avenue, New York, New York 10016

LIBRARY OF CONGRESS CATALOG CARD NUMBER: 75-23586

ISBN: 0-8247-6308-4

CURRENT PRINTING (last digit): 10 9 8 7 6 5 4 3 2 1

PRINTED IN THE UNITED STATES OF AMERICA

CONTENTS

CONTRIBUTORS

W. MARVIN DAVIS, Department of Pharmacology, School of Pharmacy, The University of Mississippi, University, Mississippi

WILLIAM L. DEWEY, Department of Pharmacology, Medical College of Virginia, Richmond, Virginia

RICHARD DRAWBAUGH, Department of Pharmacology and Toxicology, College of Pharmacy, and Department of Psychology, University of Rhode Island, Kingston, Rhode Island

PETER F. EAST, Searle Laboratories, Department of Biological Research, Chicago, Illinois

SEYMOUR EHRENPREIS, New York State Research Institute for Neurochemistry and Drug Addiction, Ward's Island, New York

M. R. FENNESSY, Department of Pharmacology, University of Melbourne, Parkville, Victoria, Australia

MAX FINK, Health Sciences Center, State University of New York at Stony Brook, Stony Brook, New York

GERALD GIANUTSOS, Department of Pharmacology and Toxicology, College of Pharmacy, University of Rhode Island, Kingston, Rhode Island

STEVEN R. GOLDBERG, Laboratory of Psychobiology, Department of Psychiatry, Harvard Medical School, Boston, Massachusetts, and New England Regional Primate Center, Southborough, Massachusetts

LOUIS S. HARRIS, Department of Pharmacology, Medical College of Virginia, Richmond, Virginia

EIKICHI HOSOYA, Department of Pharmacology, Keio University, School of Medicine, Shinjuku, Tokyo, Japan

RAYMOND W. HOUDE, Analgesic Studies Section, The Sloan-Kettering Institute for Cancer Research, New York, New York

MARTIN HYNES, Department of Pharmacology and Toxicology, College of Pharmacy, University of Rhode Island, Kingston, Rhode Island

YASUKO F. JACQUET, New York State Research Institute for Neurochemistry and Drug Addiction, Ward's Island, New York

NAIM KHAZAN, Department of Pharmacology and Therapeutics, University of Cincinnati Medical Center, and Department of Pharmacology, Merrell-National Laboratories, Cincinnati, Ohio*

HARBANS LAL, Department of Pharmacology and Toxicology and Department of Psychology, University of Rhode Island, Kingston, Rhode Island

JAMES R. LEE, Department of Pharmacology, University of Melbourne, Parkville, Victoria, Australia

W. JOSEPH POTTS, Searle Laboratories, Department of Biological Research, Chicago, Illinois

KENNETH E. RUBENSTEIN, Syva Research Institute, Palo Alto, California

RICHARD S. SCHNEIDER, Syva Research Institute, Palo Alto, California

ERIC J. SIMON, Department of Medicine, New York University Medical Center, New York, New York

JASBIR SINGH, Alcoholism Services Unit, Department of Psychiatry, Charity Hospital of Louisiana, New Orleans, Lousiana**

STANLEY G. SMITH, Department of Pharmacology and Department of Psychology, The University of Mississippi, University, Mississippi

SYDNEY SPECTOR, Roche Institute of Molecular Biology, Nutley, New Jersey

EDWIN ULLMAN, Syva Research Institute, Palo Alto, California

STANLEY L. WALLENSTEIN, Analgesic Studies Section, The Sloan-Kettering Institute for Cancer Research, New York, New York

E. LEONG WAY, Department of Pharmacology, School of Medicine, University of California, San Francisco, California

EDDIE WEI, School of Public Health, University of California, Berkeley, California

---

*Present address: Department of Pharmacology and Toxicology, University of Maryland School of Pharmacy, Baltimore, Maryland.

**Present address: Alcoholism Out-Patient Treatment Clinic, Singh Behavior Therapy Clinic, Metairie, Louisiana.

PREFACE

As members of an institute in which multidisciplinary studies on narcotic drugs are being carried out, we are fortunate in having colleagues familiar with a wide variety of experimental procedures. Nevertheless, the selection of a particular method, even after much discussion, often seems arbitrary, and even simple techniques have led to unexpected problems. We have therefore assembled this collection of articles on narcotic methodology in the hope of providing a more rational basis for experimental design, both for ourselves and for others in the field.

Although no attempt has been made to survey all possible techniques, we have tried to present representative biochemical, pharmacological, and behavioral methods for the measurement of narcotic drug effects. Methods for studying these drugs in man and in laboratory animals as well as at the tissue and molecular level have been included.

Our major concern was whether a given topic would provide useful information for research workers during the early stages of a drug investigation. Particular emphasis has been placed on providing critical evaluations of assay methods, including descriptions of major pitfalls. We also wished to present more detailed descriptions of newer techniques and certain procedures where success or failure depends on strict adherence to protocol.

If this volume eliminates, at least to some extent, the frustrating job of tracking down an experimental procedure from one research report to another and then finding that the description is inadequate or the method inappropriate to the task at hand, our efforts will have been justified.

Seymour Ehrenpreis
Amos Neidle

Methods in Narcotics Research

Part I

METHODS OF DRUG ADMINISTRATION

Chapter 1

A METHOD FOR CHRONIC INTRAVENOUS DRUG ADMINISTRATION IN THE RAT*

STANLEY G. SMITH

Department of Pharmacology
Department of Psychology
The University of Mississippi
University, Mississippi

W. MARVIN DAVIS

Department of Pharmacology
School of Pharmacy
The University of Mississippi
University, Mississippi

*Preparation of this manuscript was supported by USPHS Grant DA 00018-07 from the National Institute of Mental Health and by the Research Institute of Pharmaceutical Sciences, School of Pharmacy, The University of Mississippi, University, Mississippi.

I. INTRODUCTION

The development of chronic intravenous infusion methods for drug self-administration has provided new means for the analysis of narcotic dependence [1-4]. Unfortunately, many laboratories are hindered in taking advantage of these advances because they lack information on cannula construction, surgical techniques, and behavioral apparatus required for self-administration. This chapter is designed to acquaint the interested scientist with these methods and techniques and with some of the required equipment.

II. CANNULA CONSTRUCTION

Chronic intravenous jugular cannulas are used in drug self-administration procedures for infusion of fluids into the precava, near the right atrium of the heart. Infusing the drug solution by this route of administration produces rapid onset of its pharmacological action.

To achieve self-infusion in rats we currently employ two distinct types of jugular cannulas. The first cannula, type I (Fig. 1a), is for short-term research, 2-3 weeks in duration. The second cannula, type II (Fig. 1b), is for long-term experimentation of 3 weeks to 6 months.

A. Type I Cannula

At each stage in assembly of the cannula the reader should refer to Fig. 1a to clarify the instructions in the text. To construct this cannula the following materials are required: polyethylene 20 (PE 20) tubing; Silastic

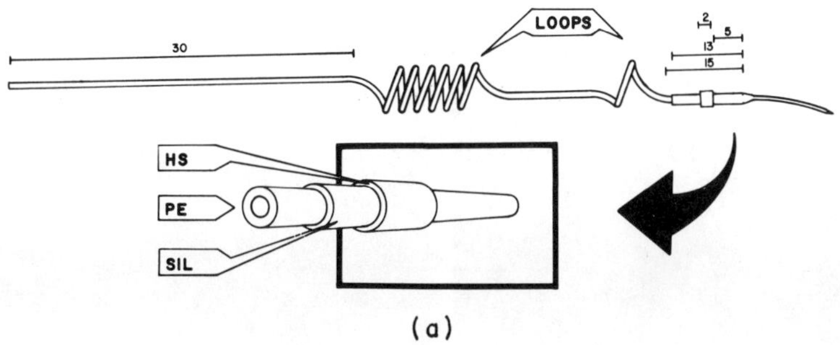

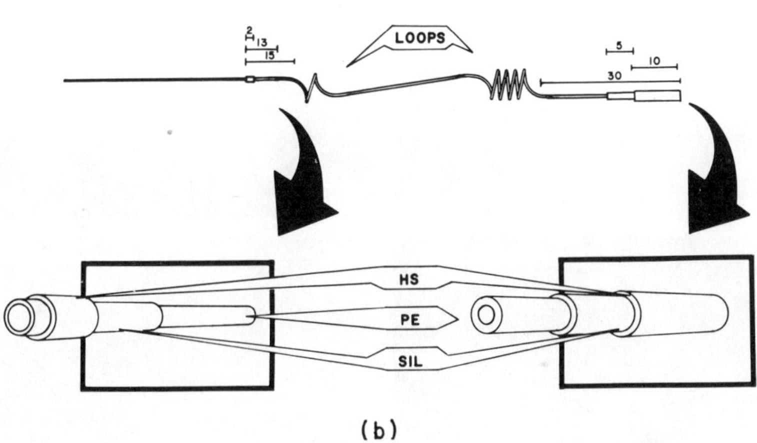

FIGURE 1. (a) Schematic representation in side and extended view of the type I cannula. Measurements from the end of the polyethylene (PE) tubing to the start of the loops are presented. Also shown are distances for placement of Silastic (SIL) and heat-shrinkable (HS) tubing from the end of the PE. (b) Schematic representation of the type II cannula. Views and measurements are similar to those for the type I cannula.

tubing, 0.020 in. i.d. x 0.037 in. o.d.; 1.0-cc tuberculin syringes with 22- and 26-gauge needles; surgical scissors or a scalpel blade; 4-in. x 4-in. (8-ply) surgical gauze sponge; chloroform; pieces of spring wire from 0.007 in. through 0.015 in. in diameter and 30 cm in length; a steel or glass rod 4 mm in diameter; Eastman 910 adhesive; 3/64-in. heat-shrinkable tubing; and a hot-air apparatus. The latter item, shown in Fig. 2a, consists of a 4-in.-long 15-gauge hypodermic needle with the tip ground off. The head of

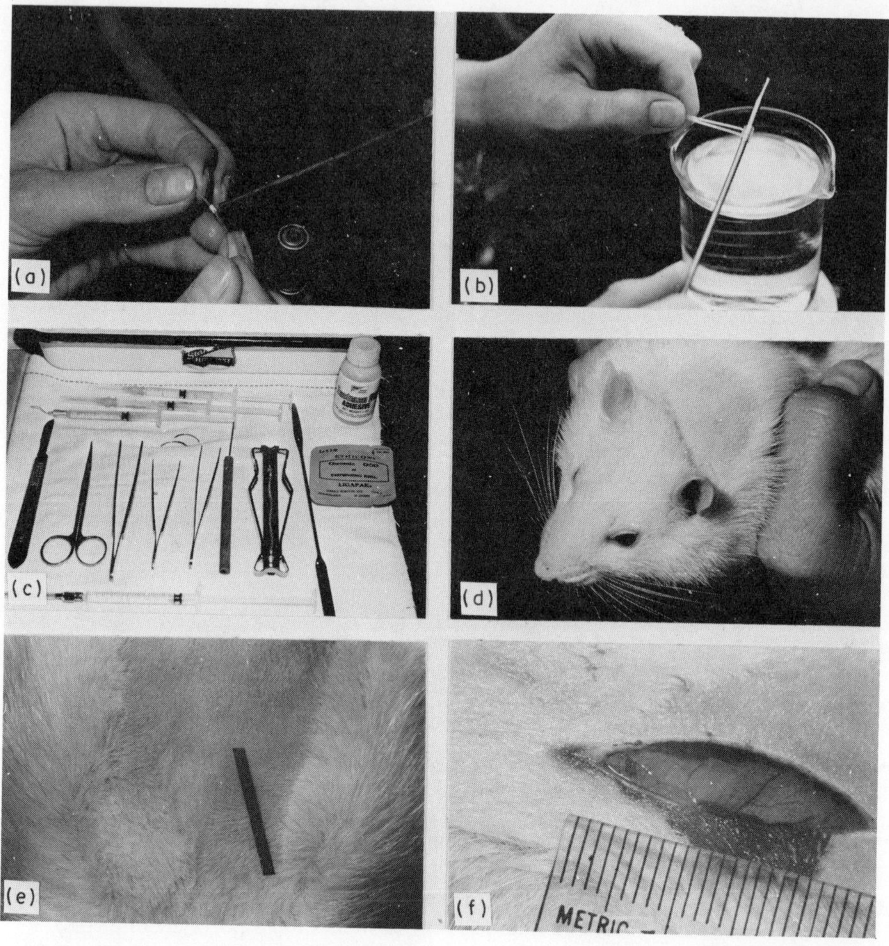

FIGURE 2. (a) The hot-air apparatus. The long metal tubing starting at the right is a 15-gauge needle. The gas burner is seen immediately below the needle. As depicted, the HS should be held directly in front of the tip of the needle. (b) The PE tubing is wound around a rod before immersion successively in hot and cold water to produce loops. (c) Surgical instruments required for cannula implantation. (d) The area to be shaved on the back of the neck. (e) The shaved area on the chest and neck area with the position of the right jugular indicated by the black line. (f) The skin incision to expose the jugular vein.

the needle is attached to an air source by a piece of 1/4-in. x 3/32-in. latex laboratory tubing. A small gas burner placed beneath the needle is used to heat the air flowing through the needle. These components are attached to a ring stand by suitable laboratory clamps.

Cut a 15-cm length of PE 20 tubing and a 4-cm length of 0.020-in.-i.d. x 0.037-in.-o.d. Silastic tubing with sharp surgical scissors or a scalpel blade. Remove all traces of dirt, dust, or oil from PE, Silastic tubing, and fingers by wiping with surgical gauze moistened in chloroform. The next step is to make loops in the PE 20 by wrapping it around a glass or steel rod 4 mm in diameter and then immersing it in boiling water for a few seconds, followed by immersion in cold water (see Fig. 2b). Make four to five loops starting 30 mm from one end and one loop at 15 mm from the other (Silastic to be placed over the 15-mm end).

After completing the loops, place the Silastic into a container of chloroform. Chloroform causes the Silastic to swell to approximately twice its normal size. The enlarged Silastic will fit neatly over the PE 20. Caution: Do not cut the PE 20 with a bevel for easier placement of the Silastic over the PE. A bevel may partly occlude the liquid flow at the PE-Silastic junction, and it can also work through the Silastic and injure the vein wall.

After the PE 20 has dried and the Silastic has expanded, place a few drops of Eastman 910 adhesive completely around and 1 mm back from the end of the PE 20 on which the Silastic is to be slipped. The Eastman 910 adhesive is easily applied from and stored in a 1-cc disposable tuberculin syringe with attached 25-gauge disposable needle. Keep the plastic needle cover over the needle when not in actual use. Remove the Silastic from the chloroform and push it 13 mm up onto the PE 20. When placing Silastic over PE, use a turning motion as this will ensure that the adhesive is spread completely around the PE to provide a full seal. The operation of placing the adhesive on the PE and guiding the Silastic onto it must be carried out quickly, as the cement dries rapidly. Also, the chloroform is volatile, and as it evaporates the Silastic shrinks. After joining the PE and Silastic, allow the chloroform and cement to dry for 2-5 min.

The final step in construction of the cannula is putting the 3/64-in. heat-shrinkable (HS) tubing over the Silastic and PE 20 and reducing it to help secure a liquid-tight bond between the two pieces of tubing. First, find the largest diameter spring wire that easily fits into the lumen of the PE 20 tubing. Then place it into the lumen of the Silastic, moving it up into the lumen of PE tubing until it is 5 mm beyond the Silastic. Cut a 2-mm piece of HS tubing and place it around the Silastic. Slide it up until it is 5 mm beyond the junction of PE 20 and Silastic (see Fig. 1a). The HS tubing is then reduced to form a liquid-tight junction between PE and Silastic by holding it in the stream of hot air flowing from the 15-gauge needle, as shown in Fig. 2a. The cannula is moved back and forth and rotated until the HS fits tightly against the Silastic. Caution: Do not direct the hot-air stream directly onto the PE 20 during this process or it will melt. After the HS is reduced to the desired size, immerse the cannula in cold water for 30 sec. Do not pull the spring wire out of the tubing until after immersing it in cold water, for the PE under the HS tubing will be pliable, and if pinched off before cooling, it may occlude the lumen of the tube.

To test the cannula for leaks, place a saline-filled 1-cc syringe with attached 25- or 26-gauge needle into the lumen of the PE (the end opposite to the Silastic), fill the entire cannula with saline, close off the end of the Silastic by pinching it between two fingers, and then inject 0.02 ml more saline into the cannula while checking for leaks.

B. Type II Cannula

The second cannula (type II) is shown in Fig. 1b. The materials needed for construction of this cannula are nearly identical to those used for the type I cannula except that PE 10 and Silastic size 0.012 in. i.d. x 0.025 in. o.d. are used instead of the larger PE and Silastic. The construction of this cannula is very similar to the type I assembly. Cut a 15-cm piece of PE 10 tubing and a 5-cm length of 0.012-in.-i.d. x 0.025-in.-o.d. Silastic tubing, and then proceed through the steps outlined above for the type I cannula.

One step in the construction of the type II cannula is different from that of type I, and two additional steps are required for its final completion. First, when the PE 10 and Silastic are joined, the HS is not placed 5 mm beyond their junction, but is placed right at their junction (see Fig. 1b). After completing the final steps indicated for the type I cannula, the spring wire is removed from the Silastic end and inserted into the lumen of the opposite end of the PE. The wire is inserted 20 mm. A 15-mm length of Silastic (small size) is expanded in chloroform and placed 15 mm down over the PE 10, i.e., until flush with the end of the PE 10. Finally, a 10-mm length of HS tubing is superimposed on the Silastic and reduced to produce a liquid-tight junction between the PE and Silastic.

C. Cannula Storage

For final cleaning dip the entire cannula into a mild, warm soap solution (preferably Ivory Flakes). Rinse the cannula in warm, clean water. Flush the lumen of the type I cannula with a syringe and 26-gauge needle. To flush the type II cannula put a 5-cm piece of 0.031-in. x 0.160-in. silicone rubber tubing over a 15-gauge needle, insert the cannula (the end with 10-mm HS) into the lumen of the tubing, and rinse. Then place the cannula in a 1:750 Zephiran antibacterial solution (1 oz of Zephiran concentrate in 1 gal distilled water) for 3 hr. Then place the cannula in a dust-free container such as a clean plastic bag, plastic wrap, or Saran Wrap. At the end of the storage period, just prior to surgery, rinse and flush the cannula with saline. Finally, if for some reason you cannot go through the above washing procedures, rinse the cannula well with Zephiran, then with saline, and flush before implanting it into the rat.

III. SURGICAL PROCEDURES

A. Procedure for Type I Cannula

For surgery you will need a 1:750 Zephiran solution; a 1:750 Zephiran/antirust solution (containing also 8.8 g sodium nitrate and 15.8 g anhydrous sodium carbonate per gallon of solution) used only for final cleaning of surgical instruments; 0.9% saline solution and 0.9% saline with 500 μg/ml heparin solution; ethyl ether (anesthesia grade) or methoxyfurane (Metofane); small animal scales; small animal clippers; a 1-gal widemouth glass jar (institutional size salad dressing or pickle jar); 4-in. x 4-in. surgical gauze sponges; a scalpel with size 10 blade; two pairs of fine-point dissection forceps; one pair of blunt-tipped medium point forceps; one pair of curved microdissecting scissors; spatula; suture needles; suture silk 3-0 and Chromic surgical gut size 3-0 or 4-0; 9-mm wound clips and applier; 1-cc syringes with 20-, 22-, 23- and 25-gauge 1-in. needles; a millimeter ruler; Eastman 910 adhesive; a solution of atropine sulfate; procaine penicillin G suspension; nitrofurazone powder (Furacin, 0.2%); and a 5-in. length of 1/4-in. x 3/32-in. rubber tubing.

The surgical instruments are placed in a pan of Zephiran/antirust solution for 5-10 min. Rinse the instruments with plain Zephiran or 70% alcohol and place on a clean surface (see Fig. 2c). The cannulas are placed in plain Zephiran solution. In the same solution place 8-cm lengths of Ethicon suture silk 3-0 and Chromic 3-0 or 4-0 surgical gut, about 12 of each. It is important to soak the surgical gut because it softens and becomes much easier to manipulate.

Place 2 ml of methoxyflurane (Metofane) or 5 ml of anesthetic ether (do not use petroleum ether by mistake as damage to lungs will result) into a 1-gal widemouth glass jar. Place absorbant material such as 4-in. x 4-in. sponge gauze in the bottom of the jar. Do the same with a small widemouth bottle (2-oz capsule bottle) filled with gauze. Give an intraperitoneal injection of 2.5-5 mg of atropine sulfate per rat.

Place a rat into the gallon jar and allow it to become unconscious or to reach the point at which a brisk shake of the jar does not arouse it. Do not turn your attention from the rat at this point or you may kill it (at one moment it may be standing and at the next be ready to be removed). If you should let the rat go until respiration has failed, quickly remove it from the jar, place a length of 1/4-in. x 3/32-in. rubber tubing over the nostrils, and blow short puffs rather than a long stream of air so as not to inflate the stomach or overinflate the lungs. This usually will revive the rat.

Once an animal is ready to remove from the jar, do so quickly. Then shave the back of the neck just behind the ears with small animal clippers (Fig. 2d); turn the rat on its back and shave the upper chest and lower neck as closely as possible (Fig. 2e). With the rat in supine position (on its back) wipe the shaved areas with gauze soaked in Zephiran solution; put its nose into the opening of the small widemouth bottle to maintain anesthesia.

Look at the exposed chest (Fig. 2e) and you will note rapid pulsations beneath the skin from the right and left jugulars on either side of the chest region. A black line is traced over the right jugular to outline its position in Fig. 2e. Make a 1- to 2-cm skin incision (just through the skin), being careful not to cut into the chest muscle, about 2 mm toward the centerline from, and parallel with, the right jugular (see Fig. 2f) using either sharp surgical scissors or a scalpel.

Use a blunt incision to expose the external jugular vein. Blunt incision is accomplished by first placing the closed surgical scissors points on the chest muscles, then opening them with slight downward pressure (Fig. 3a). Repeat this procedure and spread the muscles apart until you can see the jugular; in Fig. 3b note the dark triangular section, that is, the upper portion of the undisturbed right jugular. It will have a dark purple color. Caution: Do not allow the points of scissors to come into direct contact with the jugular vein. Open and close the scissors immediately alongside the vein in order to clear away connective tissue, but never directly on it, as profuse bleeding could result from even a slight nick. Once the jugular is relatively free of connective tissue, gently lift the vein a few millimeters with semiblunt forceps while simultaneously inserting fine-pointed forceps underneath the vein (Fig. 3c) in order to clear away fat and connective tissue (Fig. 3d). Place a trocar under the vein (Fig. 3e).

Fill the cannula with saline from a 1-cc syringe and attached 25-gauge needle; leave the syringe connected to the cannula. Measure the cannula from the HS tubing to the tip of the Silastic. For a 200- to 250-g rat cut the Silastic to 19 mm, for 250-300 g cut to 22 mm, and for 300-400 g cut to 25 mm. Cut the Silastic on a 45° angle (with scalpel) for easy insertion into the lumen of the vein.

Tie a loop around the vein with surgical silk or gut leaving a 1.5-cm loop. Push the loop as far caudad as possible on the exposed vein, then repeat with a second loop at the most cephalad part of the exposed vein (Fig. 3f). Place on a second syringe a 20-gauge 1-in. needle bent as shown in Fig. 4a. Insert the needle into the lumen of the vein (Fig. 4a). Remove the needle and insert a type I cannula into the vein via the needle puncture site as far as the HS tubing (Fig. 4b). Pull the first (caudad) loop of suture silk closed around the vein immediately beyond the vein puncture (Fig. 4c) so as

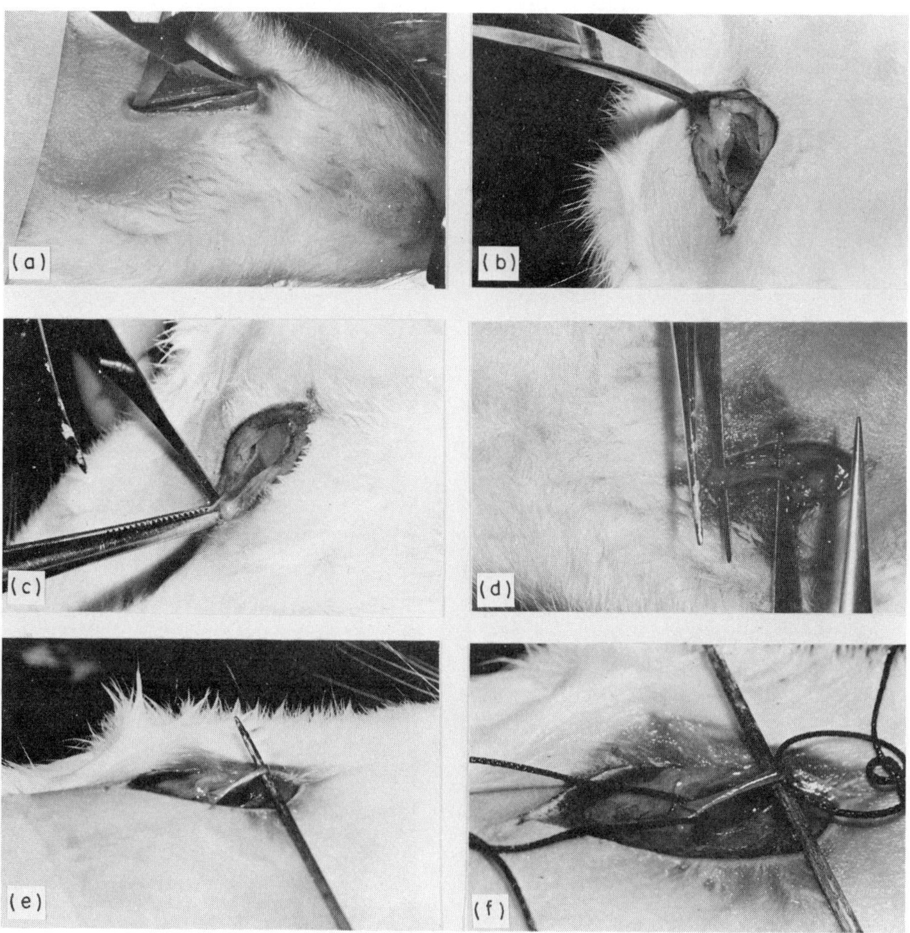

FIGURE 3. (a) Blunt incision with scissors through the muscle overlying the jugular vein. (b) The exposed jugular vein following blunt incision is seen as a dark mass in the center of the incision. (c) Hold the jugular with medium forceps while inserting the fine forceps beneath it. (d) Clean tissue away from the jugular with one forceps while holding it with another. (e) Placement of the trocar under the vein. (f) The caudad (left) and cephalad (right) loops of surgical silk placed around the jugular vein.

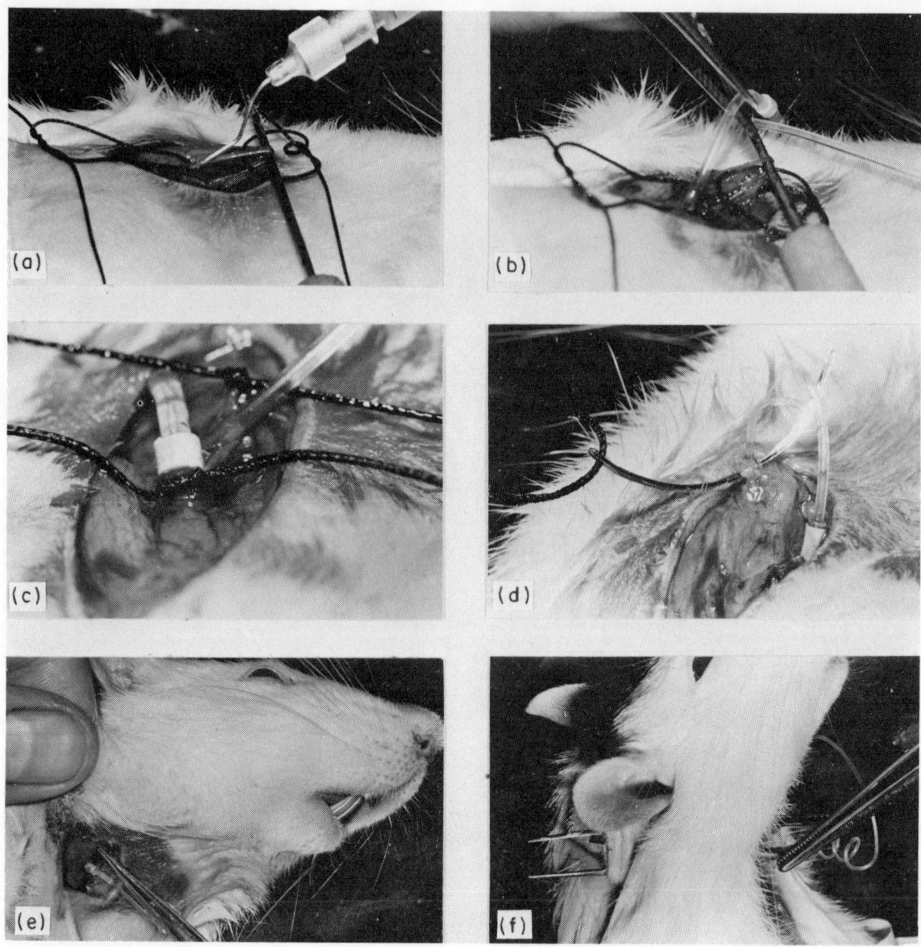

FIGURE 4. (a) The bent needle about to be inserted into the lumen of the jugular vein. (b) Hold the cannula with the forceps and insert it into the lumen of the vein. (c) The cannula is placed into the vein up to the HS tubing with two ties in place around the vein. (d) The cannula is sutured to the neck muscles immediately behind the first loop on the cannula. (e) The forceps is inserted into the muscles parallel to the jugular to start the blunt dissection for the cannula in its subcutaneous course to the upper neck. (f) The blunt dissection forceps are left in place, then spread slightly to permit passage of the cannula from the lower incision to the exit at the upper neck.

to tie the silk tightly around the vein and cannula. Next, tie off the vein below the puncture and the HS tubing (Fig. 4c). Now suture the cannula to the neck muscles (Fig. 4d). Make sure this tie is located just past the single loop. Place one drop of Eastman 910 adhesive on the junction of cannula, suture, and neck muscle.

Lay the rat on its side and with sharp forceps make a blunt incision on a line from the jugular through the muscle tissue (Fig. 4e) to the underside of the skin. Then push the forceps beneath the skin to a point on the back of the neck where a puncture wound is made through the skin. Spread the forceps slightly, and run the cannula between the forceps and out of the puncture wound (Fig. 4f).

Return the rat to a supine position, apply nitrofurazone (Furacin) powder, suture the muscle together with Chromic gut (Fig. 5a), and then close the skin incision with gut or with wound clips (Fig. 5b). Place the rat in the prone position and close the skin (puncture wound) on the back of the neck using a gut suture. With the same piece of suture tie the cannula to the skin of the neck, passing through the first of the series of loops (Fig. 5c). Place two drops of Eastman 910 on the suture and cannula at the puncture wound.

Inject 50,000-75,000 units of procaine penicillin G intramuscularly in a hind leg. Inject saline into the cannula, reverse the syringe slowly to draw blood, and again clear the cannula with saline. Either put a plug over the end of the cannula, or put a saddle on the rat and attach the cannula to it.

B. Procedure for Type II Cannula

This procedure is identical to that for a type I cannula with the following exceptions: (a) A 25-gauge 1-in. needle is bent for use in puncturing the vein; (b) a 5-cm length of 0.031-in. x 0.160-in. silicone rubber tubing attached to a 15-gauge needle is needed to connect onto the type II cannula to flush and fill it with saline (note description in Sec. II, C); (c) the length of Silastic tubing put into the vein (i.e., from HS tubing to beveled tip) is 31-33 mm for 200- to 250-g rats, 33-34 mm for 250-300 g, and 35-37 mm for 300 g and above; (d) the vein is not tied off above or below the puncture following insertion of the cannula, but rather, one drop of Eastman 910 adhesive is placed directly on the junction of HS tubing and vein (Fig. 5d); (e) suture silk is used instead of gut to tie the cannula to the neck muscle. Make sure the internal silk sutures are completely enclosed within the neck cavity when closing the wound with gut sutures or infection may result.

IV. OPERATIVE AND POSTOPERATIVE PROBLEMS

A rigidly aseptic technique is not required for the two surgical procedures discussed, but cleanliness should be maintained throughout. The

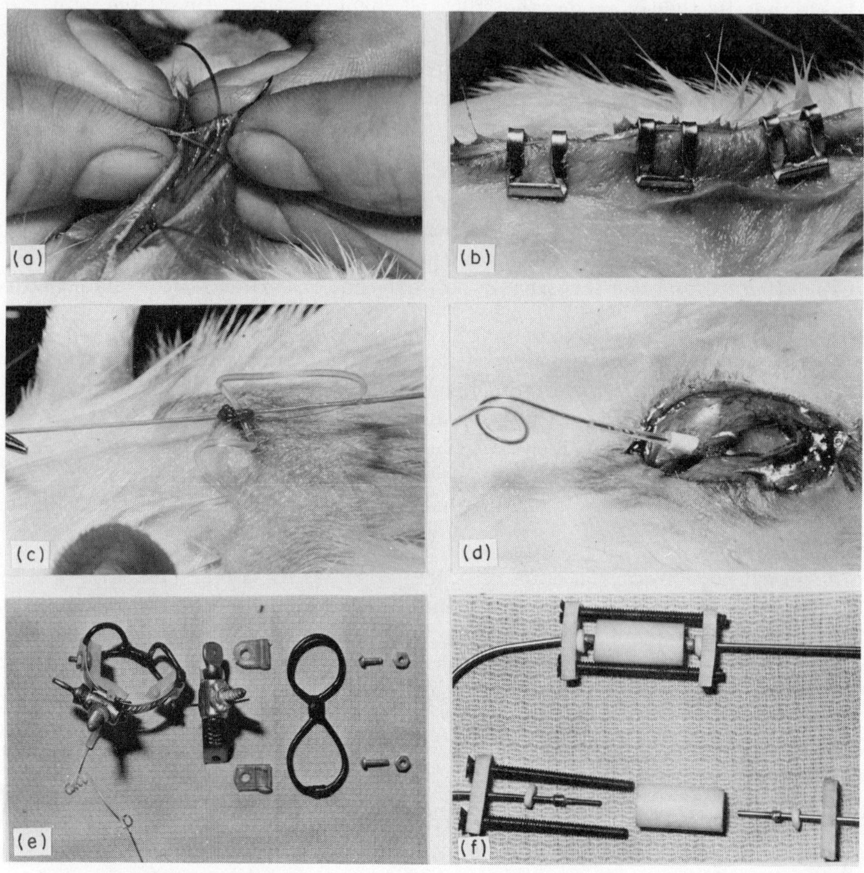

FIGURE 5. (a) Closure of the chest muscles with suture gut. (b) Skin closure by means of 9-mm auto-clips. (c) Closure of the skin wound on the back of the neck plus a tie through the first loop of the exposed cannula using the same length of surgical gut. (d) The type II cannula is inserted into the jugular up to the HS tubing and glued in place without ties. (e) An assembled rat saddle and a view of the disassembled component parts. (f) An assembled liquid swivel and a view of the disassembled component parts.

surgical instruments and the surgical surface should be washed between successive rats with Zephiran solution. If infections should occur, whether beneath the skin or on the skin surface, apply Furacin to the skin surface at the incision site.

Blood loss may occur during the surgery after puncturing the jugular; always replace this fluid loss with a similar amount of saline. Once the jugular has been punctured and the cannula is being inserted into the jugular, it should float easily down the vein. With the type I cannula this is not a problem. However, if pronounced resistance is met or if blood cannot be withdrawn with the smaller type II cannula, it is likely that the small cannula tip has entered the subclavian vein. Therefore, withdraw the Silastic to within a few millimeters of the tip and reinsert.

Once the cannula is in the vein, check its patency by infusing a small amount of saline and then carefully and slowly reversing the plunger to draw blood. If blood rises freely in the cannula, reverse the plunger and clear the cannula with saline. This should be done each time a suture is tied around the cannula to be sure the tie is not occluding the cannula. Sometimes during the surgery and afterward you will not be able to draw blood. If this happens, changing the head and neck position of the rat or flexing the upper portion of the body may resolve the problem. With the type I cannula, infuse the rat twice a day with 1.0 ml of saline containing 500 μg of heparin sodium to avoid clot formation in the cannula.

During the procedure of inserting the cannula, at least for the type II cannula, it is important to be sure that the cannula fits completely into the vein all the way to the HS. Should only 2 mm of the Silastic remain outside the vein, the cannula can work its way out of the vein during the experiment. If the cannula has been pulled from the vein at some time after the operation, attempts to infuse the rat will cause squealing and violent head movements. Also, a subcutaneous swelling near the vein on the neck should be observable. If the animal is important for continued research, reenter the neck wound, remove the old cannula, tie off the vein above and below the puncture, and insert a new cannula in the left jugular.

During surgery remove the anesthetic bottle from the nose of the rat from time to time to allow the level of anesthesia to become lighter. Do not allow this to continue beyond the point at which a rat shows kicking movements with either hind leg. Conversely, should an animal begin to kick with either hind leg during surgery, move the anesthetic bottle closer to its nose.

Finally, if at any point after surgery you feel the cannula is out of the vein or for some reason is not presenting the drug solution properly, inject a small dose of an ultrashort-duration barbiturate such as Surital. If the cannula is delivering the drug solutions properly, the rat should become ataxic within 15-20 sec after injection.

V. GENERAL APPARATUS

A. Animal Saddle

The animal saddle is used to permit connection of a cannulated rat to an infusion system. Many different types of animal saddles have been devised. Some researchers have used subcutaneous saddles [2], while others [3] use some form of external saddle as we do. The external saddle that we are presently using is shown in Fig. 5e.

Construction of this saddle requires the following materials: two plastic 1/8-in. cable clips; a stainless-steel hose clamp, cut off as shown; a piece of 16-strand fixture wire bent into a figure eight; two 1/8-in. x 1/2-in. stove bolts and nuts; strips of self-adhering plastic foam tape (weather stripping) 3/8-in. wide x 1/4-in. thick; a 2-in. length of 18-gauge stainless-steel hypodermic tubing; two 1-in. lengths of silicone rubber tubing and a 3/4-in. no. 12 pan-head tapping screw. When attempting to solder the pan-head screw and the hypodermic needle tubing to the clamp, use stainless-steel solder flux and stainless-steel solder or they will not adhere. The materials listed above (except for silicone rubber tubing and hypodermic tubing) may be purchased at local hardware, auto parts, or builders' supply outlets.

As Fig. 5e has been found to serve as a sufficient aid to the assembly of the saddle, we shall not give detailed instructions. Saddles for rats are also available commercially from BRS/LVE.

B. Liquid Swivel

The liquid swivel (Figs. 5f and 6a) is essential for automatically administering drug solutions to relatively unrestrained animals. The first type of swivel shown (Fig. 5f) was devised by Dr. William F. Crowder of the Department of Psychology at The University of Mississippi. It is easy to assemble and inexpensive (costing less than $5.00 to construct) compared to those available commercially (a cannula feedthrough swivel, BRS/LVE model 192-03, is currently priced at $95.00).

The following materials are required to construct the Crowder liquid swivel: two pieces of 18-gauge stainless-steel hypodermic needle tubing; a 1/4-in. x 3/4-in. piece of Teflon rod (the center must be drilled out with a 0.043- or 0.045-in. drill bit); two pieces of Teflon sheet, 3/8 in. wide x 3/4 in. long x 1/8 in. thick; two 1/4-in. (or larger) x 1/8-in. buttons made from the Teflon rod (drilled out with the same drill size as for the rod); two 1/8-in. tips from two taper pins (these are also drilled out to accept needle tubing as shown); and two 1/8-in. x (1 1/2)-in. screws. All of these materials except the needle tubing (available from Small Parts, Inc.; see

Appendix B) and the taper pins (available from BRS/LVE) may be obtained from hardware and builders' supply stores.

When soldering the two drilled-out pieces of taper pin to the needle tubing, stainless-steel solder flux and solder are required. Again, we will not describe the assembly steps, as our experience has shown that a picture plus the list of material has proved to be sufficient aid for others to construct the liquid swivel. The Crowder type of swivel is connected to the rat saddle by means of a length of needle tubing and alligator clip (see Sec. V, C for connection details).

A second type of liquid swivel (Fig. 6a) may be assembled from commercially available parts. A rotating adapter (left side of figure; Becton-Dickinson model 30-80, 625A) is combined with a Tuohy adapter (center of figure; Clay-Adams model 7575, A-1029). A 10-cm piece of 15-gauge stainless steel needle tubing (available from Small Parts, Inc.) is bent into an L shape and soldered into the female luer lok as shown (right side of figure). The leash for this swivel is discussed in the section on leash assembly.

A third type of swivel is now available from Sage Instruments (model 120). It is similar to the second swivel described above in that the upper end is a female luer fitting; however, the other end terminates in a tube the size of a 19-gauge needle. The overall length of this swivel is 1 3/4 in., making it very easy to work with.

C. Leash Assembly

The leash is an important part of the fluid delivery system. It comprises the securing link and/or the fluid channel from the swivel to the rat. The type to be used depends upon the kind of swivel the experimenter intends to employ.

The first type of leash is made from a 27-cm length of 18-gauge stainless-steel tubing with an 8-cm length of stainless-steel spring and a 1/2-in. alligator clip attached (Fig. 6b, left side). The needle tubing of the leash is connected to the needle tubing on the saddle by a 3-cm length of 0.031-in. x 0.160-in. silicone rubber tubing. The leash is anchored to the saddle by means of the alligator clip. This kind of leash is typically used with the Crowder type of swivel described above.

The second kind of leash is employed with the swivel based on the B-D rotating adapter (Fig. 6b, right side). It is constructed from a 30-cm length of tight coil spring (BRS/LVE, no. 95282) which is soldered at one end to the Tuohy adapter and to a 1/2-in. alligator clip. A piece of polyethylene tubing (PE 20) is threaded into the lumen of the spring and up into the Tuohy adapter. The knurled nut on the Tuohy adapter is tightened. The tightening of this nut causes a rubber gasket inside the adapter to compress and press

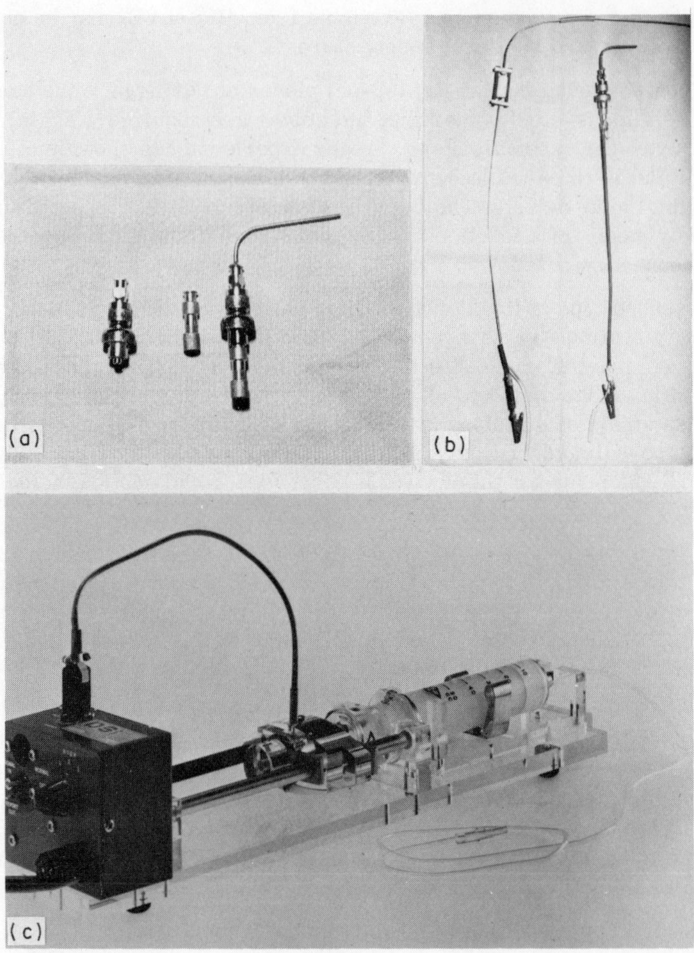

FIGURE 6. (a) A Becton-Dickinson rotating adapter (left) and Tuohy adapter (center) are fitted together along with a piece of 1.5-gauge stainless-steel needle tubing as shown (right) to form a 360-degree rotating liquid swivel. (b) The needle-tubing leash assembly for the Crowder swivel (left) and the tight spring leash assembly for the B-D or Sage swivel (right). (c) A Davis precision liquid pump. The figure includes the pump motor, the driver assembly, and the syringe (courtesy of Davis Scientific Instruments).

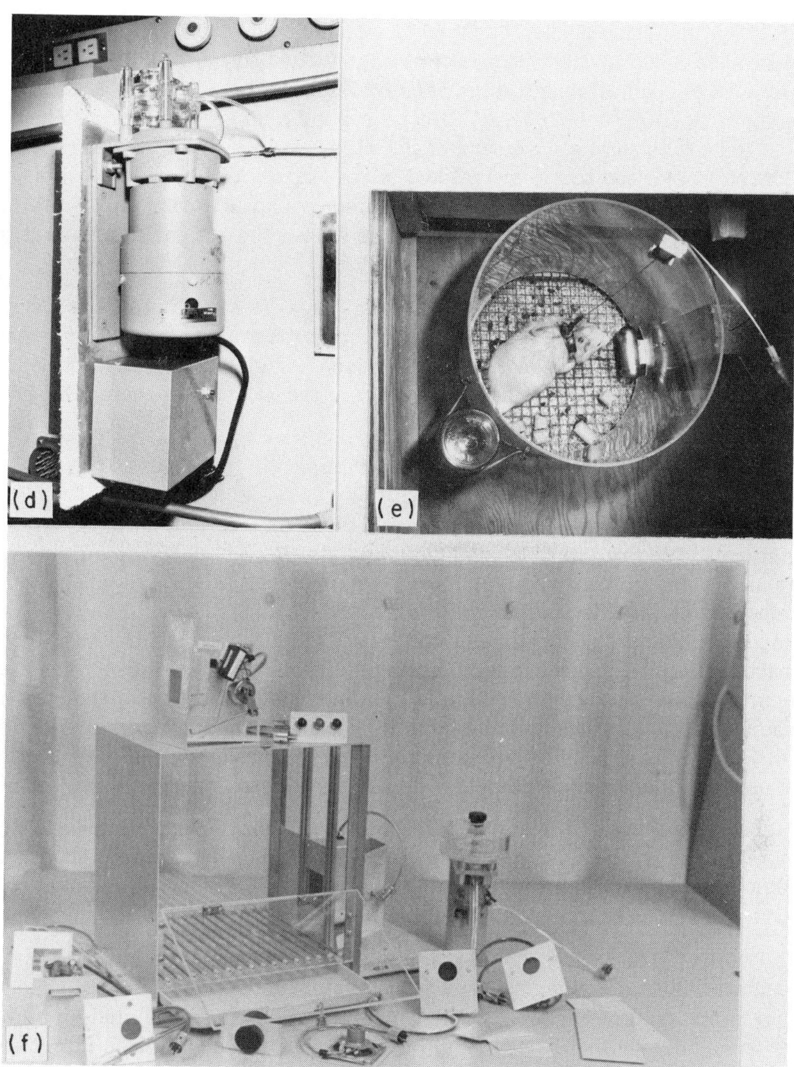

FIGURE 6 (cont.). (d) A continuous-flow roller-head liquid pump. (e) A self-administration chamber. A clear Plexiglas cylinder which encloses the rat is shown. The chamber contains a response lever, food, and water. Immediately above the chamber and extending into it is the infusion system. (f) A Coulborn interchangeable-component chamber (courtesy of Coulborn Instruments, Inc., and LVB Corp.).

firmly against the PE 20. The rubber washer holds the PE 20 in place and establishes a liquid-tight channel from the swivel to the PE. The opposite end of PE is then attached to the needle tubing on the saddle by a 3-cm piece of 0.031-in. x 0.160-in. silicone rubber tubing. The spring is anchored to the saddle by means of the alligator clip. With the spring leash soldered at one end to the swivel and held securely to the saddle by an alligator clip at the other, tension is exerted only on the spring, not on the PE 20. Also, by having the PE 20 inside the spring the rat cannot reach it to claw or chew holes in it.

The leash for the third type of swivel (Sage) is similar to the second model. It differs in that a Tuohy adapter is not required and PE 100 serves as the liquid channel to the rat. Also, since a Tuohy adapter is not used, the protective spring is soldered directly to the 19-gauge needle tubing.

D. Liquid Pumps

Liquid pumps are used to dispense a fixed unit volume of drug solution to the rat. We are currently using pumps similar to the type available from Davis Scientific Instruments and Sage Instruments. The Davis and Sage pumps are essentially motorized syringe drivers (Fig. 6c). This type of pump has some unique features which are highly desirable for self-administration research. Standard-size syringes are used with an electromagnetic stepping motor to push the plunger of the syringe. The size of the step can be adjusted so that the liquid dispensed per operation can vary from 0.001 to 0.5 ml. Thus, liquid dispensing in small but precisely metered portions can be achieved with this pump.

The second type of pump is the continuous reservoir, roller-head system (Fig. 6d). Cole Parmer Instruments markets such a pump. It is self-priming and has four interchangeable head sizes. This pump allows liquid delivery at rates from 1.0 to 1400 ml/min.

Finally, Dr. James R. Weeks has recently developed a new low-cost pneumatic syringe driver system. The system is easy to assemble and all components are commercially available. The components include a miniature pneumatic cylinder used to move the plunger on a Hamilton microliter syringe. Fluid is drawn into the syringe by a modified two-way valve. The injection volume is adjustable down to 0.02 ml at an accuracy of ±10%. Information on this system can be obtained from Dr. James R. Weeks, Experimental Biology Division, Upjohn Company, Kalamazoo, Michigan.

In deciding which type of pump to use the researcher should consider whether continuous 24-hr delivery of large volumes is desired. If this is the case, then the continuous reservoir pump should be used. If delivery of small, precisely measured volumes is required, whether over short or long periods, the motor-driven syringe or Weeks' pneumatic pump would be best suited to the task.

E. Chambers

The experimental chamber is the environment in which the self-administration research is carried out (Fig. 6e). These chambers can be obtained from BRS/LVE, Lafayette Instruments, Davis Scientific Instruments, and Coulborn Instruments, Inc. (LVB Corp.). The latter two companies are of special interest because they provide chambers with many optional components. For example, Coulborn offers a chamber which may include either regular response levers or special retracting levers as well as various types of visual displays or auditory equipment (Fig. 6f). Coulborn equipment permits the experimenter to mix or match components at his convenience. Some companies have chambers supplied with attached food dispensers. These are not necessary for self-administration research, and the added expense may be avoided by choosing chambers supplied without these features.

F. Electronic Control Equipment

Drug self-administration research, like most behavioral research, is conducted with automatic electronic controlling equipment. That is, once the rat is attached to the infusion system, all experimental conditions are accomplished automatically with electromechanical (Fig. 7a) or solid-state (Fig. 7b) controlling equipment. The data may be recorded by means of event counters (Fig. 7c), printout counters (Fig. 7d), or paper-record event recorders (Fig. 7e).

With automated controlling and recording equipment a very precise presentation of the experimental conditions and measurement of their effects can be accomplished. Also, this equipment provides a means for continuous 24-hr experiments without the necessity of the researcher being present to administer the drug or other experimental conditions. Automation also provides precise control, which avoids operator variability associated with manual operation of such conditions.

For researchers not familiar with electromechanical or solid-state controlling equipment, many of the behavioral equipment companies provide training in the use of their equipment without charge and will help with the selection and ordering of appropriate equipment. Good introductory text books are available for both electromechanical and solid-state controlling equipment [5-7].

VI. TYPES OF DATA OBTAINABLE

It is difficult to depict in this limited space all the data that can be obtained from self-administration procedures, for they are as varied as

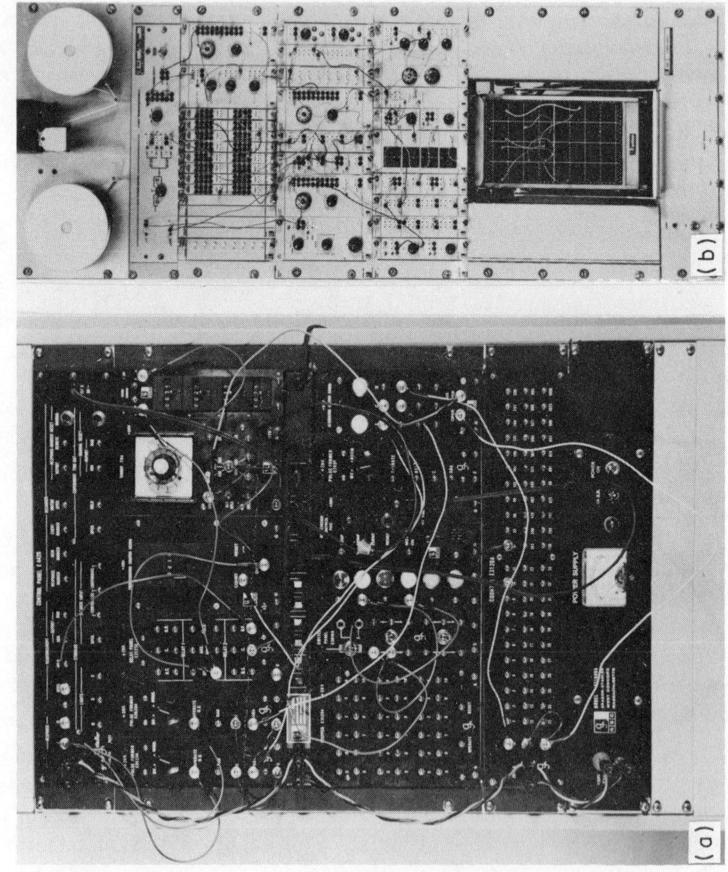

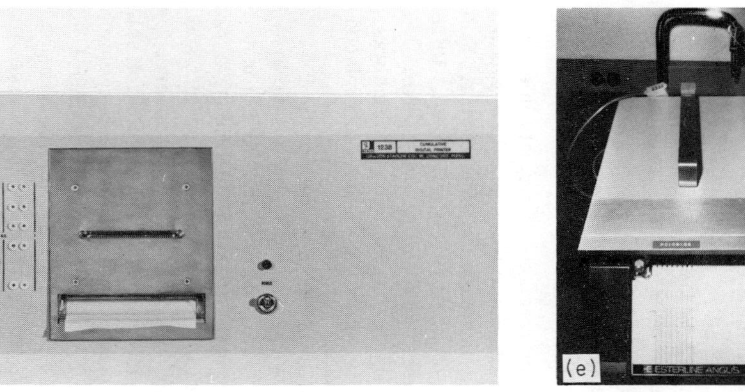

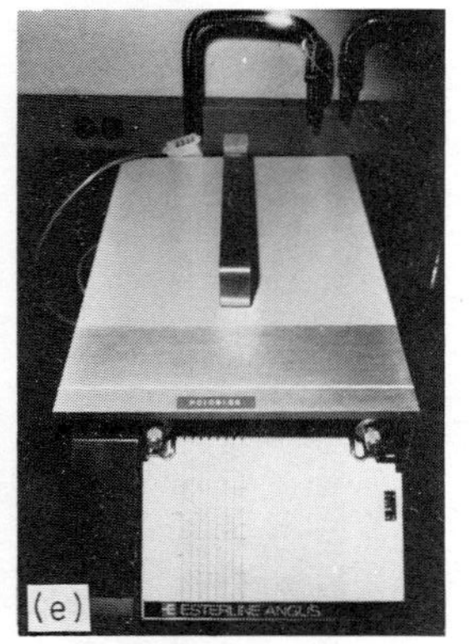

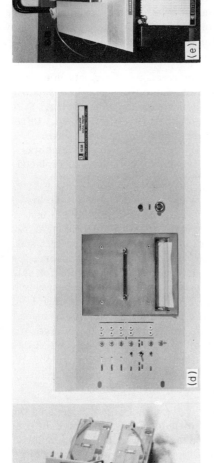

FIGURE 7. (a) A rack of electromechanical programming equipment which controls infusions and records the number of responses during a self-administration test session (courtesy of Grason-Stadler). (b) A solid-state programmer for controlling self-administration procedures (courtesy of Coulborn Instruments, Inc., and LVB Corp.). (c) An event counter that can be used to record the number of responses or the number of infusions (courtesy of Coulborn Instruments, Inc., and LVB Corp.). (d) A printout counter that can be used to record on roll paper the number of responses and/or the number of infusions. The printout counter can be programmed to record after each event (response or infusion), after a fixed number of events, or after a certain time interval (e.g., number of infusions per hour). (e) A paper event recorder. A roll of paper moves under pens (4-20) filled with ink. Each response and/or infusion is recorded as a pen deflection. Since the paper moves at a fixed speed, the time at which a discrete response or infusion occurs can be identified.

the ingenuity of the individual experimenter conducting the research. However, we shall present a few simple techniques and the resulting data.

A. Primary Positive Reinforcement

Primary positive reinforcement refers to the presentation of a drug following some arbitrary response by an animal which increases the probability of recurrence of the preceding response. In this case, the depression of a response lever which closes an electrical circuit is immediately followed by an intravenous injection of morphine.

To demonstrate primary positive reinforcement, four rats in experimental chambers were connected to the infusion system via their saddles. Each rat was allowed 1 hr to adapt to the new experimental setting. Following this period a 6-hr baseline measure (operant level) was taken. During the baseline period each accidental depression of the response lever produced an intravenous infusion of 0.018 ml of 0.9% saline, which was delivered in 0.2 sec. On the following five days the saline was replaced with a 60 μg/kg infusion of morphine sulfate.

The results of these operations are shown in Fig. 8. Note the low level of lever pressing for saline by each rat. This is expected, for a saline infusion should have essentially neutral effects. Responding during this period is a result of random exploratory movements by the rats and the resulting accidental contacts with the lever. In contrast, observe the large increases in lever pressing when morphine was substituted for saline. Responding for drug originates from a baseline of exploratory behavior like that observed during the saline session; however, instead of a neutral saline infusion, an infusion of morphine occurs. About 10-20 infusions, depending on the unit dosage, are required for a rat to discriminate that a lever press is followed by a satisfying or "rewarding" physiological state. When this occurs, increases in responding proportional to the unit dose are observed. Since we observed an increase in responding for morphine compared to saline, we infer that morphine produces a reinforcing effect.

Weeks and Collins reported a study of the effect of unit dosage on the maintenance of self-administration for morphine [8]. They gave different groups of rats 6 days of access to morphine. The unit dosages employed were 0.01, 0.032, 0.10, 0.32, 1.0, 3.2, and 10 mg/kg/injection. The results for the sixth day of self-administration are shown in Fig. 9a [8]. The data indicate that the average number of infusions per group was inversely related to the unit dosage maintaining self-administration behavior. That is, the lower the dose per infusion, the higher the number of infusions. This would be expected since the lower the dose, the shorter the duration of pharmacological action. Thus, in order to maintain a satisfying physiological effect the rat must respond again and again to produce or maintain the pharmacological action.

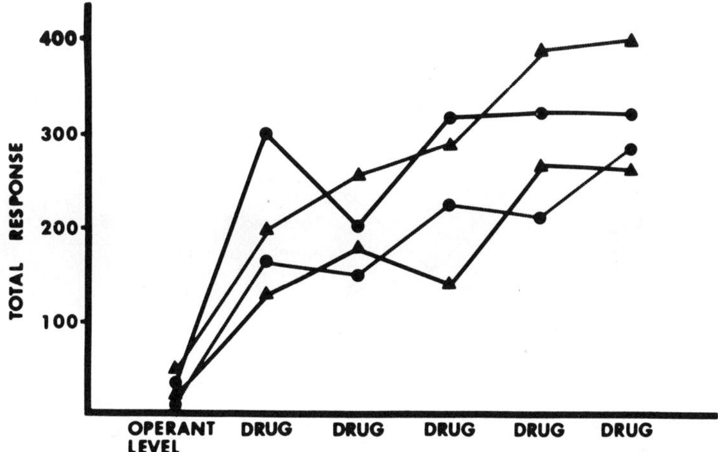

FIGURE 8. Results for a period of access to saline (baseline) and for access over 5 days to 60 μg/kg/injection (acquisition of self-administration behavior). The data from four rats are plotted using various symbols to differentiate individuals.

Analysis of the data also indicates that although subjects on lower doses (i.e., 0.32 mg/kg/injection and below) took larger numbers of infusions, they took a considerably smaller amount of morphine. This is expected since the development of tolerance, requiring a consequent elevation of intake, would be greater with the higher unit doses. Also, subjects receiving low doses would have to respond 30-1000 times to equal just one injection at the higher unit dose (i.e., a rat receiving 0.01 mg/kg/injection must respond 1000 times to equal one injection of 10 mg/kg).

The authors further showed that a number of rats displayed physical dependence following termination of 6 days of morphine self-administration (Fig. 9b [8]). All subjects became dependent at the higher dosages, while a dose-related decrease in incidence of dependence was observed at the lower dosages. The latter finding is important since it indicates that physical dependence is not a prerequisite for the maintenance of self-administration behavior.

B. Effects of Tolerance

In the setting of human drug taking, repeated injection of an opiate leads to tolerance and an increased requirement for the drug. A similar development of tolerance can be observed with rats. Tolerance may be

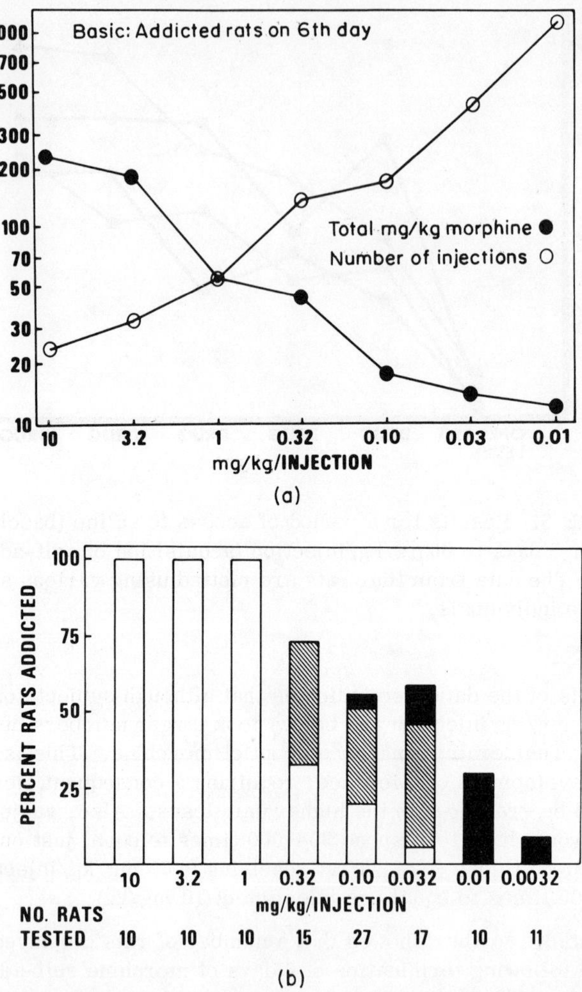

FIGURE 9. (a) Results for the sixth day of morphine self-administration for seven groups of rats differentiated on the basis of unit dose self-administered (mg/kg/injection). Data are presented for the mean total mg/kg of morphine self-administration and the mean total number of self-injections for each dose group (courtesy of Dr. James R. Weeks). (b) Data indicating the proportion of rats showing dependence after 6 days of morphine self-administration using the criteria of withdrawal weight loss (open bars) and injection rate compared to controls (solid bars) or both (striped bars). These data are from the same subjects represented in Fig. 9a (courtesy of Dr. James R. Weeks).

seen in data from three rats allowed to self-administer 1 mg/kg/injection of morphine for 6 weeks. A baseline measure was taken on the rats (day 1) followed by 41 days of access to morphine. The data (Fig. 10a) indicate that the rats gradually increased the amount of drug self-administered.

Tolerance can also be induced acutely by passive injections of the drug class later to be self-administered [9]. The latter procedure was shown by researchers at The University of Mississippi [10]. Two groups of rats were given either six intravenous saline injections, each separated by 8 hr, or an equal number of injections of morphine (150 mg/kg). Thirty-six hours after the last infusion the rats were allowed 24-hr access to morphine. The results indicated that the subjects which had been given predrug injections self-administered 2.5 times as much morphine as did those pretreated with saline.

C. Antagonism of Primary Reinforcement

A currently popular area of narcotic research is that related to the development and testing of antagonists. This popularity stems from the fact that antagonists block the pharmacological action of the opiates and produce a decline in drug-seeking behavior. This effect can be shown with self-administering animals.

For demonstration three subjects were placed in self-administration chambers, attached to the injection system, and allowed 1 hr to adapt to the experimental setting. Following adaptation the operant level (baseline) of lever pressing was measured for a 3-hr period. During the operant level period each lever press was followed by a 0.2-sec intravenous infusion of a 0.9% saline solution in a volume of 0.018 ml. On the following day a 60 μg/kg dosage of morphine was substituted for saline. Two additional morphine sessions were run at the same time on successive days. After the third day of morphine self-administration, six additional sessions were allowed; however, 15 min prior to each of the latter sessions a subcutaneous injection of 25 mg/kg of naloxone hydrochloride was administered.

The results are shown in Fig. 10b. Shown are the baseline data for three rats (panel A), their acquisition of morphine self-administration behavior (panel B), and the effects of naloxone on their self-administration of morphine (panels C and D). The data indicate that the subjects developed morphine self-administration, and then the behavior was lost following the injection of the opiate antagonist. Although not studied here, the potency of antagonists and their duration of action could easily be studied with the paradigm demonstrated above. Thus, self-administration procedures provide methods that could be used to characterize narcotic antagonists.

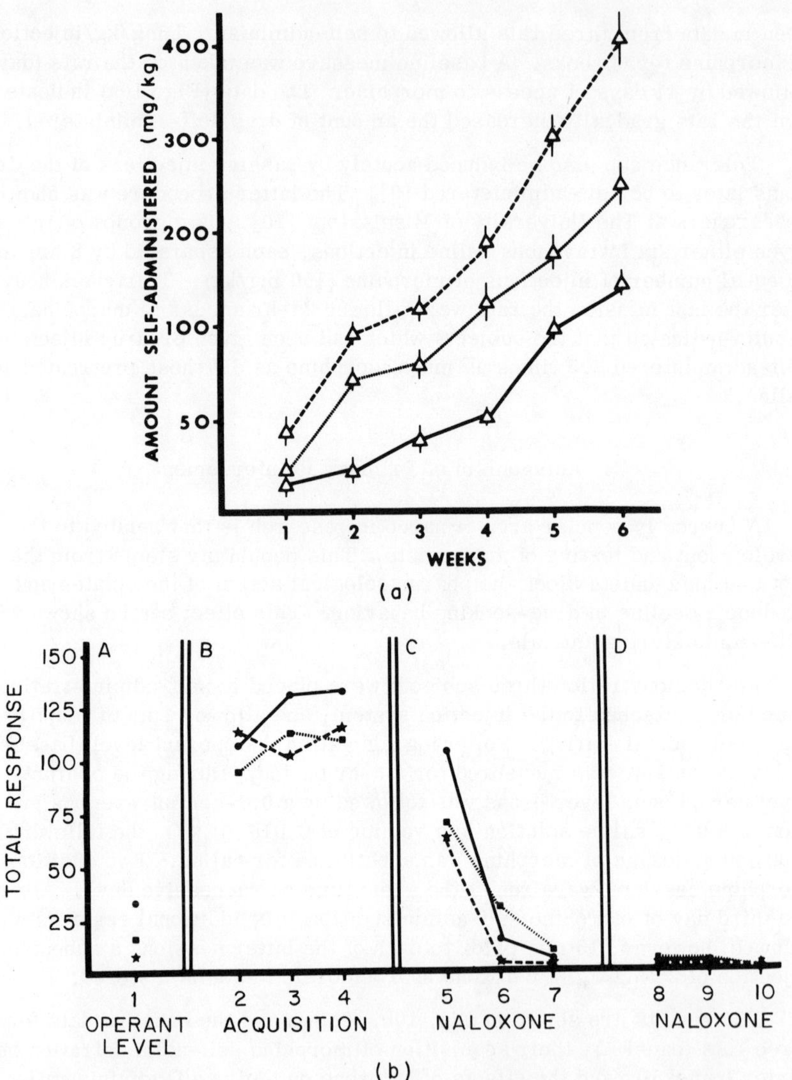

FIGURE 10. (a) The number of injections taken by three rats during operant level (baseline) and 6 weeks of access to morphine are plotted. Each rat is represented by a different symbol. Following the initial acquisition, increases in the number of injections are noted as tolerance develops. (b) Data from three rats during a saline-injection baseline (panel A), during acquisition of morphine self-administration (panel B), and during a study of the effect of a 25 mg/kg subcutaneous injection of naloxone given before access to morphine self-administration (panels C and D).

These descriptions of self-administration procedures are only intended to provide a limited introduction to this method. For a complete picture of research on opiate self-administration the reader should see the comprehensive review by Smith and Davis [11].

APPENDIX A: MATERIALS AND SOURCES

1. Drugs

Atropine sulfate ampules (1 or 5 mg/ml) or powder: Eli Lilly and Company, Indianapolis, Indiana 46206

Benzalkonium chloride (Zephiran 17%): Winthrop Laboratories, 90 Park Avenue, New York, New York 10016

Ethyl ether, USP ether for anesthesia: Mallinckrodt Chemical Co., P.O. Bos 5439, St. Louis, Missouri 63160

Methoxyflurane (Metofane): Pitman-Moore, Inc., 1241 Main St., Cuyahoga Falls, Ohio 44221

Nitrofurazone powder (Furacin): Eaton Laboratories, P.O. Box 191, Norwich, New York 13815

Procaine pencillin G (300,000 units/ml): Eli Lilly and Company

Sodium heparin (100 USP units/ml): Eli Lilly and Company

Sodium thiamylal (Surital): Parke, Davis and Company, Detroit, Michigan 48232

The drugs listed are likely to be readily available through a local or regional drug wholesale distributor for institutional purchases.

2. Surgical Supplies

Disposable needles and syringes (1-cc tuberculin syringes, 15- through 26-gauge needles): Becton-Dickinson, Rutherford, New Jersey 07070

Polyethylene tubing (PE 10 and 20): Clay Adams, 299 Webro Rd., Parsippany, New Jersey 17054

Silastic tubing: V. Mueller and Company, 6600 West Touhy Ave., Chicago, Illinois 60648

Silicone rubber tubing: Cole-Parmer Instruments Company, 7425 N. Oak Park Ave., Chicago, Illinois 60680

Surgical gauze sponge, 4-in. x 4-in.: Various manufacturers, local drug and hospital suppliers

Surgical instruments (scalpels; forceps; scissors; suture needles, 3/8-in. circle, cutting edge size 16; trocar): Aloe Medical, P.O. Box 9346, Melrose Station, Nashville, Tennessee 37204, and Clay Adams

Suture silk 3-0 and surgical gut (Chromic, type C 3-0): Ethicon, Inc., Somerville, New Jersey 08876

Wound clips and applier (9-mm): Clay Adams

In addition to the listed sources, most of these items are likely to be available through a nearby hospital supply company. In the southern United States a good general supplier for all surgical and related equipment is McNees Medical Supply Co., 4711 Highway 55 North, Jackson, Mississippi 39206.

3. Miscellaneous Supplies and Materials

Eastman 910 adhesive (1-oz bottle): F. W. Wright Company, 9999 Mercier Ave., Dearborn, Michigan 48121 and Armstrong Cork Company, Lancaster, Pennsylvania 17604

Heat-shrinkable tubing (FIT-221, White, 3/64-in. and 3/32-in.): Allied Electronics Corporation, 2400 W. Washington Blvd., Chicago, Illinois 60680

Hypodermic needle tubing, Stainless Steel: Small Parts, Inc., 6901 N. E. Third Ave., Miami, Florida 33138

Small animal clippers: Preiser Scientific, 1500 Algonquin Parkway, Louisville, Kentucky 40201

Spring wire (0.007-0.015 in. diameter): Central Steel and Wire Company, P.O. Box 5310A, Chicago, Illinois 60680

Teflon (rods and sheets): Norrell Plastics Inc., 3496 Winhoma Dr., Box 30279, Memphis, Tennessee 38130, or a general plastics supplier.

APPENDIX B: EQUIPMENT SUPPLIERS

Becton-Dickinson, Rutherford, New Jersey 07070

BRS/LVE, 5451 Holland Drive, Beltsville, Maryland 20705

Cole-Parmer Instruments, 7425 North Oak Park Ave., Chicago, Illinois 60680

Coulborn Instruments, Inc., Box 2551, Lehigh Valley, Pennsylvania 18100

Davis Scientific Instruments, 11116 Cumpston Street, North Hollywood, California 91601

Grason-Stadler, 56 Winthrop Street, Concord, Massachusetts 01742

Lafayette Instrument Company, Box 1279, Lafayette, Indiana 47902

LVB Corporation, Box 2221, Lehigh Valley, Pennsylvania 18001

Sage Instruments Inc., 230 Ferris Ave., White Plains, New York 10603

Small Parts Inc., 6901 N. E. Third Ave., Miami, Florida 33138

ACKNOWLEDGMENTS

The authors wish to express appreciation to Edith Pritchard, Wilma Beeler, and Charlotte Delcambre for their secretarial assistance and to William C. Martin of the Science Education Resources Center of The University of Mississippi for the drawings and photographs.

The authors would like to acknowledge particularly Dr. James R. Weeks, the originator of intravenous self-administration methodology, as the procedures described here are extensions of his techniques. The first author is especially appreciative of having received his original training in the use of intravenous methods from Dr. Weeks.

The authors wish to express special appreciation to Ms. Toreen E. Werner, who is in charge of surgery in our laboratory and who has made many helpful suggestions and contributions during the development of cannulas and surgical procedures. We are indebted to Ms. Werner also for her critical reading of this manuscript.

REFERENCES

1. J. R. Weeks, Experimental morphine addiction: Method for automatic intravenous injections in unrestrained rats. <u>Science 138</u>:143-144 (1962).

2. R. Pickens and J. Dougherty, A method for chronic intravenous infusion of fluids in unrestrained rats. In <u>Reports from the Research Laboratories of the Department of Psychiatry</u>, Report PR-72-1. Minneapolis: Univ. of Minnesota, 1972.

3. J. R. Weeks, Long-term intravenous infusion. In <u>Methods in Psychobiology</u> (R. D. Myers, ed.). New York: Academic Press, 1972.

4. J. D. Davis, A method for chronic intravenous infusion in freely moving rats. <u>J. Exp. Anal. Behav. 9</u>:385-387 (1966).

5. M. L. Hetzel and C. W. Hetzel, <u>Relay Circuits for Psychology</u>. New York: Appleton-Century-Crofts, 1969.

6. W. T. Jones, Introduction to Solid State Programming. Lehigh Valley, Pa.: LVB Corp., 1975.

7. Bits of Digi: An Introductory Manual to Digital Logic Packages. Beltsville, Maryland: BRS/LVE, 1969.

8. J. R. Weeks and R. J. Collins, Primary addiction to morphine in rats. Fed. Proc. Fed. Amer. Soc. Exp. Biol. 30:2336 (1971).

9. W. R. Coussens, W. F. Crowder, and S. G. Smith, Acute physical dependence upon morphine in rats. Behav. Biol. 8:533-543 (1973).

10. P. W. Wirth, R. T. Case, and W. F. Crowder, Acute dependence and acquisition of morphine self-administration in rats. Paper presented at the meeting of the Southeastern Psychological Association, New Orleans, 1973.

11. S. G. Smith and W. M. Davis, Self-administration research in the behavioral analysis of opiate dependence. In A Behavioral Analysis of Drug Dependence (H. Lal and J. M. Singh (eds.). New York: Futura, 1974.

Chapter 2

INTRACEREBRAL ADMINISTRATION OF OPIATES

YASUKO F. JACQUET

New York State Research Institute
for Neurochemistry and Drug Addiction
Ward's Island, New York

I. INTRODUCTION

It is widely agreed that morphine and other opiates exert their varied pharmacological effects primarily through their action on the central nervous system (CNS) [1]. However, until recently, little was known about sites in the CNS which mediated opiate effects.

A promising technique in the search for anatomic sites of opiate action is the intracerebral injection technique using chronically implanted intracerebral cannulas. This technique has been used extensively and fruitfully in neuropsychological studies mapping the animal brain for sites involved in motivation [2-4]. The intracerebral injection method has the advantage of bypassing the blood-brain barrier, allowing the experimenter to deliver precise quantities of drug to the intended site(s). This feature is especially advantageous in the search for anatomic sites of morphine action, since very little of the systemically administered morphine gains access to the CNS [5,6].

Unfortunately, this technique has been used in only a few morphine studies, and the small number of morphine studies using this technique to date show only moderate agreement regarding the precise anatomic localization of morphine action. This is probably due, in part, to errors arising from methodological difficulties inherent in this technique.

This chapter was written to help overcome this deficiency. It describes the details of a modified intracerebral injection technique which I gradually evolved during a prolonged period of struggling with problems arising from this technique. The modifications were designed to overcome the shortcomings of the microinjection method as they became manifest to me, and appear to yield reliable results. Although the discussion centers on morphine, the method can be used to deliver other opiates, as well as other neurochemicals, to discrete brain sites.

II. REVIEW OF INTRACEREBRAL MORPHINE INJECTION STUDIES

A. Morphine Analgesia

One of the earliest published studies of intracerebral morphine was by Tsou and Jang [7] in 1964. They used acute rather than chronic preparations. Rabbits were injected bilaterally with 2 μl saline containing 10 μg of morphine while mounted on a stereotaxic device under local anesthesia and tested for analgesia after the paralysis wore off. No details of the cannula size or injection method were given. The analgesic test consisted of radiant heat focused on the nose and thigh. Pronounced analgesia was obtained following morphine microinjection in the periventricular site of the 3rd ventricle, whereas more moderate and variable levels of analgesia were obtained following morphine injection in the periaqueductal gray. Negative sites were the dorsomedial thalamus, the caudate, septum, hippocampus, tectum, dorsomedial region of the medial geniculate body, midbrain reticular formation, and the ventrobasal complex. Topical applications of morphine in the somatosensory cortex area or intrathecal injections in the lumbar region of the spinal cord also yielded negative results. The analgesia resulting from periventricular injections of morphine could be antagonized by nalorphine. Bilateral, but not unilateral, injections of nalorphine in the periventricular site blocked analgesia caused by intravenous morphine, but intracerebral nalorphine injected into inactive sites had no analgesia-blocking effect following intravenous morphine. Intraventricular injections of morphine in which the drug remained in the lateral and 3rd ventricles and the aqueduct also resulted in analgesia, but increasing injection volume, which resulted in forcing the drug into the 4th ventricle, only weakened the analgesia. On the basis of these results, Tsou and Jang concluded that the main site of morphine analgesia resided in the central gray matter surrounding the 3rd ventricle.

Lotti et al. [8,9] injected 50 μg of morphine sulfate in 1 μl of saline throughout areas of the hypothalamus and the thalamus using the cannula system of Decima and George [10]. The outer guide cannula was 20-gauge (0.89 mm o.d.) and the injection cannula was 24-gauge (0.56 mm o.d.). These were implanted permanently in female rats, which were then tested at least 10 days following the implantation operation. The primary focus of these investigations was morphine hypothermia (see Sec. II, B), but analgesia was also assessed by observing diminution of the corneal reflex and loss of withdrawal of the tail on pinching. Analgesia was observed from sites throughout the hypothalamus.

Foster et al. [11], also using the cannula system of Decima and George [10] in chronically implanted rats, found that 25 μg of morphine sulfate in 1 μl of saline in the periventricular region of the rostral hypothalamus resulted in analgesia as measured by the hot-plate method.

Buxbaum et al. [12] found that 0.1 and 2.0 μg of morphine, in 0.5 or 1.0 μl injection volume, injected in the anterior thalamus resulted in a dose-effect response for analgesia. Analgesia was also observed following morphine injections into other unspecified thalamic and hypothalamic areas. However, no analgesia was observed after injections into the caudate, olfactory bulb, or reticular formation. No details were given regarding size of cannula or injection method.

Herz et al. [13] studied analgesia (as shown by inhibition of licking elicited by electrical stimulation of the tooth pulp) in the rabbit following intraventricular or intracerebral injections of morphine and found that 40 μg of morphine hydrochloride (20 μg bilaterally) into the hypothalamus, subthalamus, and the mesencephalon, especially in the medial parts of these structures, resulted in a marked analgesia. However, injections of morphine into the septum, the commissura fornicus, the dorsal hippocampus, and the dorsal and lateral parts of the thalamus were without effect. Contrary to the findings of Tsou and Jang [7] (who also used rabbits, but as acute rather than chronic preparations), only moderate analgesia occurred when intraventricular morphine was restricted to the 3rd ventricle, whereas there was more pronounced analgesia following morphine administration into the more caudal ventricular areas. The authors concluded from this that the most likely central sites of action were the gray areas surrounding the aqueduct and the structures on the floor of the 4th ventricle. The difference in results from those of Tsou and Jang [7] was suggested to be due to a different analgesic reaction being tested. The cannula system consisted of an outer guide with an inside diameter of 1 mm (outer diameter not given), and the injection needle extended 4 mm beyond the end of the guide cannula.

Jacquet and Lajtha [14], using 30-gauge outer cannulas (0.30 mm o.d.) and 35-gauge injection cannulas (0.13 mm o.d.) in chronically implanted rats, found that 10 μg of morphine in 0.5 μl Ringer's solution, injected bilaterally into the posterior hypothalamus and into the 3rd ventricle, resulted in significant analgesia (using the flinch-jump test with graduated electric shock to the feet as the aversive stimulus). Negative sites included the dorsomedial thalamus, septum, caudate, hippocampus, and anterior hypothalamus. In a subsequent study [15], the periaqueductal gray was also found to yield pronounced analgesia (to strong pinch and pinpricks), although this was accompanied by an explosive hyperreactivity to auditory and visual stimuli that had previously been neutral stimuli. Some recent histological studies [16,17] indicating that fibers coursing through the periaqueductal gray terminate in and near the posterior hypothalamus suggest that the periaqueductal gray and the posterior hypothalamus may be part of the same pathway mediating morphine analgesia.

In summary, although there is not precise agreement on the exact anatomic localization of morphine analgesia, these studies agree that medial diencephalic and mesencephalic structures are involved.

B. Morphine Hypothermia

Lotti et al. [8,9] in the studies described in Sec. II, A, injected 50 μg of morphine sulfate in 1 μl of saline throughout areas of the hypothalamus and the thalamus and found that the preoptic and anterior hypothalamus yielded hypothermia. Hypothermia was measured with a thermistor probe inserted at least 8 cm into the rectum. Intraventricular injections of 50 μg of morphine sulfate in 1 μl of saline failed to lower core temperature, however.

Foster et al. [11], in the study described previously, found that a fall in core body temperature occurred in response to injections of 22.5 and 45.0 μg of morphine injected into the preoptic and anterior hypothalamic nuclei, thus confirming the studies of Lotti et al. [8,9].

C. Morphine Activation of Pituitary Adrenal System

Lotti et al. [18], using the cannula system of Decima and George [10] in chronically implanted female rats, found significant reductions in adrenal ascorbic acid when 50 μg of morphine sulfate (in 1 μl of saline) was injected into the mid-, but not rostral or caudal, hypothalamus. A smaller amount of morphine, 5 μg (in 1 μl of saline), injected into the same area resulted in a significant increase in mean plasma corticosterone level. The authors concluded that the pituitary adrenal activation resulting from systemic morphine administration in rats is mediated by an action of morphine upon the mid-hypothalamic regions (including the whole or part of the anterior, paraventricular, ventromedial and dorsomedial nuclei of the hypothalamus).

D. Morphine Dependence

Wei et al. [19,20], using 20-gauge outer cannulas in chronically implanted rats, injected 40-200 μg of naloxone (in crystalline form) in morphine-dependent animals and found that the medial thalamus and rostral mesencephalic structures precipitated abstinence symptoms (i.e., two or more escape attempts, or three or more wet shakes within 10 min following naloxone injection). From this, the authors concluded that medial thalamic nuclei and closely adjacent structures may be the primary sites for the development of opioid dependence.

III. EVALUATIONS OF INTRACEREBRAL INJECTION METHODOLOGY

How precise and specific is the technique of intracerebral drug injection via chronically implanted cannulas? This question has been raised repeatedly and attempts have been made to answer these critical questions.

For example, Routtenberg [21] raised the possibility that drugs may diffuse widely through the brain into ventricular spaces, and ventricular transport of the drug to distant sites may occur. Subsequently, Routtenberg et al. [22], using histochemical fluorescence to trace spread of injected catecholamines (in crystalline form), found that there were three types of diffusion following dopamine injection: (a) a spherical spread around the cannula tip approximately 2 mm in diameter, (b) diffusion along axonal fibers in an orthodromic direction, and (c) spread to the ependymal wall and choroid plexus of the ipsilateral and contralateral ventricle.

Montgomery and Singer [23], in rebuttal, criticized Routtenberg et al. for using much higher doses than those used in typical microinjection studies. The high dose in crystalline form presumably increased osmotic pressure and increased diffusion of the injected drug. In a subsequent study, however, Routtenberg and Bondareff [24], using solutions of norepinephrine at lower doses, found diffusion to consist of a spherical spread of at least 1 mm in diameter around the cannula tip, and also movement of the chemical up the shaft of the cannula, as well as axon-related movement. Bondareff et al. [25], using 24-gauge guide cannulas in chronically implanted rats, and injecting 0.5, 1.0, and 5.0 μg of dopamine or norepinephrine per 1 μl of saline via polyethelene tubing attached to the top of the cannula, found that spread of these catecholamines was directly related to (a) concentration of drug and (b) osmolarity of injected solution. It was found that 1 μg of dopamine in 1 μl of saline spread rostrocaudally about 2 mm. Again, some leakage was observed along the shaft of the cannula. In some cases, spreading of the catecholamine into the ventricle was noted when the cannulas were placed close to the ventricular wall. When the cannula placement was more remote from a ventricle, the fluorescence ended before reaching the ependymal epithelium.

Grossman and Stumpf [26] found, on the basis of autoradiography using a technique that limited spread of radioactivity during processing and film mounting (thus eliminating a potential artifact), that the spread of labeled crystalline atropine was approximately 1.0-1.8 mm in diameter in spherical form around the cannula tip. In many cases, there was a tendency for the radioactivity to appear in a pear-shaped area, extending some distance up the shaft of the cannula. Ventricular spaces nearest the site of atropine injection, however, failed to show concentrations of radioactivity. Some radioactivity showed up in the vascular system during 5-12 minutes following the injection, indicating possible transport of drug away from the injection site. Some radioactivity was also noted in distant contralateral and ipsilateral sites, but the levels were much lower than that which would be sufficient to produce behavioral effects.

Singer and Montgomery [27] discounted the probability of significant ventricular involvement in intracerebral injection studies. They pointed out that intraventricular injections of neurochemicals result in markedly different behavioral and physiological effects or show different latencies and dose-response relationships from the effects of the same substance when injected directly into specific nonventricular sites.

In this connection, it is interesting to note that Booth [28] pointed out that large-sized cannulas (e.g., the 20-gauge cannulas even now widely in use) resulted in lesions over 1 mm wide, and that a comparison of large and small cannulas indicated that greater tissue damage lowered the threshold for response and reduced the maximum response. Bondareff et al. [25] pointed out the possibility of extracellular spaces serving as a possible route for diffusion of injected drug. Intracerebral lesions often result in brain swelling, which may be due to an increase in extracellular space. When the volume of extracellular space was decreased by pretreatment with dexamethasone, which is known to ameliorate brain swelling associated with intracerebral trauma, there was decreased spread of injected catecholamines [25]. These results indicate the desirability of minimizing trauma to the brain by using as small a cannula as possible and allowing enough time for postsurgical recovery.

The question of drug diffusion in significant amounts following intracerebral injection encompasses the following possible routes: (a) along the shaft of the cannula, (b) along fiber tracts, (c) through brain tissue to ventricles and from there to distant sites, (d) vascular absorption and transport to distant sites, and (e) along extracellular spaces.

On the other hand, the highly specific anatomical localization of neurochemical effects makes it unlikely that significant drug diffusion occurs following microinjection. Booth [28], for example, reported distances between effective and ineffective sites of as little as 0.10 mm. I also found that inaccuracy in cannula placement of as little as 0.25 mm produced erratic results.

The variables which appear to be relevant to the problem of attenuating drug diffusion are listed below:

1. Size of Cannula

This is a critical variable in obtaining accurate anatomical localization of drug effects. The outer diameter of a 20-gauge cannula (currently widely used) is 0.89 mm. This is larger than many of the structures in the rat brain that have been the subject of chemical stimulation studies. For example, the ventromedial hypothalamic nucleus is approximately 0.75 mm wide at its widest extent; a 20-gauge cannula, if implanted squarely on target (which is difficult), would also be impinging on adjacent areas. Under these circumstances, it would be difficult to ascribe the resulting drug effects to chemical stimulation of this structure exclusively, since adjacent stimulated structures may also contribute to the observed effect. Surprisingly, however, such claims have been made using such large cannulas in the rat. I recommend the use of a 30-gauge cannula as the guide cannula and placement of the tip of this cannula 1 mm dorsal to the actual site. A 35-gauge wire stylet is kept in place in the 30-gauge cannula, with the stylet tip extending 1 mm from the tip of the guide cannula. The injection cannula, also 35-gauge, is calibrated to extend 1 mm beyond the guide cannula. Thus, only the smaller gauge stylet and injection cannula are allowed to penetrate the actual site, minimizing the area of tissue damage.

2. Crystal vs Fluid

Montgomery and Singer [23] pointed out that crystals must dissolve in the endogenous fluid before they can have any effect. This results in high and uncontrolled concentrations resulting from the dissolving crystals and possibly high osmotic pressure. Another disadvantage is that the exact dose cannot be specified, and therefore a dose-response relationship (which is an essential part of any pharmacological investigation) cannot be obtained. Therefore, drugs should be injected in the form of fluids.

3. Volume

It is quite obvious that volume is a critical variable in diffusion. Myers [29] recommends that for the small rat brain the volume should be limited to no more than 0.5 μl. Greater volume may result in tissue damage as well as diffusion.

4. Osmolarity

Bondareff et al. [25] obtained a positive relationship between osmolarity of injected substance and spread of catecholamines through brain tissue. Thus, the osmolarity of the injected solution should be controlled.

5. Injection Method

Some methods involve attaching polyethylene (PE) tubing to the top of the guide cannula. However, this increases the likelihood that the injected fluid will travel up along the shaft of the cannula following the path of least resistance. In the case of an injection needle which is cut to the same length as the guide cannula, the same objection holds. The injection needle should extend 1 mm beyond the guide cannula tip to minimize this possibility. However, in order to avoid making an injection into a fresh stab wound, the stylet which normally sits in the guide cannula to prevent its occlusion should also extend 1 mm beyond the cannula tip. The injection should be made slowly, and an interval allowed to elapse before pulling out the injection needle so that the drug is absorbed by the tissue and not pulled back into the cannula shaft.

6. Lipophilic vs Hydrophilic Drug

This is probably a factor in how quickly the drug is absorbed by the vascular system and redistributed. Morphine, being hydrophilic, is probably not absorbed by the vascular system and redistributed in significant quantities within a reasonable time following injection.

IV. INTRACEREBRAL INJECTION METHOD

The intracerebral microinjection technique is a method by which the drug is delivered via a stainless-steel cannula to a population of brain cells, as distinct from the iontophoretic injection method whereby the drug is delivered via a micropipette and electrophoresis to a single cell. The advantage of the intracerebral microinjection method over systemic drug injection is that relatively precise quantities of drug can be delivered to discrete brain areas. However, the intracerebral injection method may give rise to unreliable and/or spurious results due to several possible sources of error inherent in the technique. The procedure to be described in detail in the following pages is a modification of existing intracerebral microinjection techniques which was developed by the author to minimize these sources of error. The most important feature of the method to be described consists of using a fine-gauge cannula, 30-gauge, as the outer guide, which is placed 1 mm dorsal to the site itself. The injection site is penetrated only by the much smaller injection needle, which is 35-gauge. The use of such fine-gauge cannulas and needles necessitates greater care in carrying out the surgical implantation and drug injection, but is worth the trouble for the greater accuracy and reliability of results achieved.

The surgical procedures involved in stereotaxic implantation of the cannulas are not discussed in this chapter; this would merely be redundant since excellent presentations are already available (e.g., Myers [29]). The only additional recommendations are the following: (a) All cannulas, stylets, and skull screws should be sterilized before implantation to minimize the possibility of bacterial infection in brain tissue and (b) use a Luminated Micromagnifier (obtainable from Circon Microsurgical; see Appendix) to enhance the visibility of the various components of this microinjection method, and a pair of fine-pointed microforceps (obtainable from Clay Adams, see Appendix) to facilitate handling of these small objects.

A. Construction of Cannula, Stylet, and Injection Needle

1. Cannula

Thirty-gauge cannulas are now available from Plastic Products, Inc. (see Appendix). Previous to this, these cannulas were custom-made for our laboratory. The basic construction of these cannulas is quite simple. Thirty-gauge stainless-steel tubing, available from Small Parts, Inc. (see Appendix), is cut to predetermined lengths (18 mm for my lab, which is sufficiently long to reach most sites in the rat brain) and mounted in a cylindrical pedestal (either plastic or metal) which is threaded on the exterior to accept a screw-on plastic dust cap. For bilateral implantation of medial sites, such as most hypothalamic sites, two such cannulas can be mounted side-by-side in parallel with a separation of 1.5 mm (from the center of one cannula to the other) as in Fig. 1d. The 30-gauge cannulas are recessed below the surface of the pedestal by approximately 0.5 mm, and access to the opening of the 30-gauge cannula is by a cone-shaped opening that allows easier access (see Fig. 1a).

2. Stylet

The stylets that fit the 30-gauge cannulas are not commercially available and have to be made. The 30-gauge cannulas have an inner diameter of 0.15 mm and will accept a 35-gauge needle with an outer diameter of 0.13 mm. A stylet, made of stainless-steel wire of similar diameter (0.005 in., obtainable from Cole Parmer Instrument Co., see Appendix), is kept in the cannula at all times other than when the animal is being injected in order to prevent the cannula from clogging. The head of the stylet is mounted with a small glass bead to prevent it from entering further in the brain (Fig. 1b). To make the stylet, cut 35-gauge wire approximately 2 mm longer than the desired length. A glass bead is mounted on the head of the stylet in the following manner. A microliter glass capillary tube (obtainable from Drummond Scientific Co.; see Appendix) is cut in 2-mm lengths. This is done by running a glass-cutting blade (obtainable from Fisher Scientific) 4 or 5 times across the surface where it is to be broken off, then threading the capillary tube with a wire before breaking off the piece of glass tubing with a pair of forceps. The threaded wire prevents the small piece of glass tubing from flying off. This piece of glass tubing is then melted onto the top of the stylet wire. Set the piece of the 2-mm glass tube on the very tip of the wire stylet with only 1 mm of the glass tubing overlapping the tip of the wire; then carefully hold this to a medium flame from a Bunson burner until the glass tubing turns completely red and melts into a circular bead on the wire stylet. Care must be taken to make the glass bead small enough so that when the stylet is inserted into the cannula, the head sits comfortably within the circumference of the enlarged cone-shaped opening of the 30-gauge tubing (see Fig. 1a). In this way, the stylets cannot be moved or twisted inadvertently when the cap is screwed on the cannula ensemble.

The next step is to cut the stylets to a predetermined length accurately. The length of the stylets should match the length of the injection needle so that the injection is made in an already existing wound and not in a freshly made one. In order to minimize diffusion of chemical to other sites via the outer wall of the cannula, the injected drug is ejected 1 mm from the tip of the cannula. When the injection occurs closer to the tip of the cannula, there is a tendency for the injected drug to "travel" up the shaft of the cannula following the path of least resistance. Therefore, the injection needle is 1 mm longer than the cannula, i.e., 19 mm, and the stylets should accordingly be 19 mm in length (see Fig. 1b).

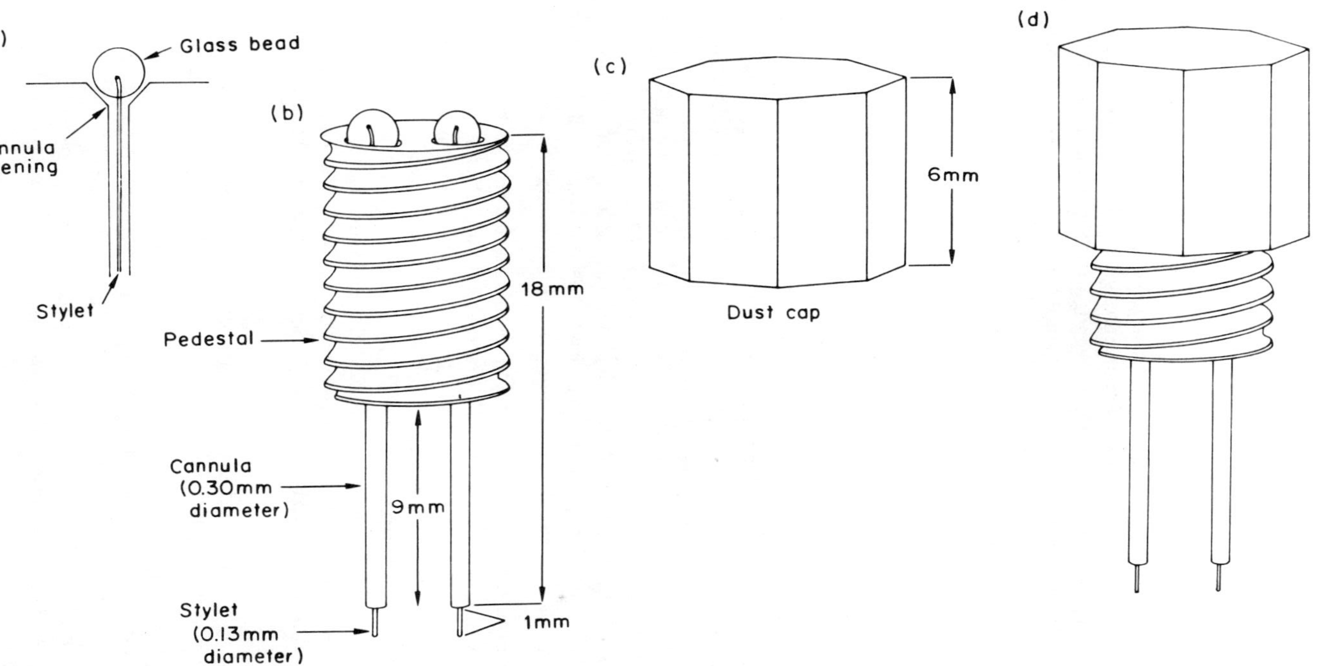

FIGURE 1. A side view of a bilateral cannula. (a) The cone-shaped access to the cannula opening to accommodate the glass bead mounted on the head of the stylet. (b) A bilateral cannula with stylets in place (note the 1-mm extension of the stylet from the end of the cannula). (c) The dust cap that screws onto the bilateral cannula. (d) A bilateral cannula with stylets and dust cap.

3. Injection Needle

The needle consists of a short piece of 35-gauge stainless-steel tubing which is mounted on a shorter piece of 30-gauge stainless-steel tubing. The 35-gauge tubing is thin-walled and apt to constrict with any slight pressure, and so should be handled as little as possible. It is therefore mounted on the thicker-walled 30-gauge tubing so that the needle can be handled at this end without constricting the needle. These tubings can be obtained from Small Parts, Inc. (see Appendix). The 35-gauge tubing is cut to 1-in. lengths using a pair of scissors. The 30-gauge tubing is cut to half-inch lengths using a pair of wire cutters. Care must be taken in cutting the 30-gauge tubing since it will close up when pinched. One method is to insert a 0.005-in. wire into the tubing before cutting and then bevel the opening by holding it against a grinding wheel at a slight angle. The 1-in. length 35-gauge stainless-steel tubing is inserted into the half-inch 30-gauge stainless steel tubing a distance of approximately 6 mm, leaving 19 mm to extend from the 30-gauge tubing (see Fig. 2). In this way, when inserted into the 18-mm, 30-gauge cannula, the injection needle should protrude exactly 1 mm beyond the cannula tip.

The two pieces of stainless-steel tubing are bonded together by application of a bonding agent. Place a small drop of Eastman 910 (obtainable from any photographic supply store) on a clean dish. Dip the tip of a pin into the bonding fluid and then quickly run the pintip around the junction of the two tubings. Be spare in applying the Eastman 910; an overly liberal drop is apt to "run" up the shaft of the 35-gauge tubing and plug the opening. Allow the junction to air-dry, taking care that it is not in contact with any surface while drying. Allow a minimum of 2 min for complete drying.

To calibrate the length of the injection needle, set aside one cannula as the "calibration cannula" or "standard" (marking it to distinguish it from the other cannulas). This is to prevent "drift" in measurement. All stylets and needles are calibrated using this standard. The stylets and needles should be exactly 1 mm longer than the standard, extending 1 mm beyond the tip. Use a Luminated Micromagnifier (with a 3X magnifying lens) when calibrating needles and stylets to insure accuracy. It should be emphasized that errors as small as a quarter of a millimeter may result in unreliable results.

The life of any given injection needle is limited. Therefore, it is advisable to prepare a batch of 20 or more and to have some in reserve at all times.

B. Injection Method

The animal is allowed at least 1 week, and preferably 2 weeks, for postsurgical recovery. This interval allows the surgical wound to heal, and renewed bleeding is minimized.

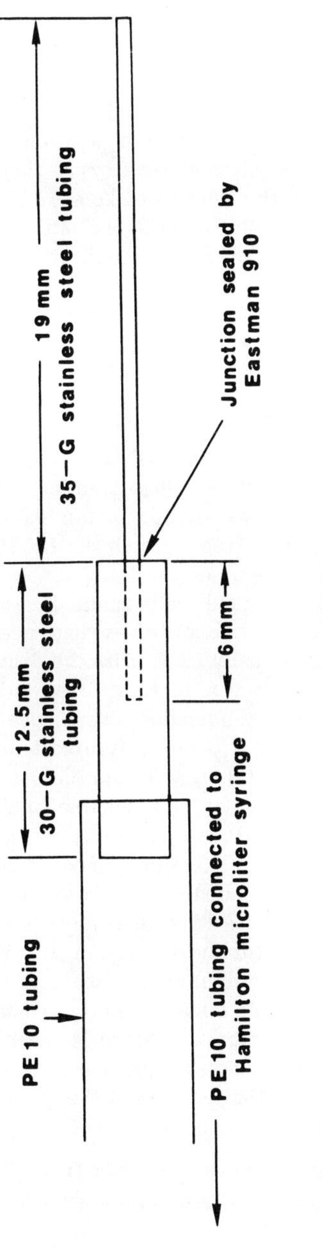

FIGURE 2. The injection needle, constructed of 35-gauge stainless-steel tubing, mounted on a shorter piece of 30-gauge stainless-steel tubing and bonded together by application of Eastman 910; PE 10 tubing connected to a Hamilton microliter syringe is then connected to the needle.

Fill a 10-μl Hamilton syringe (with permanently mounted 30-gauge needle, 1 in. in length and with a 22° angled tip) mounted on a Chaney adaptor, with a mixture of 70% alcohol and 30% distilled water. Be sure that there are no bubbles in the alcohol solution when filling the syringe and pump the syringe several times to remove all air pockets from it. Using a separate, previously sterilized syringe filled with the drug solution, fill PE 10 tubing (approximately 20 cm in length) with the drug solution (being sure to rinse the tubing thoroughly and air-dry the tubing if used before). Hold the PE 10 tubing against the light to make sure there are no air bubbles in the tubing. Run 4-5 drops from the free end of the PE 10 tubing. Take the injection needle (being sure always to handle it by the 30-gauge end and not the 35-gauge end, which tends to plug easily after the slightest pressure) and fit the free end of the PE 10 tubing over the 30-gauge end. The overlap should be about 2-3 mm. Make sure that the PE 10 tubing fits securely over the 30-gauge stainless-steel tubing, and that there is no leak. Run 2-3 drops of the drug through the needle. Fluid should flow freely but slowly from the needle with a slight pressure. When the 35-gauge needle becomes plugged or partially constricted, as it easily becomes, resistance can be felt when pressure is applied to the syringe plunger. When this happens, discard the needle and fit on a new needle. After loading the PE 10 tubing and the injection needle with the drug, detach the PE 10 tubing from the syringe. Next, retract the plunger on the Hamilton syringe (already filled with the 70% alcohol) by 0.2 μl. This will result in a small air bubble being lodged in the tip of the Hamilton microliter syringe needle. Now attach the free end of the PE 10 tubing already filled with the drug solution to the Hamilton microliter syringe needle tip, making sure to slip it over securely to cover the entire angled tip of the needle. Next, push in the Hamilton syringe plunger by 0.4 μl. An air bubble, approximately 4 mm in length, should then appear in the PE 10 tubing. Trace the outline of the bubble on an underlying sheet of paper. It may be advisable to tape the Hamilton syringe to the sheet of paper to prevent it from moving and thus losing the reference point for the air bubble. The movement of the air bubble indicates whether the drug reached the intended site, or was blocked by an obstruction in the needle, or escaped via a leak elsewhere in the system. The recommended injection volume for the rat is 0.5 μl. With a 0.5 μl volume injection, the air bubble should travel approximately 10 mm in the PE 10 tubing. The size of the air bubble should remain constant. If the air bubble becomes compressed, this is a sign that there is trouble somewhere in the injection system. There is either a plugged needle, which is the most likely explanation, or a leak at the junction of the PE 10 tubing and the Hamilton syringe needle tip.

For the actual injection, remove the stylet from the cannula and insert the injection needle as far as it will go. Since we have previously calibrated both the cannula and the injection needle, we are now confident that the injection needle tip extends exactly 1 mm from the cannula tip, and therefore the injection needle tip sits precisely in the intended site, assuming that the stereotaxic implantation of the cannula was accurate.

Slowly depress the plunger on the Hamilton syringe at the rate of about 0.1 μl per 10-12 sec. An injection of 0.5 μl should take about 1 min. Once the injection is over, allow the injection needle to stay in the cannula for another minute or so. This is to allow the tissue to absorb the drug, so that the drug will not be pulled back into the cannula barrel by the suction created by the removal of the injection needle. Make sure that the air bubble in the PE 10 tubing has travelled the appropriate distance before pulling out the needle and replacing the stylet and the dust cap on the cannula.

The final step in the injection procedure is to flush out the injection needle immediately following the injection. Attach the 30-gauge end of the injection needle to PE 10 tubing which is in turn attached to a syringe filled with the 70% alcohol; allow 4-5 drops to be pushed out of the needle before placing the needle back into a dust-free container. If drug solution is allowed to sit in the needle for any length of time, this will result in a plugged needle.

To unplug a needle, place it in a water-filled beaker and boil for about 5 min. Sometimes this will serve to dislodge or dissolve any foreign matter plugging the shaft. However, if the plugging is due to the needle wall becoming constricted, there is little that can be done to undo this damage.

C. Immobilization of the Rat to Allow Injection

The cannula opening into which the injection needle is inserted is small and difficult to see. Moreover, the needle is very pliable and bends easily. Once bent, the needle becomes plugged and therefore useless. Thus, it is essential to have a relatively immobile animal for the injection procedure. However, a rat tends to struggle violently when an experimenter attempts to hold it immobile. This often results in the rat injuring itself, or equally undesirable, ferocious attempts by the rat to bite the restraining hand. Often the experimenter is obliged to hold the rat so tightly that anoxia results, and the rat loses consciousness, or worse, expires. At best, the restraining procedure results in the rat becoming fearful, as shown by piloerection, excessive urination, and defecation. This increased physiological activation undoubtedly affects the subsequent behavior to be measured, confounding these effects with the effects of the injected drug.

There is a simple method which obviates these difficulties, and keeps the rat calm and immobile. Complete quiescence is induced in the rat by snugly wrapping its body in four or five layers of soft cloth, keeping only its head exposed. For the first layer, use a disposable Teri-Towel (obtainable from National Scientific Co., Inc.; see Appendix). Care must be taken to include all four limbs in the wrapping and to keep the towel wound tightly, but not so tightly as to interfere with breathing. Then, on top of the towel, apply another layer or so of soft cloth. Secure the wrapping with belts of Velcro (see Fig. 3). At first, the rat becomes emotional when immobilized in this manner. This is evident by the loose stools and large number of feces which are evacuated during this time. Therefore, it is necessary to habituate the animal to this procedure before any actual injection is carried out. In my laboratory, the rat is given this treatment once a day for three days in a row before actual injection. By the fourth wrapping, the rat has become habituated to the procedure and shows little emotional reaction when wrapped. More importantly, such a wrapped animal is docile and rarely attempts to bite even when a finger is put within range. In this manner, a rat can be injected successfully by one person without assistance, without anesthesia, and without any adverse consequences to the experimenter or to the rat (see Fig. 4).

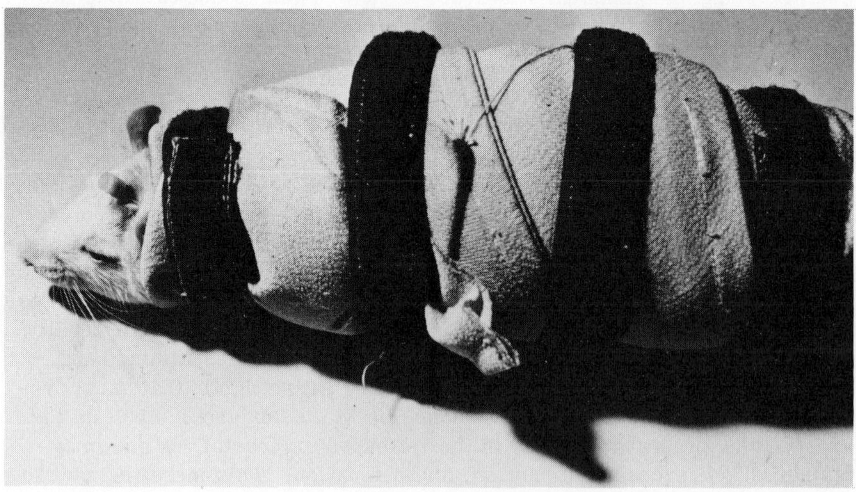

FIGURE 3. A rat "wrapped" in a disposable Teri-Towel and an additional layer of soft cloth, and secured by four belts of Velcro.

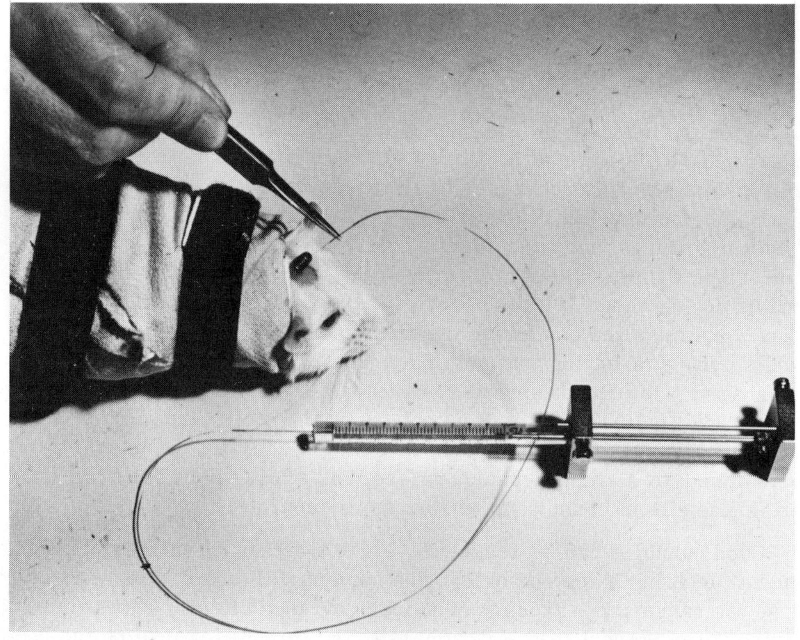

FIGURE 4. A "wrapped" rat undergoing intracerebral injection.

D. Histological Confirmation of Injection Site

When the animal is ready to be sacrificed, the animal is anesthetized and then injected in each cannula with 0.5 μl of a solution containing blue dye (0.19% Evans blue dye in distilled water, and previously Millipore-filtered 5 times). After waiting 10 min to allow for absorption of the dye into tissue, the animal is perfused according to standard methods (e.g., those described by Wolf [30]), then decapitated, and the brain is removed with the cannula still in place in the brain with an intervening piece of the skull still attached. This is accomplished by cutting away the outer skin and eyes, removing the lower jaw with a pair of large scissors, and stripping all tissue from the skull with a pair of forceps. Next cut away the eye sockets and nasal bridge with a bone cutter; then remove the two ear canals by inserting the angled edges of the bone cutter around the junction of the ear and skull and gently lifting out the ear without crushing. Then remove the rest of the skull except that part underneath the cement holding the cannula to the skull. Place the brain with the attached skull and cemented cannula in a 10% formalin bath for a day or so. This will allow the brain to firm up, and thus, if the cannula is disturbed accidentally within the brain, the damage is minimized. After a day or so in the formalin bath, the brain is ready for histological examination.

Place the brain on the freezing stage of a microtome. However, in order to slide the brain at an angle which corresponds to that used in the reference atlas, it is necessary to start with one surface correctly angled. A variable-inclined plane (described by Herberg and Franklin [31]) is used to cut the brain at the correct angle before it is placed on the freezing stage. For the purpose of anatomic localization of injection site, the slices need be no finer than 100 μm. Usually, the dye spreads across 10-15 slices, and the slice containing the most ventral penetration (usually the middle one) is taken for anatomic placement. The spread of dye is typically egg-shaped, i.e., most spread rostrocaudally (probably corresponding to the axonal diffusion noted by Routtenberg et al. [22]), 0.8 mm spread along the vertical dimension, and 0.5 mm spread along the lateral dimension. Standard staining techniques (see Wolf [30]) can be followed to ascertain the site of cannula placement more accurately.

Used cannulas can be recycled. Place the cannula with its surrounding cement block in an acetone bath. The cement will dissolve in a day or so. Rinse the cannula in a fresh acetone bath and then blot dry with paper towel. A thin coat of cement may still adhere to the threaded tracks on the pedestal. This should be removed using a pair of fine-pointed forceps.

V. ADVANTAGES OF INTRACEREBRAL INJECTION

What are the advantages of intracerebral injections over other methods of studying morphine action?

First, one can identify anatomic sites in the CNS which mediate morphine action. Using the techniques described above, Jacquet and Lajtha [14,15] were able to identify two sites in the CNS which reliably yield analgesia following morphine injection. These were the posterior hypothalamus (Fig. 5) and the periaqueductal gray matter (Fig. 6). The latter site, in addition to yielding analgesia following morphine administration, also yielded an explosive hyperreactivity which was specific to certain stimuli (auditory and visual). Figure 6 shows that these two effects were correlated with morphine dose. The posterior hypothalamus and the periaqueductal gray appear to be part of the same pathway mediating morphine analgesia. The latter, in addition, appears to mediate hyperreactivity due to an overlapping pathway. (For an example of the hyperreactivity, see Fig. 7.)

Second, one can assess analgesic potency of opiates interacting directly with receptor sites in the CNS. Jacquet and Lajtha [15] found that relative analgesic potency of opiates following intracerebral administration does not

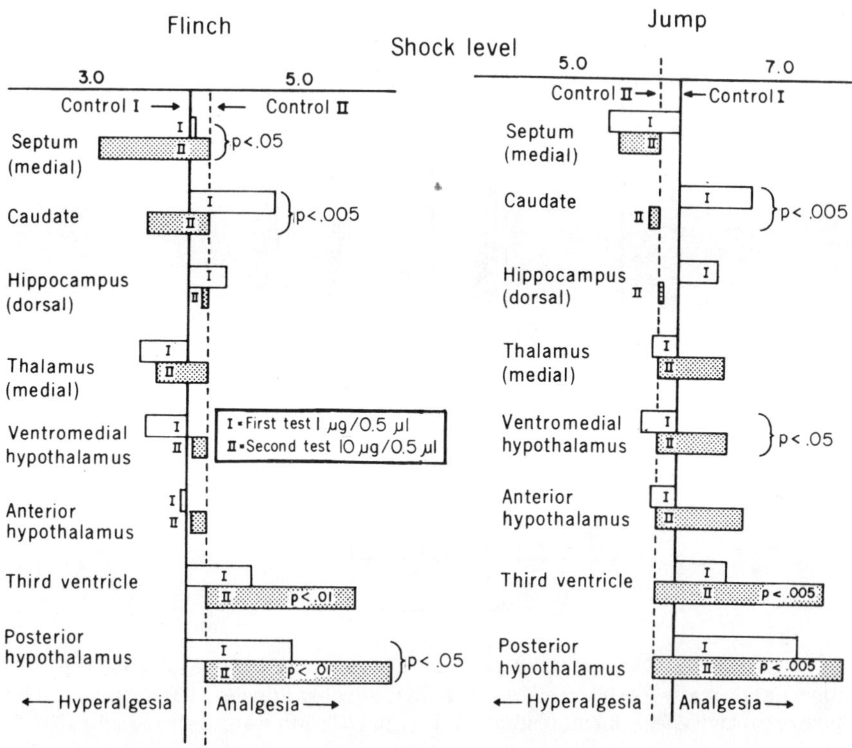

FIGURE 5. Flinch and jump thresholds of eight experimental groups and one control group (total n = 78). The baselines for the control group are shown by the center vertical lines, the solid line for the first day (I) and the broken line for the second day (II). The open bars are data representing the first day (1 μg morphine); the stippled bars are data for the second day (10 μg). The bars to the left of the baseline represent hyperalgesia, while those to the right represent analgesia. Probability (p) values within bars represent significant differences from the control; those outside of bars represent significant differences between doses (that is, between tests I and II). (From Jacquet and Lajtha [14].)

parallel their analgesic potency following systemic administration. This is similar to results obtained by Kutter et al. [32], who found differences in analgesic potencies following intraventricular vs intravenous injections of opiates. This is probably due to the blood-brain barrier which allows lipophilic drugs to readily penetrate into the CNS, but prevents penetration by the more hydrophilic drugs, such as morphine. Our results indicate

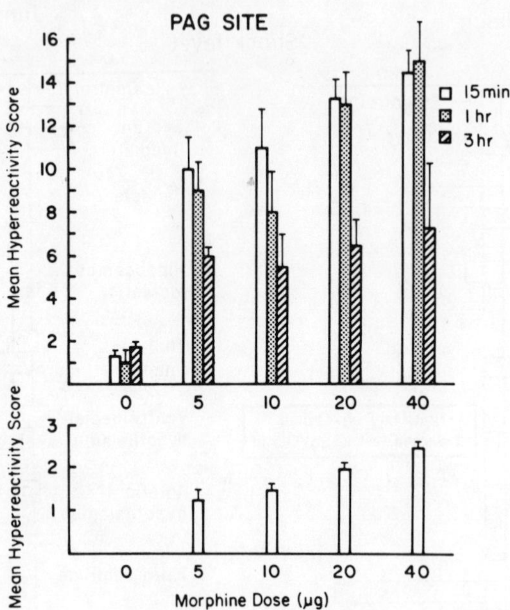

FIGURE 6. Dose-related scores of hyper- and hyporeactivity of periaqueductal gray (PAG) animals after intracerebral doses of morphine. The hyperreactivity was measured at 5, 10, and 15 min after intracerebral administration, and the highest score achieved was assigned to the animal. The hyporeactivity was measured at 15, 60, and 180 min after intracerebral administration. Separate groups are shown at each morphine dose, each group consisting of four to six animals. (The injection volume was always 0.5 μl for each bilateral site.) (From Jacquet and Lajtha [15].)

that when this barrier is bypassed, morphine is a much more potent analgesic than such lipophilic opiates as levorphanol, which is estimated to be 2-10 times as potent in the systemic route.

Third, one can assess whether naloxone acts at the same site to block morphine analgesia. Jacquet and Lajtha [15] found that when naloxone is injected in the sites previously found to mediate morphine analgesia, it caused a diminution in the analgesia. If naloxone was injected just prior to the morphine in the same site, the onset of the analgesia was blocked, but for only 10 min. Evidently, naloxone is very short-acting, with blocking action being much shorter than the duration of morphine action. If injected following morphine, naloxone reversed the morphine analgesia but, again, for only 10 min.

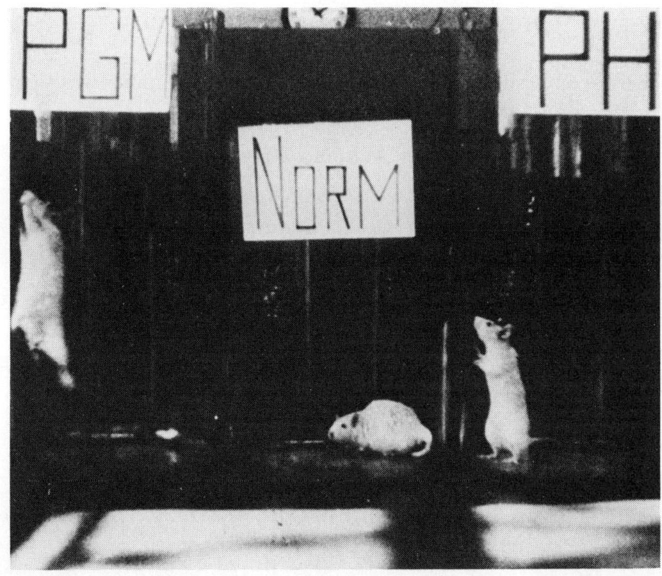

FIGURE 7. In response to a sharp noise (i.e., striking the side of the glass jar with a metal hemostat), the rat, previously injected intracerebrally with 10 μg of morphine bilaterally (total dose, 20 μg), makes a vertical leap, often as high as 36 in.

Fourth, one can assess whether tolerance occurs in CNS sites. In the same study [15] it was found that analgesic tolerance to ip morphine was manifested by rats that had received prior intracerebral morphine. This would indicate that tolerance is due to local changes occurring in the CNS rather than to changes occurring in the blood-brain barrier or due to changes in peripheral metabolism or elimination.

Finally, one can compare local chemical stimulation with local electrical stimulation. Morphine injection in the periaqueductal gray gave rise to effects similar to those caused by electrical stimulation at this site. Previous reports [33,34] have shown that electrical stimulation of the periaqueductal gray produces profound analgesia, to the extent of permitting surgery without anesthesia in the rat. We also were able to excise a small tumor from the dorsal region of the neck in a rat given 10 μg of bilateral morphine in the periaqueductal gray without any sign of pain. This suggests that the same pathway which gives rise to analgesia is activated by both electrical stimulation and by morphine stimulation.

APPENDIX: MATERIALS AND SOURCES

Luminated micromagnifier: Circon Microsurgical, Santa Barbara Airport, Goleta, California 93017 (catalog no. MS 5600)

Fine-pointed microforcep: Clay Adams, Parsippany, New Jersey 07054 (catalog no. A-1909)

0.005-in. Stainless-steel wire: Cole Parmer Instrument Co., 7425 N. Oak Park Ave., Chicago, Illinois 60648 (catalog no. 1425)

Thirty-gauge cannulas: Plastic Products, Inc., P. O. Box 1214, Roanoke, Virginia

Thirty-gauge and 35-gauge stainless-steel tubing: Small Parts, Inc., 6901 N. E. 3rd Ave., Miami, Florida 33138

Precision capillary tubes (0.4 mm i.d.): Drummond Scientific Co., Broomall, Pennsylvania 19008

Glass-cutting blades: Fisher Scientific Co., P. O. Box 537, Pittsburgh, Pennsylvania 15230 (catalog no. 11 348 8)

Eastman 910 adhesive: Fleck Photographic Co., W. 39th St. and 5th Ave., New York, New York 10036

Hamilton 10-microliter syringe with permanently affixed needle (1-in. length with 22° bevel): Hamilton Co., 4960 Energy Way, P. O. Box 7500, Reno, Nevada 89502 (catalog no. 701N)

Chaney adaptor: Hamilton Co. (catalog no. 14700 CH)

Intramedic polyethylene tubing (PE 10 tubing): Clay Adams

Teri-Towels: National Scientific Co., 25200 Miles Ave., Cleveland, Ohio 44146

REFERENCES

1. J. H. Jaffe, Narcotic analgesics. In _The Pharmacological Basis of Therapeutics_ (L. S. Goodman and A. Gilman, eds.). New York: Macmillan, 1970, pp. 237-275.

2. S. P. Grossman, Eating or drinking elicited by direct adrenergic or cholinergic stimulation of hypothalamus. _Science 132_:301-302 (1960).

3. L. Stein and J. Seifter, Muscarinic synapses in the hypothalamus. _Amer. J. Physiol. 202_:751-756 (1962).

4. N. E. Miller, K. S. Gottesman, and N. Emery, Dose response to carbachol and norepinephrine in rat hypothalamus. _Amer. J. Physiol. 206_:1384-1388 (1964).

5. S. J. Mulé, Physiological disposition of narcotic agonists and antagonists. In Narcotic Drugs: Biochemical Pharmacology (D. H. Clouet, ed.). New York and London: Plenum Press, 1971.

6. W. H. Oldendorf, S. Hyman, L. Braun, and S. C. Oldendorf, Blood-brain barrier: Penetration of morphine, codeine, heroin, and methadone after carotid injection. Science 178:984-986 (1972).

7. K. Tsou and C. S. Jang, Studies on the site of analgesic action of morphine by intracerebral micro-injection. Sci. Sinica 13:1099-1109 (1964).

8. V. J. Lotti, P. Lomax, and R. George, Temperature responses in the rat following intracerebral microinjection of morphine. J. Pharmacol. 150:135-139 (1965).

9. V. J. Lotti, P. Lomax, and R. George, Acute tolerance to morphine following systemic and intracerebral injection in the rat. Int. J. Neuropharmacol. 5:35-42 (1966).

10. E. Decima and R. George, A simple cannula for intracerebral injections in chronic animals. Electroencephalogr. Clin. Neurophysiol. 17:438-439 (1964).

11. R. S. Foster, D. J. Jenden, and P. Lomax, A comparison of the pharmacologic effects of morphine and N-methyl morphine. J. Pharmacol. Exp. Ther. 157:185-195 (1967).

12. D. M. Buxbaum, G. G. Yarbrough, and M. E. Carter, Dose-dependent behavioral and analgesic effects produced by microinjections of morphine sulfate into the anterior thalamic nuclei. The Pharmacologist: 12:210 (1970).

13. A. Herz, K. Albus, J. Metys, P. Schubert, and H. Teschemacher, On the central sites for the antinociceptive action of morphine and fentanyl. Neuropharmacology 9:539-551 (1970).

14. Y. F. Jacquet and A. Lajtha, Morphine action at central nervous system sites in rat: analgesia or hyperalgesia depending on site and dose. Science 182:490-492 (1973).

15. Y. F. Jacquet and A. Lajtha, Paradoxical effects following morphine microinjection in the periaqueductal gray matter in the rat. Science 185:1055-1057 (1974).

16. C. C. Chi, An experimental silver study of the ascending projections of the central gray substance and adjacent tegmentum in the rat with observations in the cat. J. Comp. Neur. 139:259-272 (1970).

17. B. L. Hamilton, Projections of the nuclei of the periaqueductal gray matter in the cat. J. Comp. Neuro. 152:45-48 (1973).

18. V. J. Lotti, N. Kokka, and R. George, Pituitary-adrenal activation following intrahypothalamic microinjection of morphine. Neuroendocrinology 4:326-332 (1969).

19. E. Wei, H. H. Loh, and E. L. Way, Neuroanatomical correlates of morphine dependence. Science 177:616-617 (1972).

20. E. Wei, H. H. Loh, and E. L. Way, Brain sites of precipitated abstinence in morphine dependent rats. J. Pharmacol. Exp. Ther. 185: 108-115 (1973).

21. A. Routtenberg, Drinking induced by carbachol: Thirst circuit or ventricular modification. Science 157:838-839 (1967).

22. A. Routtenberg, J. Sladek, and W. Bondareff, Histochemical fluorescence after application of neurochemicals to caudate nucleus and septal area in vivo. Science 161:272-274 (1968).

23. R. B. Montgomery and G. Singer, Histochemical fluorescence as an index of spread of centrally applied neurochemicals. Science 165: 1031-1032 (1969).

24. A. Routtenberg and W. Bondareff, Histochemical fluorescence as an index of spread of centrally applied neurochemicals. Science 165: 1032 (1969).

25. W. Bondareff, A. Routtenberg, R. Narotzky, and D. G. McLone, Intrastriatal spreading of biogenic amines. Exper. Neurol. 28:213-229 (1970).

26. S. P. Grossman and W. E. Stumpf, Intracranial drug implants: an autoradiographic analysis of diffusion. Science 166:1410-1412 (1969).

27. G. Singer and R. B. Montgomery, Specificity of chemical stimulation of the rat brain and other related issues in the interpretation of chemical stimulation data. Pharmacol. Biochem. Behav. 1:211-222 (1973).

28. D. A. Booth, Localization of the adrenergic feeding system in the rat diencephalon. Science 158:515-516 (1967).

29. R. D. Myers, Methods for chemical stimulation. In Methods in Psychobiology (R. D. Myers, ed.), Vol. 1. London and New York: Academic Press, 1971, pp. 247-280.

30. G. Wolf, Elementary histology for neuropsychologists. In Methods in Psychobiology (R. D. Myers, ed.), Vol. 1. London and New York: Academic Press, 1971, pp. 281-299.

31. L. J. Herberg and K. B. J. Franklin, A variable inclined plane for blocking the rat's brain. Physiol. Behav. 10:617-618 (1973).

32. E. Kutter, A. Herz, H. Teschemacher, and R. Hess, Structure-activity correlations of morphine-like analgesics based on efficiencies following intravenous and intraventricular application. J. Med. Chem. 13:801-805 (1970).

33. D. V. Reynolds, Surgery in the rat during electrical analgesia induced by focal brain stimulation. Science 164:444-445 (1969).

34. D. J. Mayer and J. C. Liebeskind, Pain reduction by focal electrical stimulation of the brain: an anatomical and behavioral analysis. Brain Res. 68:73-93 (1974).

Part II

METHODS FOR STUDYING THE PHARMACOLOGICAL EFFECTS OF NARCOTICS

Chapter 3

A SYSTEMATIC APPROACH TO THE EVALUATION OF POTENTIAL NEW DRUGS FOR DEPENDENCE LIABILITY AND FOR EFFICACY IN THE TREATMENT OF NARCOTIC ADDICTION

PETER F. EAST and W. JOSEPH POTTS

Searle Laboratories
Department of Biological Research
Chicago, Illinois

I. INTRODUCTION

In an industrial setting, a research program to investigate problems of drug dependence is, like drug abuse itself, a many-headed Hydra; as soon as one problem is resolved, two more take its place. The system described in this chapter is largely the result of attempts to deal with a few of these problems. The techniques described were usually developed to meet a specific need and were subsequently modified to serve broader objectives.

Two major objectives are met through the efforts of our drug dependence program: (a) to identify nonnarcotic and nonaddictive antidiarrheal and antitussive agents with clear separation of these actions and (b) to identify agents that would be useful in the treatment of narcotic dependence. The latter could be narcotic agonists to ameliorate the withdrawal syndrome and/or permit maintenance therapy, or antagonists that are currently used to discourage narcotic use. In both cases the agent would, ideally, be nonnarcotic and nonabusable.

A third objective is to do basic research concerning drug abuse and dependence, which calls for investigation of behavior and its biochemical correlates. The basic research effort not only provides support and generates chemical leads for the first two objectives, but also is directed at increasing understanding of the mechanisms involved in the tolerance and the dependence phenomena. Selection of suitable techniques from the mass of information dealing with problems of drug dependence can be a difficult process. This chapter, while not intended as a review, will attempt to present, in a logical and practical sequence, those techniques which we have found most useful in achieving these objectives.

II. THE METHODS

A. Mouse Narcotic Dependence Model

Groups of 40 mice (Charles River, HAM/ICR), 18-25 g, are injected intraperitoneally (ip) at 8-hr intervals for 11 days with the narcotic agent of interest, to produce physiological addiction. When morphine sulfate is used as the addicting agent, the initial dose of 4 mg/kg is increased with each successive injection by 4 mg/kg through day 9 (injection no. 27), resulting in a final dose of 108 mg/kg. The mice are maintained at this level for seven further injections to day 11. Groups of 10 mice are at this point arbitrarily selected for control or drug treatment and receive either saline or the compound of interest at an initial screening dose of 25 mg/kg by intragastric (ig) injection on the morning of day 11.

Saline-treated (control) abstinence is characterized in morphine-dependent mice by repetitive vertical jumping [1-4]. Alteration of this phenomenon is used to assess the narcotic or withdrawal blocking activity of unknown compounds or standards. The severity of the withdrawal may be quantified by the number of jumps made by narcotic-dependent mice, and for this purpose acrylic chambers 8 in. x 12 in. x 24 in. high are used to house groups of five mice during the withdrawal period. Vertical motion is detected by photocells mounted 5 in. above the chamber floor which detect the change in light intensity caused by mice jumping in front of them. Electromechanical counters score cumulative counts, which are recorded for each group of five mice at hourly intervals for 15 hr. Saline-treated, narcotic-addicted animals consistently produce 500-600 jumps in this time, whereas treatment with narcotic antagonists increases, and treatment with narcotic agonists decreases, withdrawal jumping.

B. Hot-Plate Tests for Analgesia: Mouse

Three modified versions of the method described by Eddy and Leimbach [5] are used to detect narcotic agonist or antagonist activity of unknown compounds by their effect on the reaction time to a thermal (nociceptive) stimulus. In each case, groups of 10 male mice (Charles River, HAM/ICR), 18-25 g, are tested three times at 20-min intervals to determine the time in seconds to respond to being placed, individually in a restraining cylinder, on a hot plate (55 ± 0.3°C) either by licking a foot or jumping. Mice taking longer than 15 sec to respond are discarded. The median of the three pretreatment response times is used for later comparisons in all three versions of the test.

1. In the initial screening procedure, saline or the compound of interest is administered ip immediately following the third pretrial. Thirty minutes later, the mice are retested on the hot plate to determine inherent analgesic activity of the test compound. This trial is followed by administration of morphine sulfate at a standard dose of 40 mg/kg ip and by further hot-plate trials 15, 30, 60, and 90 min later. If a mouse fails to respond within 30 sec after being placed on the hot plate, the trial is terminated and the analgesic effect is considered to be maximal.

2. To evaluate narcotic antagonist activity, morphine sulfate at a standard dose of 40 mg/kg ip is administered after the third hot-plate trial. Fifteen minutes later, the mice are retested on the hot plate to determine the new response time for each mouse. Saline or the compound of interest is then administered ig or ip at a dose of 25 mg/kg and the mice are retested on the hot plate at 15, 30, 60, and 90 min postinjection.

3. To evaluate analgesic (antinociceptive) activity, the standard hot-plate procedure is used. Following the third hot-plate trial, saline or the compound of interest is administered ip or ig. Each mouse is then retested at 15, 30, 60, 90, and 120 min following drug administration.

In determining analgesic activity, a positive response is taken to be a reaction time at any of the succeeding trials which is double the pretrial median time. A dose of test compound is considered active if 50% or more of the treated group respond positively.

To determine activity in the antagonist tests, the group mean response time from those animals treated with both morphine and the test compound is compared with the mean from the group receiving both morphine and saline. Statistically shorter mean response latencies at any three retest times are taken to indicate activity. The standard narcotic antagonists, naloxone and nalorphine, both block and reverse morphine analgesia in these procedures.

C. α-NOAA-Induced Jumping: Mouse

Weissman [6], reported that α-naphthyloxyacetic acid (α-NOAA) was effective in eliciting repetitive vertical jumping in normal mice following ip administration of doses from 237 to 1000 mg/kg. While unable to determine the pharmacological mechanism mediating the effect, he suggested that it would provide a useful control to determine the specificity of drugs found to suppress the jumping of morphine withdrawal in dependent mice.

The effect of α-NOAA was readily confirmed and a dose of 500 mg/kg ip was selected as standard. This dose reliably elicits repetitive jumping for 15-20 min following injection. In practice, saline or the compound of interest is administered ip or ig to groups of 10 mice, 30 min prior to treatment with α-NOAA. The animals are then placed individually into the recording cages previously described for morphine withdrawal. Total jumps for each mouse are recorded for a 1-hr period.

This procedure provides a simple check, using existing equipment, to determine the sedative or tranquilizing activity of a compound by measuring its effect on a response which is qualitatively similar to the morphine abstinence response in mice.

D. Mouse Writhing Test for Analgesia

Groups of 10 male mice (Charles River), 18-25 g, are pretreated with saline (0.1 ml/10 g body wt) or the compound of interest at an initial dose of 25 mg/kg ig. Fifteen minutes after drug treatment the mice are challenged with administration of phenylquinone at a dose of 2.5 mg/kg ip.

Control (saline-treated) mice react to the phenylquinone challenge with a characteristic writhing response consisting of an arching of the back with concurrent stretching of the hind quarters. The number of separate "writhes" are counted for each mouse over a 10-min period starting 5 min following phenylquinone administration. Known analgesics, including aspirin and morphine, suppress or block this response in a dose-related manner. The test is particularly useful, however, in detecting the analgesic activity of compounds such as nalorphine which have mixed narcotic agonist and antagonist activity [7].

E. Rat Narcotic Dependence Model

Three methods are currently in use to produce narcotic dependence in rats.

1. The depot injection method utilizes a sustained release preparation of morphine and other compound with known or suspected narcotic activity. The compound is prepared by dissolving it in a mixture of paraffin oil and a suspending agent (Arlacel 80). This solution is then emulsified with an equal volume of saline. As the standard for comparison, morphine sulfate is injected subcutaneously (sc) at a dose of 150 mg/kg in a volume of 10 ml/kg to form a depot [8].

Typically, rats receiving this sustained release depot injection rapidly become extremely sedated by the continuous high level of systemic narcotic. Twenty-four hours following the injection, physical dependence to morphine can be demonstrated by the administration of low (1.0 mg/kg) sc doses of the narcotic antagonist naloxone, which precipitates severe withdrawal symptoms. This technique is useful in the follow-up testing of compounds showing antagonist activity in the mouse withdrawal jumping, and also as a rapid means of detecting narcotic-like activity in the rat.

2. The ip infusion technique is equally effective in producing a physically dependent animal. In this case, rats are prepared with indwelling catheters that terminate in the peritoneal cavity and are externalized by way of a cranial attachment. After recovery from surgery, the rats are housed in individual cages and connected via swivel systems to syringe pumps which provide a continuous infusion through the ip catheter. This technique is a slight modification of that described by Teiger [9].

Morphine is infused for 7 days at a constant rate of 6 ml/24 hr at an increasing daily dose: day 1, 25 mg/kg/day; day 2, 50 mg/kg/day; day 3, 100 mg/kg/day; and day 4 through day 7, 200 mg/kg/day. Termination of the morphine infusion on day 8 causes the appearance of withdrawal signs within 4 hr. Drugs known to substitute for morphine (agonists) suppress or defer the onset of the withdrawal. Withdrawal symptoms observed and scored in both of these rat addiction models include weight loss, hypothermia, diarrhea, irritability, jumping, ptosis, chewing and gnawing, body shakes (wet dog), and tremor. A numerical score is assigned to each of the behavioral symptoms, the sum of which, over the recording period, provides a standard measure of the severity of the withdrawal. In addition, electroencephalogram (EEG) recording electrodes may be implanted during the surgical preparation to allow analysis of changes in the EEG both before and during withdrawal.

3. A third technique for producing a rat model of narcotic addiction/withdrawal involves the twice daily administration of increasing doses of narcotic standards or the compound of interest. Injections may be either ip or ig. The standard dosage regimen for morphine addiction begins with a dose of 4 mg/kg which is increased by 4 mg/kg with each injection until a dose of 72 mg/kg is reached on day 9. Four more injections are given at this dose and the rats are then allowed to undergo withdrawal on day 12. In rats addicted to morphine on this schedule, withdrawal symptoms appear 14-16 hr after the last injection and can be reliably reproduced. The severity of the withdrawal is scored over a 48-hr period, using the behavioral and physiological symptoms described previously.

F. Rat Self-Administration Model

Male rats (Charles River), 200-250 g, are trained to perform a continuous avoidance schedule (Sidman). Each animal is individually housed in a multicompartment, sound-attenuating test cage with ad lib food and water. Two levers, each with an associated cue light, are mounted on one wall approximately 3 in. from the grid floor. The animals are trained to defer a 1-sec shock (0.4 mA) by depressing the right lever. Each lever press defers the shock for 40 sec. Failure to lever press within 40 sec results in the onset of the shock, which is repeated at 8-sec intervals until another lever press occurs.

Rats are trained to a stable baseline with at least 90% of the total lever presses occurring in the response-shock (RS = 40 sec) interval as opposed to the shock-shock (SS = 8 sec) interval. Multiple shocks occur only rarely and then only at the start of each session, which is of 2-hr duration twice daily.

Having attained stable baseline performance, each rat is surgically prepared with either an intravenous (iv) or ig chronic indwelling catheter which is externalized via a cranial attachment. On recovery from surgery, the cannula from each rat is connected in a manner similar to the ip infusion rats with the difference that the syringe pumps are operated by relay programming activated by the second (left) lever in each test cage. Saline is made available for self-administration and automatic injections are given every 6 hr if no lever press occurs during that time. Six days are allowed for postoperative recovery before restarting the Sidman avoidance schedule; a further 3 days are usually needed for restabilization of the shock avoidance baselines.

Drug solutions are at this time substituted for saline in the pumps. Depression of the left lever then results in the infusion of either morphine or the compound of interest. Drug availability is restricted to two 5-min periods per hour indicated to the rat by the cue light above the lever.

This model combines a "work" situation with drug self-administration and has the potential to clarify the interaction of possibly abusable drugs with performance of a stress-producing task. It also allows observation of the effects of self-administered drugs on complex behavior, thus revealing their more "subtle" effects.

G. Monkey Self-Administration Model

Rhesus monkeys of either sex weighing 2.5-5.0 kg are surgically prepared, using aseptic techniques, with a chronic indwelling catheter in the internal jugular vein. Upon recovery from surgery, each monkey is fitted with a custom-designed nylon mesh jacket that protects the catheter from the animal. The monkeys are minimally restrained within the test cage by a spring and swivel system that is connected between the jacket and the cage wall. The system also carries and protects the catheter's tubing connection to a syringe pump.

A lever is mounted on the cage wall in a position easily accessible to the animal. Relay programming activated by depression of the lever causes operation of the syringe pump, which infuses a constant volume of liquid per lever press. Initially, each lever press results in a saline infusion of 0.1 ml/kg and the animal is allowed several days of saline self-administration to determine the baseline for lever pressing. After stabilization, the saline in the syringe pump is replaced with morphine or the compound of interest (if soluble).

Almost all monkeys prepared in this way and given free access to iv morphine very rapidly learn to self-administer it. Those that do not can be induced to lever press by simple shaping techniques and will then achieve relatively stable rates of lever pressing within 3-4 weeks. Self-administered daily doses vary with the unit dose per infusion but are usually within the range of 15-75 mg/kg/day morphine sulfate [10,11].

A variation of this technique allows the study of insoluble compounds. In this case, the animals are prepared with an indwelling esophageal cannula which is externalized in the same manner as the iv cannula but is connected instead to a solenoid controlled valve that allows delivery of compounds kept in suspension by constant stirring. Using either technique, if an animal fails to initiate self-administration of any compound, repeated automatic infusions are given to determine whether cessation of drug infusions after some predetermined time would result in the onset of withdrawal symptoms.

Several other variations of the monkey self-administration model are used. They include a substitution technique that is used to determine the effect of an unknown compound on the rate of lever pressing for morphine in the addicted animal. Narcotic agonists or antagonists may be separated and defined by their effects either in suppressing or elevating the rate of lever pressing. Another variation is used to determine the narcotic dependence liability of the unknown compound by its effectiveness in suppressing the abstinence signs seen 14-16 hr following morphine withdrawal in self-administering animals.

III. THE SYSTEM

Each unknown compound is initially tested simultaneously in two procedures. Figure 1 demonstrates this and subsequent steps in the system. The morphine-dependent mouse withdrawal (W/D) jumping test (a) is a relatively nonspecific procedure. It offers, however, the advantage of sensitivity to both narcotic agonists and narcotic antagonists and clearly distinguishes between them. The mouse hot-plate procedure (b_1) detects antinociceptive activity and interference with the analgesic effect of morphine.

The combination of data generated in these two procedures provides the information for the decision regarding further testing. Inactivity of a compound in both tests in obviously not of interest and further testing would not be performed. If activity is observed in either or both of the procedures, additional studies are indicated. If a test compound demonstrates narcotic antagonist properties by precipitating withdrawal jumping and reducing morphine analgesic effects, this activity would be confirmed in detail in the second hot-plate procedure (b_2) by challenging morphine analgesia. The writhing test (d) detects weak agonist activity which may be present in compounds that appear to be antagonists in a, b_1, and b_2 (e.g., nalorphine, which has mixed agonist/antagonist properties). Pure antagonist activity in all the tests to this point would encourage further testing in the rat models (e_1, e_2) in two ways: first, to confirm the narcotic antagonist activity in another species and, second, to determine activity in preventing narcotic dependence.

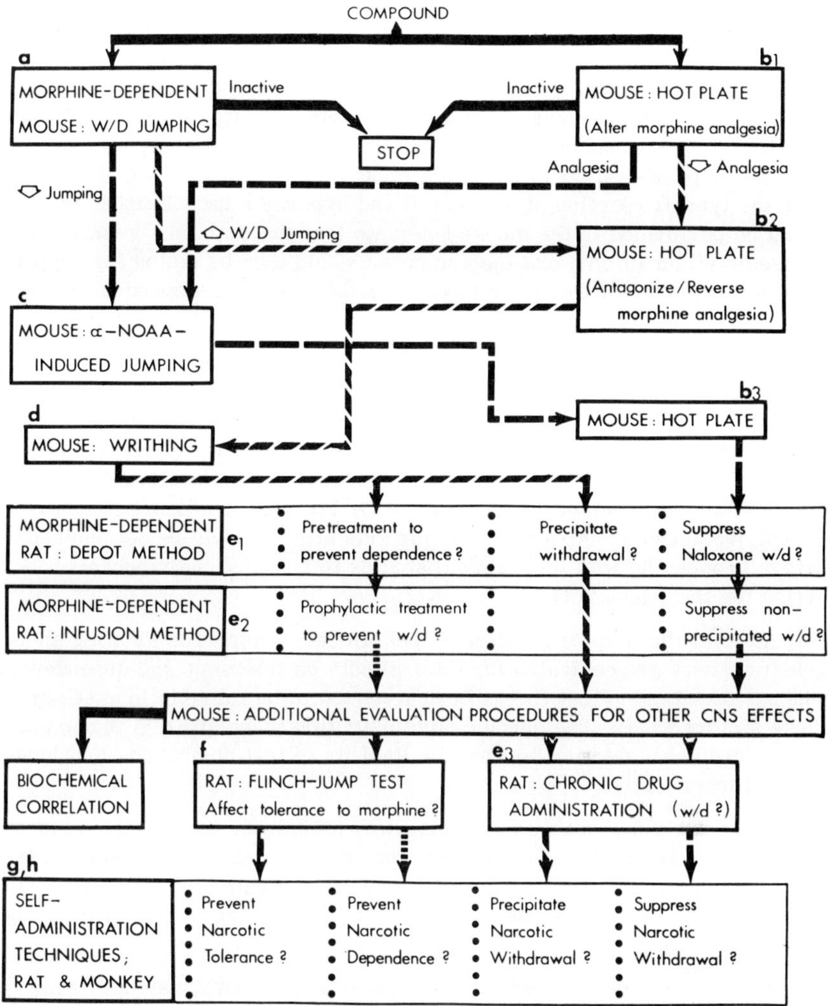

FIGURE 1. Summary and sequence of tests for evaluation of test compounds. Code letters refer to description in text.

If a test compound demonstrates analgesic or withdrawal suppressant effects (a and b_1), it would then be tested to determine antagonist activity against α-NOAA-induced jumping in mice (c). Failure of the test compound to suppress this jumping would indicate specific narcotic withdrawal suppression activity and a lack of sedative action. Effective suppression of α-NOAA jumping would not, however, be sufficient reason to discontinue testing at this point. Weissman [6] found reserpine, chlorpromazine, and chlordiazepoxide to be effective in this procedure only at doses that also produced clear depressant symptoms. We have verified these findings and also have found morphine to be highly effective in suppressing α-NOAA jumping (unpublished observations) although only at those doses that produce the typical reaction of Straub tail and hyperactivity. Further testing would be performed in the mouse hot-plate test (b_3) to better identify the analgesic effect (if any) and the compound would then be tested for suppression of morphine withdrawal symptoms in the morphine-dependent rat (e_1, e_2).

Test compounds that are still of interest after evaluation in the rat morphine-dependent models (e_1, e_2) are subjected to a series of tests designed to discover other CNS activity. These include hexobarbital potentiation, roto-rod, and general locomotor-activity tests for sedative and stimulant effects, a passive avoidance procedure for minor tranquilizer activity, and an electroconvulsive shock or Metrazol challenge for anticonvulsive activity. Absence of major side effects would be determined before proceeding with biochemical studies to examine the mechanism of action for the effect [12].

After evaluation for additional CNS effects, compounds showing antagonist activity are evaluated for their effects on tolerance and dependence. The rat flinch-jump test (f) has been reported to be valuable in assessing these factors [13]. The chronic administration technique (e_3) is used at this point to estimate the dependence liability of test compounds that have shown agonist activity.

The final and probably most important techniques to classify compounds with potentially beneficial effects are the self-administration tests in the rat and monkey. These procedures allow determination of the four activities shown in Fig. 1 (g, h) and also allow estimation of the abuse liability of the compound.

The procedures outlined in this chapter are in many instances based on standard techniques which are well known in the literature. The sequence of activities as outlined has evolved over a period of several years and is based on empirical work in our laboratories.

The particular sequence which may be of use to other investigators will depend on their needs and interests. The procedures and the sequence indicated here provide us with both research and development capabilities in the critical area of drug abuse evaluation.

REFERENCES

1. F. Huidobro and C. Maggiolo, Some features of the abstinence syndrome to morphine in mice. Acta Physiol. Lat. Amer. 11:201-209 (1961).

2. F. Huidobro and C. Maggiolo, On the intensity of the abstinence syndrome to morphine induced by daily injections of nalorphine in white mice. Arch. Int. Pharmacodyn. Ther. 158:97-112 (1965).

3. D. H. Tedeschi, P. J. Fowler, W. H. Crowley, J. F. Pauls, R. Z. Eby, and E. J. Fellows, Effects of centrally acting drugs on confinement motor activity. J. Pharm. Sci. 53:1046-1058 (1964).

4. E. L. Way, H. H. Loh, and F.-H. Shen, Simultaneous quantitative assessment of morphine tolerance and physical dependence. J. Pharmacol. Exp. Ther. 167:1-8 (1969).

5. N. B. Eddy and D. Leimbach, Synthetic analgesics. II. Dithienylbutenyl- and dithienylbutylamines. J. Pharmacol. Exp. Ther. 107: 385-393 (1953).

6. A. Weissman, Jumping in mice elicited by α-naphthyloxyacetic acid (α-NOAA). J. Pharmacol. Exp. Ther. 184:11-17 (1973).

7. R. I. Taber, D. D. Greenhouse, and S. Irwin, Inhibition of phenylquinone induced writhing by narcotic antagonists. Nature (London) 4954:189-190 (1964).

8. H. O. J. Collier, D. L. Francis, and C. Schneider, Modification of morphine withdrawal by drugs interacting with humoral mechanisms: Some contradictions and their interpretations. Nature (London) 237: 220-223 (1973).

9. D. G. Teiger, A rapid method for induction of physical dependence to narcotics in the rat, resulting to marked withdrawal signs without the use of antagonists. Fed. Proc. Fed. Amer. Soc. Exp. Biol. 31: 527 (1972).

10. C. R. Schuster, Psychological approaches to opiate dependence and self-administration by laboratory animals. Fed. Proc. Fed. Amer. Soc. Exp. Biol. 29:2-5 (1970).

11. T. Yanagita, An experimental framework for evaluation of dependence liability of various types of drugs in monkeys. Proc. Int. Congr. Pharmacol., 5th 1:7-17 (1972).

12. E. L. Way, Brain neurohormones in morphine tolerance and dependence. Proc. Int. Congr. Pharmacol., 5th 1:77-94 (1972).

13. H. A. Tilson and R. H. Rech, The effects of p-chlorophenylalanine on morphine analgesia, tolerance and dependence development in two strains of rats. Psychopharmacologia 35:45-60 (1974).

Chapter 4

THE ASSESSMENT OF AND THE PROBLEMS INVOLVED IN THE EXPERIMENTAL EVALUATION OF NARCOTIC ANALGESICS

M. R. FENNESSY and JAMES R. LEE

Department of Pharmacology
University of Melbourne
Parkville, Victoria, Australia

I. INTRODUCTION

Over the centuries that man has been capable of organized thought and action, relief from pain has been one of his most persistent searches. Classically, pain can be defined as a very unpleasant sensation resulting from any intense stimulation to some region of the body.

At present the drugs available for relief of pain fall into three broad categories: the narcotic analgesics, the narcotic antagonist analgesics, and the antipyretic analgesics. Each of these drug types has undesirable effects associated with them. The narcotic analgesics have the well-documented capacity to induce tolerance and psychological and physical dependence. Most narcotic antagonist analgesics have some dependence liability and have associated undesirable psychopharmacological effects. The antipyretic analgesic drugs have been shown to be closely associated with renal damage. Consequently the search for ideal analgesic agents is continuing. This search requires the screening of chemical compounds for analgesic activity in animals. At present this search is hindered by the lack of suitable testing procedures.

The literature concerned with analgesic testing techniques has been extensively reviewed [1-8] and no comprehensive listing of references will be attempted here. We shall discuss certain criteria that an ideal analgesic test should fulfill.

The method used should predict whether the experimental drug will relieve pain in man. In man, pain is a subjective experience [2], the perception of which may be ascertained only by the individual concerned and then assessed by direct interview. Two different types of pain are experienced by man: "superficial" pain, which results from injuries such as burns or abrasions, and the "deep" pain experienced in various pathological conditions, such as bone fracture or cancer [4]. The analgesic test should be able to differentiate between actions upon these two different types of pain in man.

In animals receiving nociceptive stimuli (such as heat, pressure, electrical or chemical stimuli) it is impossible to determine whether these stimuli produce sensations that are similar to those experienced by man. Nevertheless, such stimuli produce typical changes in behavior by which the animal attempts to escape. It is not known whether these responses in animals are related to human pain, but these responses are used for the pharmacological evaluation of analgesics. The development of the narcotic antagonist analgesic drugs (e.g., nalorphine and pentazocine), together with a renewed interest in the antipyretic analgesics, has highlighted inadequacies in the classical analgesic tests employing heat and pressure as the noxious stimuli.

The following criteria have been suggested as being necessary if meaningful information is to be obtained from an analgesic test:

1. A quantitative determination of the threshold value of the noxious stimulus must be possible. In man this usually is the lowest intensity leading to a verbal report by the subjects. In animals this would be the reaction threshold.

2. Quantitative information upon differences in intensities of stimuli should be yielded. The method must also discriminate between different doses of drugs and drugs of different potencies.

3. The stimulus applied should not result in tissue damage when applied at the threshold intensity. The application of intensities above the threshold intensity, which is necessary to determine the extent of an increase in reaction threshold after analgesic administration, should not result in tissue damage or alteration.

4. Repeated application of the stimulus should not result in tissue damage or an alteration in the reaction threshold.

5. In addition, for use in screening programs, the technique must be economical and relatively rapid in performance. This tends to exclude any technique that requires surgical preparation of the animal.

Two basic techniques of quantification of the responses are used. These are the quantal response and the graded response. The quantal response is obtained by selecting suitable reaction criteria which are usually referred to as the end point. The response is then assessed as an all-or-none response. By using various doses of drug and obtaining the percentage of animals reacting, a dose of the drug that would be effective in 50% of the population can be calculated. This is the analgesic ED_{50}. Many procedures for this statistical manipulation are available but perhaps the simplest and most frequently used is that of Litchfield and Wilcoxon [9]. The graded response is obtained by measuring the amount of increase in the stimulus that is required to elicit the response. This is usually the increase in the reaction time or the increase in intensity of the stimulus.

With all types of noxious stimuli used in analgesic tests, prolonged exposure to, or excessive increase in, the intensity of the stimulus results in tissue damage. To minimize this possibility a maximum time or intensity is selected beyond which the stimulus is not applied. This is known as the cutoff time.

The methods chosen for discussion are those which in the experience of the authors are the most commonly employed. They are classified under the following headings: thermal, mechanical, electrical, chemical, and behavioral.

II. DESCRIPTION OF METHODS

A. Thermal Techniques

1. Tail Flick to Hot Water

a. Details. This method was first employed in mice [10] and rats [11]. It appears to be the simplest of the thermal techniques because no special equipment is required. The animal is held in a conical paper bag formed by folding and stapling stiff paper into a conical or pyramidal shape. The animal's tail protrudes from one side and is dipped into hot water. With the mouse, the water is maintained at 58°C and with rats, at 55°C. The control mice react by a withdrawal of the tail and the reaction time for this withdrawal after immersion is recorded. The reaction time for saline-treated mice is 1-1.5 sec and animals that do not react within this time are discarded. The cutoff point is 6 sec and mice not responding in this time are considered to be in an analgesic state. Similar criteria are used for rats. Groups of 10 mice are used for each dose level of a narcotic analgesic. The reaction time is determined every 30 min beginning 15 min after administration of the drug. At each determination two reaction times are measured and the greater is recorded. This technique has been modified to employ water at 52°C and the test repeated every 15 min [12]. Computation of an ED_{50} can be accomplished by noting the number of animals not responding in 5 sec.

b. Special equipment. No special equipment is required.

c. Sensitivity. An ED_{50} of 4.6 mg/kg for morphine has been reported. It has also been reported that 22 mg/kg codeine and 120 mg/kg phenylbutazone produce an average reaction time of 5.5 sec [10]. This method shows about the same sensitivity as the tail flick to radiant heat test.

d. Pitfalls. This technique is not widely used despite its simplicity, thus making comparison of the data with the literature difficult. Another pitfall is that the end point may be a spinal reflex [6]. In our experience the animals used should be young, as keratinization of the tail increases with age and this alters the reaction profile. Injections in the tail should also be avoided.

2. Hot Plate

a. Details. This technique was first described by Woolfe and Macdonald [13] and has subsequently been modified [14,15]. Mice, 20-25 g, or rats, 100-150 g, are placed gently on a heated (55.5-56°C) copper surface (see Sec. II,A,2,6) and the time from contact with the surface until the time the animal reacts by jumping or licking and/or kicking its hind paws is recorded. When a mouse is placed on the heated surface its first reaction is to sit on its hind legs and lick or blow on its forepaws. A few seconds later it attempts to jump out of the cylinder or reacts by licking and/or kicking the hind paws. The cutoff point is 30 sec and the mice not reacting in this time are considered to be in an analgesic state. The animals are screened and those reacting before 4 sec or after 15 sec are discarded. Groups of 10 animals are used for each dose level of the narcotic analgesic. These reaction times can be determined at convenient intervals as short as 10 min. Again, the ED_{50} for analgesia in this test can be calculated by noting the percentage of animals that do not react within 30 sec. By employing change in reaction times, a more sensitive, but less convenient, index of analgesia can be obtained.

b. Special equipment. The hot-plate test uses a hollow copper tank (20 cm x 20 cm x 5 cm) with a reflux condenser and a thermometer mounted in one corner. The tank contains a 50:50 volume of ethyl formate and acetone (boiling point, 55.8°C), the temperature of which is maintained by a heated water bath.

c. Sensitivity. The sensitivity of this method for testing the analgesic activity of narcotic analgesics compares favorably with other acceptable thermal methods. Reports have appeared of ED_{50} values for morphine being as low as 4 mg/kg. However, in our laboratory, the ED_{50} has consistently, over a period of years and in all seasons, been between 8.5 and 10 mg/kg.

d. Pitfalls. When the animal is placed on the hot plate it quickly learns that a noxious stimulus is to be applied and may jump immediately after being placed on the plate. This has been documented as the influence of learning on morphine analgesia and tolerance [16-18]. The observer must be very attentive, as the licking of hind paws can be very rapid in execution. The type of response at threshold stimulation indicates that a supraspinal reflex may be involved, as the animal must locate the source of the stimulus and react appropriately. Finally, tissue damage may occur if the animals are left in contact with the plate for too long.

3. Tail Flick to Radiant Heat (Fixed Intensity, Variable Duration)

a. Details. This technique was first described by D'Amour and Smith [19] for rats and Andrews and Workman [20] for dogs as an adaptation of the Hardy et al. [21] technique in man. With rats, an electric light source (1000 W) is placed so that a biconvex lens focuses the light onto a plastic plate having a hole 1.5 cm in diameter. The rat is held so that the tail is beneath the hole. An asbestos shutter can be placed over the plastic plate. The intensity of the light is varied so that the rat reacts by flicking the tail within about 5 sec after the removal of the asbestos shutter. In a subsequent study, this was modified by the introduction of a point system so that a graded effect of a drug could be obtained [22]. A cutoff time of 10 sec was used. This technique has been modified by employing a red hot wire 3 mm from the tail [23]. With the dog and the guinea pig the same basic system is used in which the end point is a skin flick. The reaction time is normally measured at 15-min intervals after drug administration. An ED_{50} can be calculated from the number of animals that do not respond within 10 sec.

b. Special equipment. A powerful light source (1000 W) and a rheostat arrangement for the variation of intensity of the light are required. The biconvex lens should be about 10 cm in diameter. The hot-wire modification of the technique requires less special apparatus.

c. Sensitivity. The minimally effective dose of morphine is about 4 mg/kg whereas that of codeine is 28 mg/kg. The analgesic action of nalorphine and pentazocine has also been detected [24]. Hart [25] claims that by modifying the procedure to allow the lamp to remain on at a very low intensity during the nontest time, the reliability of the results is increased. However, data were not presented to support this assertion, except that the reaction time may vary as much as 1.7 sec in consecutive readings. However, it has been reported that the response time for a single group of 18 untreated rats varied from 5 to 14 sec [26]. On the other hand, Winter [6] reported that 90% of the responses in 19 groups of 6 rats were within 0.7 sec of the average within a group.

d. Pitfalls. The rats used in this technique should be young so as to minimize the effect of keratinization upon heat sensitivity. When skin flick is employed the color of the skin should be consistent to standardize the heat absorption. Tail vein injections should be avoided in the tail-flick procedure. The other pitfalls to be considered are whether the observed reaction is of a spinal origin and whether the effect of the analgesics themselves on body temperatures will modify the reaction time.

4. Tail Flick to Radiant Heat (Fixed Duration, Variable Intensity)

a. Details. The basis of this technique was first described by Hardy et al. [21]. It consists of focusing the light from a 500- or 1000-W projection bulb on a 3.5 cm^2 area of skin. The lamp is on for precisely 3 sec every minute. The current delivered to the bulb is varied so as to produce the threshold pain in man or a skin flick in animals. When the desired response is obtained the experimental subject is removed and a radiometer is used to determine radiation. The normal interval between the threshold determinations is 30 min. The area of skin is usually blackened in an attempt to standardize the heat absorption by the skin. The data from this technique are very difficult to quantify by an ED_{50} calculation, and it has been pointed out that of four reports which had appeared by 1948, no two analyzed the data in the same manner [1].

b. Special equipment. A radiometer is required to measure the radiation delivered at the threshold intensity. An electronic timing device is necessary to enable the precise timing of the exposure and a rheostat device is required to vary the intensity of the light delivered.

c. Sensitivity. This technique has not been used extensively in animals. Consequently, it is difficult to assess its sensitivity.

d. Pitfalls. The absorption of heat by the skin is subject to such variations as the degree of blackening of the skin, the temperature of the skin, which may rise with repeated exposure to the lamp, and the area of skin selected. The amount of energy emitted by the lamp alters with the age and usage of the bulb and hence requires repeated standardization of the apparatus.

When human subjects are used, all the difficulties of human perception of pain are encountered. These include factors such as the subject's state of mind, particularly with respect to anxiety. The anxiety of the subject can be altered by the experimenter's attitude to the subject, the subject's understanding of the procedure, and previous experience of the technique.

As with all heat procedures, the danger of skin damage is always present. In man, the threshold level of radiation can give rise to blistering [21] and, in guinea pigs, a two- to threefold increase in the threshold stimulation causes blistering [27]. Because of this factor, it is usual to approach the threshold from below the threshold level of radiation, but this may introduce a systematic error in the determination [28].

B. Mechanical Techniques

1. Tail Clip

a. Details. This technique, first described by Haffner [29], has subsequently been modified [30,31]. It is the simplest of the mechanical techniques to employ and one of the most widely used of the analgesic techniques. The animals used are generally the rat or mouse, although other animals such as the cat and monkey have been utilized. An artery clip, with the branches enclosed in thin rubber tubing, is applied to the tail. The animal reacts by locating the clip and making continuous attempts to remove it. The animals are first screened and those not attempting to remove the clip after 15 sec are rejected. The drug is administered and the test repeated at 30, 60, 90, and 120 min after administration of the analgesic. Animals not responding after 30 sec are scored as positive. A cutoff time of 30 sec is used. An ED_{50} is readily calculated from these data.

b. Special equipment. No special equipment is required.

c. Sensitivity. Analgesic ED_{50} values for morphine were found to be 5.7 mg/kg subcutaneously and 7.8 mg/kg intraperitoneally in mice [30] and 1.1 mg/kg subcutaneously and 1.8 mg/kg intraperitoneally in rats [32]. The monkey is not a very suitable subject as the reactions in these animals are slow [33] and no accurate measurement of the pain threshold can reasonably be made.

Collier [4] reported that, when an end point of 10 sec was used, morphine given subcutaneously to mice had an ED_{50} of 7.1 mg/kg, whereas that of d-propoxyphene was 37 mg/kg; codeine, 28 mg/kg; aminopyrine, 99 mg/kg; and phenazone, 290 mg/kg. No analgesic activity of nalorphine or acetylsalicylic acid was detected.

d. Pitfalls. The main problem in performing this test is in standardizing the point of application of the clip to the tail of the animal. A convenient method for minimizing the variation arising from this factor is to clearly mark the point of application of the clip on the tail and on the clip. Repeated application of the clip to the tail can cause swelling which results in an altered reaction profile in the test. Perhaps the greatest source of variation is in the opening tension of the clip. An apparatus to determine this is shown in Fig. 1. Although this is a relatively crude technique, it has wide application as a basic screening test.

2. Compression Tests

a. Details. A metal rod with a sharpened tip [34] or one with a blunt tip [35] has been applied to the rat tail. This has been modified so that the pressure is applied to the rat paw after the injection of yeast to produce inflammation [36]. With tail compression, the rats are positioned so that the pressure is applied about 1 cm from the base of the tail [34] or 2.5 cm from the tip of the tail [35]. The pressure is increased until the rat attempts to escape or vocalization occurs. The pressure is then recorded. In subsequent determinations the pressure is applied to the same place on the tail. The following cutoff pressures have been used: (a) 500 g [34], (b) 25 g above the predrug pressure levels [37], and (c) 680 mm Hg [35]. The predrug end-point pressure is 10-30 g with a sharpened tip and about 68 mm Hg with the blunt tip.

A modification of this procedure has been described in which the rat is placed so that the tail is inserted through a rectangular bracket. One side of the rectangular bracket is moved in by means of a calibrated screw to compress the rat's tail against the other side of the bracket. That portion of the tail, 2.5 cm from the tip, is placed under the movable plate. The screw is tightened until the plate is just touching the tail. The knob of the screw is then turned until a squeak response is obtained and the number of turns required is recorded. A positive analgesic effect is noted when the number of turns required after the analgesic equals or exceeds twice the predrug reading [38].

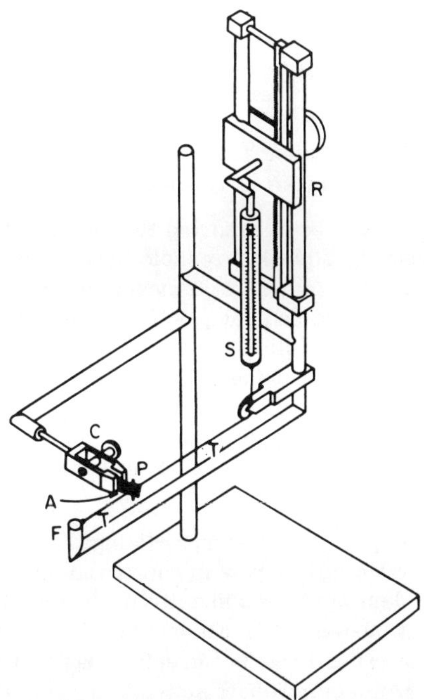

FIGURE 1. Apparatus for measuring the opening tension of an artery clip. The artery clip (A) is held in the clamp (C) so that its jaws can be pulled apart by the threads (T). One thread is attached to a fixed point (F) and the other to the hook of a spring balance (S). A pin (P) is inserted between the jaws of the artery clip. The racking mechanism (R) is operated so as to pull the jaws open; the tension at which the pin drops is read on the spring balance. (Reprinted from Collier [4], p. 198, by courtesy of Academic Press.)

The inflamed rat paw pressure technique requires injection of 0.1 ml of a 20% suspension of brewers' yeast into the plantar surface of the hind foot of the rat [36]. Pressure is then applied to the inflamed foot and the pressure required to produce a response of escape or vocalization is recorded. The pressure required on a yeast-inflamed foot is about 55 mm Hg 24 hr after the yeast injection. The other hind foot (control) required a pressure of 157 mm Hg.

b. Special equipment. An apparatus suitable for use with most of these methods is commercially available. Alternatively, an apparatus for producing uniformly increasing pressure can be constructed. This consists of two syringes connected by an inelastic flexible tube filled with a fluid.

A manometer is connected to a side arm in the tubing. One of the syringes is clamped vertically (plunger downward) and the end of the plunger forms the compression point. The other syringe is uniformly compressed until the desired response is obtained and the manometer reading is then noted. A mechanical drive is convenient for a uniform rate of compression, but a device for instantaneous release is required.

c. Sensitivity. It has been reported that a dose of 3 mg/kg of morphine was sufficient to raise the squeak threshold by a factor of 3 in the pointed rod technique [5], whereas a dose of 8 mg/kg of morphine was effective in measurements on the uninflamed rat paw [39]. In the yeast-inflamed rat paw pressure technique, the following doses of drugs produced a rise in the threshold pressure [36]: morphine, 1.5 mg/kg; levorphan, 0.125 mg/kg; codeine, 6.25 mg/kg; aminopyrine, 25 mg/kg; and sodium salicylate, 25 mg/kg. Sodium salicylate and phenylbutazone, in doses up to 100 mg/kg, were not effective in raising the threshold pressure on the control paw, i.e., the one not inflamed by yeast.

d. Pitfalls. The problem of standardizing the point of application of the pressure on the rat's tail or paw is one of the main difficulties of this technique. The problem of altered sensitivity in subsequent testing is present. With testing at 20-min intervals over five tests, the variation between readings on the same rat tail was not greater than that between different rats [25]. However, another report states that, with testing at the same point (20 mm from the tail tip) at 30-min intervals, the threshold pressure had decreased significantly by the third reading and the sixth reading was only 50% of the first reading [6]. The use of a different point on the tail also resulted in a downward trend which was attributed to this conditioning. However, when two predrug recordings were performed (2-3 hr apart) and two postinjection readings were obtained, the threshold pressure was sufficiently stable to allow the testing of drugs [6].

With the yeast-inflamed paw pressure technique, the detection of narcotic analgesics is without difficulties. With the antipyretic analgesics, however, the relative analgesic and antipyretic contributions are difficult to ascertain. An attempt to overcome this problem was performed by monitoring the volume of the inflamed paw to determine the antipyretic action of the drug [40]. No correlation was found between the rise in reaction threshold pressure caused by acetylsalicylic acid and any reduction in the inflammation-induced volume increase in the foot of the rat.

C. Electrical Techniques

1. Scrotal Stimulation

a. Details. Electrical stimulation is applied to the adult male rat scrotum, upon which six points have been described for the application of electrical stimulation [41]. These are the scrotal surface that covers the body of the testes, the tips of the testes, and the proximal or distal ends of the septum. Fine platinum electrodes are applied to two points on the scrotum, which are marked. The stimulation duration is maintained at 0.1 msec and the voltage is then increased until vocalization occurs. The current is claimed to be so small that no other harmful effect but "pain" is produced. It is claimed that by close observation superficial pain can be differentiated from deep pain. Superficial pain is said to occur when the squeak response is obtained without a cremasteric reflex. The cremaster muscle is the muscle which, on contraction, squeezes the testes into the abdominal cavity. When an increased voltage is applied the cremaster muscle is observed to contract strongly, thus exerting pressure on the testes, which in turn produces a squeak response. When voltages that normally produce a squeak response without contraction of the cremaster muscle are not effective, it is thought that the perception of superficial pain is abolished. If the cremaster muscle contracts, but no squeak response is obtained, it is assumed that the perception of both superficial and deep pain is abolished. This technique has been adapted to permit the use of both male and female rats [42]. Electrodes are attached to the genital papillae of rats and a squeak response can be obtained with stimulation of 18-22 V.

b. Sensitivity. A dose of morphine of 10 mg/kg produced a rise of 12 V in the rat squeak response to electrical stimulation of the genital papillae [42]. Effective analgesic doses of morphine, 1 mg, codeine, 6 mg, and sodium salicylate, 10 mg, reduced the response to electrical stimulation of the rat scrotum [41]. These doses appeared to be the total dose.

c. Special equipment. Platinum electrodes and an electronic stimulator are the only special equipment required.

d. Pitfalls. In this method, as with all electrical methods, the stimulus is easy to apply but difficult to control accurately [6]. A systematic study of the apparatus for delivering controlled electrical stimuli intimated that the power delivered is a much more fundamental variable when applied to the verbal reports of the intensity of shock stimuli [43]. Current is more significant than voltage.

Macht and Macht [41] employed a device called the Harvard inductorium to apply the electrical stimulus. This is an induction coil or a spark ignition coil [41]. The coil was calibrated to the voltage produced and the results reported required a control threshold stimulation that varied from 100 to 800 V. One to two hours after administration of 5 mg of morphine, the threshold response rose from 180 to 2852 V in one animal. In our opinion the data reported showed a variation that was too great to allow meaningful interpretation.

2. Tooth Pulp Stimulation

a. Details. This technique consists of attaching electrodes, usually via amalgam fillings, to the teeth of the animal [44-47]. The animals used are rabbits, guinea pigs, dogs, cats, and man. A convenient attachment electrode is formed by cutting the head off a safety pin and bending the ends in three places so that the tension of the pin causes the points to come into apposition. An indifferent electrode may be attached elsewhere on the body. The electrode is then stimulated by a square-wave electronic stimulator with the following parameters: frequency, 40 Hz; duration of impulse, 5 msec; and duration of stimulation, 0.5 sec. The voltage is then varied, increasing the strength of the stimulation by 10% of the previous reading until a response is obtained. Determination of the reaction threshold can be made at 30-min intervals. In guinea pigs, the response is a rapid backward thrust of the head. In rabbits, cavities (of uniform depth, 1 mm) are drilled in the upper incisor teeth [48]. Small circular spring electrodes are placed in the cavities from each side and electrical stimulation (20 Hz, 1 msec duration for 2 sec) is applied. The voltage administered is gradually increased until a threshold voltage is reached. Two responses to electrical stimulation of the rabbit have been described. The first response seen is a licking and chewing response which commences with a stimulation intensity of about 3 V. The second response is a mouth opening which is seen at about 20 V. Electrical stimulation of the tooth pulp of dog and man has been used [49]. The end points used were verbal reports of pain in man and head jerk or facial muscle twitch in the dog. The reaction thresholds or stimulation parameters were not specified.

b. Sensitivity. Morphine (7.5 mg/kg), pethidine (10 mg/kg), levorphanol (3.75 mg/kg), and methadone (3.75 mg/kg) produced a satisfactory rise in the threshold voltage in the guinea pig [47]. Another author reported that morphine (1.5, 2.5, and 5.0 mg/kg, intravenously) resulted in a rise of 2, 3, and 14 V, respectively, in the threshold for licking and chewing movements, whereas the threshold for the more intense stimulation (mouth opening) was significantly raised to a similar degree by morphine in doses of 2.5 and 5.0 mg/kg, but not by 1.5 mg/kg [48]. On the other hand, it was found that doses of morphine of 16-32 mg/kg given subcutaneously were required to produce a rise in the reaction threshold in the rabbit [50]. The subcutaneous administration of morphine (16 mg) produced a rise of about 0.1 V in the threshold intensity of the electrical stimulation to tooth fillings in man [51], whereas 1 mg/kg of morphine administered to dogs produced a 0.4-V rise in the threshold intensity [52].

c. Pitfalls. The problems associated with using electrical stimulation as the nociceptive stimulus have been critically reviewed by Beecher [2] and Winter [6], and extensively studied by Hill et al. [53]. Beecher [2], in particular, states that the threshold is not sufficiently reliable and, contrary to the assertions of other authors [52] that pain is the only sensation arising from the electrical stimulation of the tooth, other sensations are elicited by this technique. The presence of receptors sensitive to heat, cold, and touch have been demonstrated [54]. Another report suggested that painful mechanical manipulation of the teeth in man results in an "elevated central irritability in the sensory pathways" [55]. This elevated central irritability may be present for some years. If such a situation occurs in animals, subsequent determinations of the reaction threshold would seem to have an additional complication.

3. Tail Stimulation

a. Details. This method has been described by Grewal and others [56-68]. The end point used in this test is vocalization. More recently, the stimulation parameters in the test have been studied in which electrical stimulation is applied through electrodes (no. 20 injection needles) placed intracutaneously about 20 mm apart in the middle section of the mouse tail [56]. After studying the effects of varying (a) the frequency of stimulation from 50 to 1600 Hz, (b) the pulse width between 0.1 and 4.8 msec, and (c) the duration from 10 to 160 msec, the following parameters of stimulation were considered to be optimal: duration, 40 msec; frequency, 125 Hz; and pulse width, 1.6 msec [56,69]. The effect of the polarity of the electrodes was also studied and it was found that, with the positive electrodes in the proximal position, the vocalization threshold was 6.3 V, whereas with the negative electrode in the proximal position the vocalization threshold was 7.8 V. Subsequently, the positive electrode was placed in the proximal position. The reaction threshold was also found to vary with the body weight of the mouse. Three determinations of the vocalization threshold were made at 15-min intervals before drug administration. The vocalization threshold did not alter when seven determinations were performed at 15-min intervals. After the administration of the drug, a mouse was considered to be in a state of analgesia if the reaction threshold was more than 25% above the average predrug reaction threshold.

Another method consists of attaching electrodes made of clock springs to the mouse tail [68]. The mouse is held in a cage so that its tail protrudes. The tail is cleaned with ether, and electrode jelly is vigorously rubbed on. The electrodes are 1 cm wide and 1.5 cm apart and weighted to maintain a uniform pressure on the mouse tail. The electrical stimulus is applied at the rate of one per second (8.5 V, duration 1/26 sec). Mice are screened and those not reacting by vocalization within 5 sec are rejected. Untreated mice were found to vary by two shocks or less in their reaction threshold on retesting. After administration of the drug an increase in the reaction threshold of three shocks over the predrug number is taken as evidence that analgesia is present and an ED_{50} value can be calculated.

b. Special equipment. Paalzow [69] mentions that specially designed cages were used so that it was unnecessary to remove the electrodes from the mouse tail during the course of the experiment. However, he does not describe the cage. The present authors presume that these cages are similar to that illustrated in Burn et al. [57]. In addition, Paalzow has used two stimulators coupled in train to produce a burst of electrical square waves.

c. Sensitivity. It has been reported that morphine given subcutaneously in doses of 15, 30, and 60 mg/kg produced 18, 44, and 67% of analgesia, respectively. The analgesic ED_{50} values reported were as follows: amidone, 1.25 mg/kg; phenadoxone, 3.56 mg/kg; and pethidine, 0.33 mg/kg [68]. On the other hand, Paalzow [69] reported the following ED_{50} values: methadone, 1.2 mg/kg; morphine, 2.1 mg/kg; pethidine, 5.0 mg/kg; and codeine, 10.4 mg/kg, when administered subcutaneously. Oral administration showed a similar trend in sensitivity. In addition, oral administration resulted in the following ED_{50} values: d-propoxyphene, 61.7 mg/kg; sodium salicylate, 307.5 mg/kg; and acetylsalicylic acid, 435.5 mg/kg.

d. Pitfalls. Perhaps the most condemning attitude toward the electrical stimulation of the mouse tail is that of Reinhard and De Beer (see Burn et al. [57]), the original describers of the technique used by Grewal [68], who did not consider the technique sufficiently reproducible to be published. It has been stated that not less than 60 mice per dose of the analgesic agent should be used [68]; however, this, to us, would not seem to be compatible with an economical basic screening test for analgesia. In addition, the postinjection testing time was 15 min after subcutaneous administration, which, in our opinion, is well before the maximal analgesic action of the narcotic analgesics. Reports have appeared showing that the maximal analgesic effect of narcotic analgesics appeared 15 min after oral administration to mice which had been deprived of food overnight [57]; however, no data were presented to justify this statement. The majority of reports have demonstrated that regardless of the route of administration, maximal analgesia with these drugs lies between 30 and 45 min after administration.

Charpentier [64] reported that, when electrical shocks were applied to the rat's tail, 8 mg/kg of morphine administered intraperitoneally raised the reaction threshold by 78%, but that this increase was not statistically significant because of gross irregularities of response. Paalzow [69] reported that three dose levels of an analgesic with 20 mice per dose level were sufficient to calculate ED_{50} values with 95% confidence limits. However, he measured the reaction threshold of mice receiving different doses of analgesics at their peak effect time after administration, and this time varied. In our opinion, the analgesic action should be measured at constant times after administration if an ED_{50} value is to be calculated. The increased reliability and sensitivity of the technique as described by Paalzow [69] over that described by Grewal [68] may possibly be due in part to the increased sophistication of the electronics used. Obviating the necessity of applying electrode jelly to the mouse tail may be another improvement because electrical conduction between the electrodes on the tail of the mouse is decreased.

D. Chemical Techniques

1. "Writhing" or "Stretching" Syndrome

a. Details. In this test a 0.02% solution of phenylquinone (2-phenyl-1,4-benzoquinone) in a 5% aqueous solution of ethanol is injected intraperitoneally into mice. The phenylquinone should be first dissolved in the appropriate volume of ethanol and then diluted with distilled water. The solution should be freshly prepared each day and injected intraperitoneally in a volume of 0.1 ml/10 g of mouse [70]. In a time period between 3 and 10 min after the injection, the mouse reacts with the characteristic "writhing" or "stretching" response. This syndrome consists of rotation of the hips, a "sucking in" of the abdomen, and elongation of the body with arching of the back. An illustration of mice in this attitude is shown in Fig. 2. The syndrome continues for about 60 min after the phenylquinone injection. The mice are previously screened and those animals not exhibiting the writhing response five times in 10 min are rejected [3], and the analgesic estimation of a drug is performed on the following day. For estimation of the analgesic activity of a drug the animal is injected, preferably not by the intraperitoneal route, and at the desired time the phenylquinone is administered. The elapsed time is usually 30 min. Two methods of quantification are used: First, the percentage of animals not responding in a 20-min period after the phenylquinone is noted. These are considered to be in a state of analgesia and an ED_{50} value can be calculated. Second, the total number of writhing responses is counted in a 20-min period following phenylquinone administration. An ED_{50} is then calculated from the percent reduction in the number of writhing responses when compared with the responses in a control group. The latter method appears to be more sensitive; however, it requires closer observation.

The writhing syndrome can be induced by a large number of agents. These include acids, 5-hydroxytryptamine, histamine, acetylcholine, and bradykinin. The most frequently used are phenylquinone, bradykinin, and acetic acid. The species used include mice, guinea pigs, cats, and man, but the frequency of writhing is much less in animals other than rats and mice [8].

b. Special equipment. No special equipment is needed.

c. Sensitivity. The sensitivity of this method varies with the method of quantification used. It has been reported that counting the number of

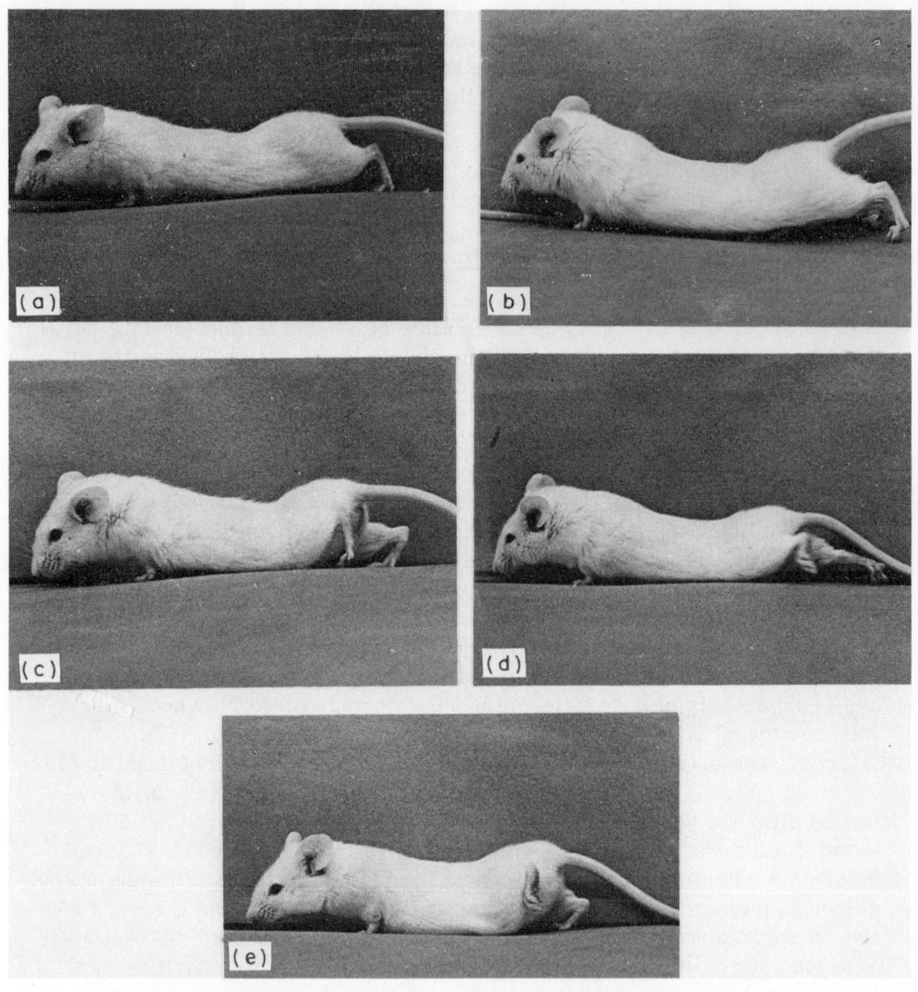

FIGURE 2. Mice 30 min after the intraperitoneal injection of acetic acid. Frames (a) and (b) show a mouse arching the back and rubbing the abdomen on the floor. Frames (c), (d), and (e) show another mouse in a writhing or stretching response that includes rotation of the hips.

writhing responses within a specific time resulted in an ED_{50} value of 68 mg/kg for sodium acetylsalicylate, whereas counting the number of mice not writhing in that time resulted in an ED_{50} value of 100 mg/kg for sodium acetylsalicylate [71]. With phenylbutazone, the ED_{50} values were 42 and 220 mg/kg, respectively. The ED_{50} value for morphine was 0.45 mg/kg when either a 0.025% solution of phenylquinone in 5% aqueous ethanol or a 6.0% aqueous solution of acetic acid was used to induce the writhing syndrome [72].

d. Pitfalls. The main disadvantage of this method is that, although all known clinical analgesics (narcotic, narcotic antagonist, and antipyretic) are detected, the following drugs, which are not generally classified as analgesics, are also detected as being positive: pentylenetetrazole, lignocaine, physostigmine, pilocarpine, atropine, antihistamines, and LSD [71].

The phenylquinone-induced writhing test results in an ED_{50} of 12.5 mg/kg for pethidine when mice are held singly and 5.1 mg/kg when mice are aggregated in groups of ten [73]. This test is simple, economical, and sensitive, to the point that it predicts analgesia for the narcotic analgesics, narcotic antagonist analgesics, and the antipyretic analgesics. However, its main disadvantage is that positive results are obtained with many types of drugs that are not clinically effective analgesics.

2. Intraarterial Test

a. Details. This test was first performed by injecting autacoids into the splenic artery of a conscious dog, which had been previously cannulated under anesthesia [74]. Of the various autacoids tested, bradykinin was found to be the most potent. About 2 μg/dog of bradykinin was required, whereas 5-hydroxytryptamine and histamine required about 50 μg/dog. The reaction consisted of tachycardia, hypertension, hypernea, vocalization, and biting.

An adaptation of this technique has been reported in which bradykinin is injected into the carotid artery of the rat [75]. Under light ether anesthesia, a polythene cannula is implanted into the right common carotid artery of the rat and the other end is passed subcutaneously to the back of the neck and fixed on the skin surface. At least 1 hr after recovery from anesthesia, bradykinin is injected slowly into the carotid cannula over a period of about 2 sec. The initial dose of bradykinin is 0.1 μg, increased in steps of 0.1 to 5 μg until a response is obtained. The response occurs 7-10 sec after administration, never later than 15 sec, after the injection of a threshold dose of bradykinin. The response consists of a lateral twist of the head toward the site of injection and an ipsilateral raising of the foreleg. Rats not responding to an injection of 0.5 μg of bradykinin were rejected. If the injection of a threshold dose was repeated at 5-min intervals for 6 hr, a constant response was observed. When the bradykinin threshold dose had been established, the analgesic agent was administered and 10 min later the threshold dose of bradykinin was again administered and repeated at 10-min intervals until no response was seen. An animal was considered to be in a state of analgesia when two consecutive stimuli had not elicited a response. An analgesic ED_{50} can then be calculated. The narcotic analgesics were administered subcutaneously and the nonnarcotics were given intraperitoneally.

b. Special equipment. No special equipment is needed apart from the facilities to perform the surgery required to implant a cannula.

c. Sensitivity. In this method, an analgesic ED_{50} value for morphine has been reported to be 1.1 mg/kg and that of aspirin to be 50 mg/kg when administered intravenously, as determined by the injection of bradykinin into the splenic artery of a conscious dog [76]. The following ED_{50} values have been reported for the intraarterial injection of bradykinin to the rat: acetylsalicylic acid, 37 mg/kg; phenylbutazone, 30 mg/kg; morphine, 2.45 mg/kg; and pethidine, 5.3 mg/kg [75]. These techniques have not found a wide acceptance and so the reproducibility and sensitivity of the results cannot be determined.

d. Pitfalls. Since these techniques are relatively new, the problems involved in their performance are difficult to assess. The complexity of the preparation indicates that they are not suitable for the routine screening of drugs but would appear to have an application in investigations concerning the neurophysiology of nociceptive stimuli. The narcotic antagonist analgesics are not detected, but intravenous amphetamine produces an ED_{50} value of 0.88 mg/kg in the splenic artery technique using bradykinin [76].

3. Blister Base

a. Details. This technique was first described by Armstrong et al. [77,78]. It consists of placing a circular plaster, 0.5-1.0 cm in diameter and containing 0.3% cantharadin, on the forearm skin of man for about 5 hr on the evening preceding the day of the experiment. A blister develops during the night and in the morning the blister fluid is aspirated, the raised epidermis cut away, and the exposed blister base bathed in physiological saline. The pain induced by these manipulations subsides in about 15 min. The exposed base is very sensitive and the application of certain substances produces a stinging pain. The substances that produce pain include acids, alkalis, hypo- and hypertonic solutions, histamine, 5-hydroxytryptamine, acetylcholine, potassium, and polypeptides. However, adrenaline and noradrenaline are inactive.

Initially, the intensity of the pain was measured by having the subjects squeeze a bulb [77]; the pressure generated was monitored as an indication of the pain produced. Later, the technique was modified to use a numerical scale for subjective pain, as follows:

0 = no pain

1 = slight pain

2 = moderate pain

3 = severe pain

4 = very severe pain

A graphic recording of the pain is obtained by having the subject move a pointer along a scale marked 0, 1, 2, 3, and 4 to indicate the intensity of the pain. The solution to be tested is placed on the blister base for 1-2 min and repeated at approximately 10-min intervals. A screen can be placed so that the subject cannot see the solutions being tested or the record produced.

b. Special equipment. Since cantharadin is the active ingredient in the reputed "aphrodisiac" obtained from *Cantharis vesicatoria* ("Spanish fly"), its use is subject to strict control, and its availability should be determined.

c. Sensitivity. Severe pain can be elicited by the application of solutions containing 0.1 μg/ml of acetylcholine. 5-Hydroxytryptamine produces pain in concentrations as low as 10 ng/ml, whereas histamine produces itch in concentrations of 1 ng/ml and pain at concentrations of 10 ng/ml.

d. Pitfalls. This technique involves most of the problems associated with human experimentation. The use of human volunteers embodies the problem of how "normal" is the "normal" volunteer.

E. Behavioral Techniques

1. Rat Flinch-Jump Test

a. Details. The technique consists of placing a rat in a box with an electrifiable grid floor and a transparent front [79]. An electric shock of controllable amperage at approximately 230 V is delivered to the grid floor from a Model 228 Applegate electronic stimulator, which provides a constant current source to minimize the effects that changes in skin resistance have on current density. Each animal is placed in the box and 14 series of electric shocks are administered. Each series of shocks consists of 10 shocks of the following amperage: 0.1, 0.2, 0.3, 0.4, 0.9, 1.4, 1.9, 2.4, 2.9, and 3.4 mA. In the first series, the shocks are delivered in increasing intensity and then descending and ascending intensities are alternated in each series. Each shock is of 1.0 sec duration and is given at 30-sec intervals. The interval between each series of shocks is 2 min.

The response of the animal is classified under two categories: The first of these is a "flinch" response, which is characterized by a "startle" or "crouch" behavior in which the animal's feet do not leave the grid. This is seldom accompanied by signs of agitation. The second response is the "jump," which is defined as occurring when the animal removes two or more feet from the grid at the time of the shock onset. This response is usually accompanied by agitation, vocalization, and running.

The intensity threshold for each of the two responses is defined as the minimum current that produces the response in 13 out of the 14 trials; i.e., if an animal jumps on 13 out of the 14 series at 1.50 mA, then this is taken as the jump threshold. For rats treated with saline, the mean flinch threshold is 0.2 mA (SD = 0.08) and the mean jump threshold is 1.04 mA (SD = 0.10) [79].

b. Special equipment. A cage with one transparent side and an electrifiable grid floor and an electronic stimulator capable of delivering a constant controllable current are required. A timing device is desirable to enable reproducible time schedules to be obtained.

c. Sensitivity. Morphine (2 mg/kg), nalorphine (0.5 mg/kg), codeine (30 mg/kg), and sodium acetylsalicylate (100 mg/kg) all produced a 100% rise in the jump threshold to a 2.0-mA current [79]. These were the lowest doses of the drugs tested. Except for nalorphine, a dose-response relationship was seen in the jump threshold. None of the drugs tested, even in the highest doses tested (morphine, 5 mg/kg; nalorphine, 2 mg/kg; codeine, 40 mg/kg; and sodium acetylsalicylate, 500 mg/kg), had any effect on the flinch threshold. Chlorpromazine and perphenazine were also found to be active on the jump threshold. Reserpine, tetrabenazine, iproniazid, and amphetamine were found to be inactive.

d. Pitfalls. The method as described requires the administration of 14 series of 10 shocks at 30-sec intervals, with 2 min between series [79]. This adds up to 91 min for each test. In a later report [80], drugs were administered 1 hr before the test procedure; consequently, these responses were measured up to 2.5 hr after drug administration. This would appear to be an excessively long time after drug administration for the measurement of analgesic action.

2. Avoidance Behavior

a. Details. In this method rats are placed in an experimental chamber (25 cm x 26.5 cm x 30 cm) constructed of aluminum sides, glass top, and a floor of stainless-steel rods placed 2 cm apart. Two levers project into the cage [81]. Electric shocks from a constant current stimulator are delivered to the floor rods, walls, and levers. The output of the stimulator varies from 0.07 to 0.65 mA in 25 discrete steps. An "add-subtract" device is used to increase the strength of the shock every 2 sec. An avoidance response is recorded when the rat presses either of the levers and the shock intensity is decreased by one step. Recordings are made of the stimulation output, the number of responses, and the amount of time spent at each of the 25 steps in the shock intensity. Rats are trained until their performance is stable both within sessions and from session to session.

Immediately after injection with the drug, the animal is placed in the experimental chamber for 100 min, only the last 90 min of which are recorded. The median shock level is then calculated. The median shock level is defined as the shock level above (and below) which the shock intensity was maintained for half the time. The mean median shock level for rats treated with saline was shock level 4.75 (shock level 1 being the weakest shock).

b. Special equipment. An experimental chamber as described above is required. Complex electronics is also required.

c. Sensitivity. Sodium salicylate (250 mg/kg) and morphine (2.5 mg/kg) significantly raised the mean median shock level. When the interval between increases in the shock level was increased from 2 to 10 sec, no significant effect of either morphine (2.5 mg/kg) or sodium salicylate (250 mg/kg) was detected.

d. Pitfalls. Any effect of a drug detected in this test could be due to a number of factors besides an effect on the perception of the stimulus. This includes effects on recent memory, effects on muscle coordination and other variables associated with training.

3. Pain-Conditioned Anxiety

a. Details. This method was described by Hill et al. [82]. The rats are maintained at about 70% of their satiation body weight by individual feeding, which promotes food seeking behavior in the experiment. They are placed in a conditioning chamber (19.2 cm x 17.8 cm x 24 cm) in which a bar is mounted as described by Skinner [83]. Bar pressing results in a food reward. Conditioned bar pressing is developed by the Skinner method on a periodic 2-min schedule that is later altered to periodic reinforcement with a 2-min mean. After about 15 days, when the cumulative record of bar pressing is smooth and a rapid bar pressing rate has been attained, conditioned anxiety is induced. This is performed by sounding a 60-cycle tone for 4 min at the end of which an electric shock is delivered to the floor grid. The electric shock is 40-60 V and lasts for 0.5 sec. The voltage of the shock is varied according to each animal's performance in the shock-tone conditioning. The mean number of bar presses during the tone sounding is 13.4% (range 0-26%) of the bar pressing rate during the 4 min immediately prior to the tone sounding. Immediately after the shock the bar pressing resumes at the pretone rate. The drugs are injected subcutaneously and the rats replaced in the home cages for 75 min. The rats are placed in the Skinner box and the bar pressing rate is recorded for 20 min. During this 20-min period the tone and the electric shock are delivered. The rate of bar pressing during the 4-min tone period, as a percentage of the 4 min immediately prior to the buzzer, is calculated. The amount of restoration of the bar pressing behavior is deduced to be an indication of the reduction of "pain-induced" anxiety.

b. Special equipment. A Skinner box, a method of applying the electric shocks, and a means of recording the bar pressing behavior are required.

c. Sensitivity. A dose-dependent restoration of the bar pressing behavior existed at doses of morphine from 4 to 11 mg/kg. The maximum bar pressing rate attained was 80% of that during the pretone period. Doses of morphine at 12 mg/kg and above impaired the bar pressing rate [82,84,85].

d. Pitfalls. This test, in particular, is confronted by an interpretation difficulty; namely, does the effect observed have any relationship to analgesia? The use of reduced-weight animals (70% of satiation weight) introduces additional variables in that the altered metabolic condition may result in indeterminable effects upon the actions of drugs, e.g., on the metabolism and disposition of the drug. In addition, any effects of the drug upon recent memory may not be detected in this test procedure. Furthermore, the time lapse between drug injection and the test itself (75 min) seems to be too prolonged for the detection of the analgesic effects of drugs. This may contribute to the seemingly large doses of analgesics used in this test.

III. COMMENTS AND CONCLUSIONS

The characterization and evaluation of the analgesics may be considered to be a difficult task because of the problems of assessing pain (in experimental animals), anxiety, and euphoria. However, most techniques, apart from the recent behavioral methods, tend to indicate a reasonable degree of analgesia comparable to that in man. For this is the most relevant aspect of animal analgesic experimentation, i.e., to predict whether a drug is clinically useful in man.

Detection of analgesic action is efficient in most antinocicpetive tests. In a screening program those tests that do not routinely predict analgesia for the narcotic antagonist analgesics and the antipyretic analgesics should be used in a cautious manner. Nevertheless, more and more evidence is evolving to show that most techniques are capable, under appropriate conditions, of predicting the analgesic activity of these compounds.

The number and nature of the tests to be used are dependent on the expertise of the pharmacologist. Experiments with mice and rats have definite advantages because the activities of reference drugs are well established and documented with tests involving both simple and complex responses. However, several analgesic tests should be employed which differ widely in the site and the mode of stimulation. Nevertheless, the nature of the test chosen should depend on the economy in time, the number of animals to be used, and the reliability of the results yielded, as well as the suitability of these results for statistical analysis.

In the authors' opinion, gaps exist that hinder, from a fundamental point, further development of the biochemical, behavioral, anatomical, and electrophysiological analyses of the different types of noxious stimulation and of the responses produced. Nevertheless, it is hoped that increased knowledge in these fields will yield safer and more reliable ways of obtunding pain.

REFERENCES

1. L. C. Miller, Ann. N.Y. Acad. Sci. 51:34 (1948).
2. H. K. Beecher, Pharmacol. Rev. 9:59 (1957).
3. E. Keith, Amer. J. Pharm. 132:202 (1960).
4. H. O. J. Collier, in Evaluation of Drug Activities (D. R. Laurence and A. L. Bacharach, eds.), Vol. 1. New York: Academic Press, 1964, p. 183.
5. R. A. Turner, Screening Methods in Pharmacology. New York: Academic Press, 1965, p. 100.
6. C. A. Winter, in Medicinal Chemistry: A Series of monographs (G. de Stevens, ed.), Vol. 5. New York: Academic Press, 1965, p. 28.
7. J. Jacob, in Drug Evaluation (P. Mantegazza and F. Piccinini, eds.). Amsterdam: North-Holland Publ., 1966, p. 278.
8. R. K. S. Lim and F. Guzman, in Pain (A. Soulairae, J. Cohn, and J. Charpentier, eds.). London: Academic Press, 1968, p. 49.
9. J. T. Litchfield and F. Wilcoxon, J. Pharmacol. Exp. Ther. 96:99 (1949).
10. J. Ben-Bassat, E. Peretz, and F. G. Sulman, Arch. Int. Pharmacodyn. Ther. 122:434 (1959).
11. P. A. J. Janssen, C. J. E. Niemegeers, and J. G. H. Dory, Arzneim. Forsch. 13:502 (1963).
12. M. W. Nott, Eur. J. Pharmacol. 5:93 (1968).
13. G. Woolfe and A. D. Macdonald, J. Pharmacol. Exp. Ther. 80:300 (1944).
14. N. B. Eddy and D. Leimbach, J. Pharmacol. Exp. Ther. 107:385 (1953).

15. P. A. J. Janssen and A. H. Jageneau, J. Pharm. Pharmacol. 9:381 (1957).

16. S. Kayan and C. L. Mitchell, Arch. Int. Pharmacodyn. Ther. 182:287 (1969).

17. G. F. Gebhart, A. D. Shermon, and C. L. Mitchell, Psychopharmacologia 22:295 (1971).

18. G. F. Gebhart and C. L. Mitchell, Arch. Int. Pharmacodyn. Ther. 191:96 (1971).

19. F. E. D'Amour and D. L. Smith, J. Pharmacol. Exp. Ther. 72:74 (1941).

20. H. L. Andrews and W. Workman, J. Pharmacol. Exp. Ther. 73:99 (1941).

21. J. D. Hardy, H. G. Wolff, and H. Goodell, J. Clin. Invest. 19:649 (1940).

22. D. L. Smith, M. C. D'Amour, and F. E. D'Amour, J. Pharmacol. Exp. Ther. 77:184 (1943).

23. O. L. Davies, J. Raventös, and A. L. Walpole, Brit. J. Pharmacol. 1:255 (1946).

24. W. D. Gray, A. C. Aosterberg, and T. J. Scato, J. Pharmacol. Exp. Ther. 172:154 (1970).

25. E. R. Hart, J. Pharmacol. Exp. Ther. 89:205 (1947).

26. D. D. Bonnycastle and C. S. Leonard, J. Pharmacol. Exp. Ther. 100:141 (1950).

27. C. V. Winder, C. C. Pfeiffer, and G. L. Maison, Arch. Int. Pharmacodyn. Ther. 72:329 (1946).

28. W. Edwards, Psychopharmacol. Bull. 47:449 (1950).

29. F. Haffner, Deut. Med. Wochensche 55:731 (1929).

30. C. Bianchi and J. Franceschini, Brit. J. Pharmacol. 9:280 (1954).

31. C. Bianchi and A. David, J. Pharm. Pharmacol. 12:449 (1960).

32. M. R. Fennessy, Brit. J. Pharmacol. 34:337 (1968).

33. P. K. Smith, J. Pharmacol. Exp. Ther. 62:467 (1938).

34. E. Eagle and A. J. Carlson, J. Pharmacol. Exp. Ther. 99:450 (1950).

35. A. F. Green, P. A. Young, and E. I. Godfrey, Brit. J. Pharmacol. 6:572 (1951).

36. L. O. Randall and J. J. Selitto, Arch. Int. Pharmacodyn. Ther. 111:409 (1957).

37. E. L. Way, H. E. Takemori, G. E. Smith, H. H. Anderson, and D. C. Brodie, J. Pharmacol. Exp. Ther. 108:450 (1955).

38. P. C. Dandiya and M. K. Menon, Arch. Int. Pharmacodyn. Ther. 141: 223 (1963).

39. C. R. Calcutt, S. L. Handley, C. G. Sparkes, and P. S. J. Spenser, in Agonist and Antagonist Actions of Narcotic Analgesic Drugs (H. W. Kosterlitz, H. O. J. Collier, and J. E. Villareal, eds.). New York: Macmillan, 1972, pp. 176-191.

40. T. M. Gilfoil, I. Klavins, and L. Grumbach, J. Pharmacol. Exp. Ther. 142:1 (1963).

41. D. I. Macht and M. B. Macht, J. Amer. Pharm. Ass. Sci. Ed. 29:193 (1940).

42. E. Contreras and L. Tamayo, Arch. Biol. Med. Exp. 4:69 (1965).

43. H. E. Hill, H. G. Flanary, C. H. Kornetsky, and A. Wikler, J. Clin. Invest. 31:464 (1952).

44. W. Koll and H. Reffert, Naunyn-Schmiedebergs Arch. Exp. Pathol. Pharmakol. 190:687 (1938).

45. A. Fleish and M. Dolivo, Helv. Physiol. Pharmacol. Acta 11:305 (1953).

46. G. K. W. Yim, H. H. Keasling, E. G. Gross, and C. H. Mitchell, J. Pharmacol. Exp. Ther. 115:96 (1955).

47. S. Radouco-Thomas, G. Nosal, C. Radouco-Thomas, and E. Le Breton, in Neuropsychopharmacology (P. B. Bradley, P. Deniker, and C. Radouko-Thomas, eds.). New York: Elsevier, 1959, pp. 391-396.

48. L. Saarnivaara, Ann. Med. Exp. Biol. Fenn. 47:113 (1969).

49. F. R. Goetzl, D. Y. Burrill, and A. C. Ivy, Bull. Northwest Med. School 17:280 (1943).

50. F. E. Leaders and H. H. Keasling, J. Pharm. Sci. 51:46 (1962).

51. A. C. Ivy, F. R. Goetzl, and D. Y. Burrill, War Med. 6:67 (1944).

52. F. R. Goetzl, D. Y. Burrill, and A. C. Ivy, J. Pharmacol. Exp. Ther. 82:110 (1944).

53. H. E. Hill, C. H. Kornetsky, H. G. Flanary, and A. Wikler, Arch. Neurol. Psychiat. 67:612 (1952).

54. D. Scott and T. R. Tempel, in Sensory Mechanisms in Dentine (D. J. Anderson, ed.). New York: Pergamon Press, 1963, p. 27.

55. O. E. Reynolds and H. C. Hutchins, Amer. J. Physiol. 152:655 (1945).

56. L. Paalzow, Acta Pharmacol. Suecica 6:193 (1969).

57. J. H. Burn, D. J. Finney, and L. G. Goodwin, Biological Standardization, 2nd ed. London: Oxford Univ. Press, 1952, 316 pp.

58. F. Cugurka, Arch. Int. Pharmacodyn. Ther. 97:206 (1954).

59. M. F. Lockett and M. N. Davis, J. Pharm. Pharmacol. 10:80 (1958).

60. M. N. Carrol and R. K. S. Lim, Arch. Int. Pharmacodyn. Ther. 125:383 (1960).

61. D. R. Maxwell, H. T. Palmer, and R. W. Ryall, Arch. Int. Pharmacodyn. Ther. 132:60 (1961).

62. P. Lund Nilsen, Acta Pharmacol. Toxicol. 18:10 (1961).

63. J. Charpentier, C. R. Soc. Biol. 155:727 (1961).

64. J. Charpentier, C. R. H. Acad. Sci. 255:2285 (1962).

65. J. S. McKenzie and N. R. Beechy, Arch. Int. Pharmacodyn. Ther. 135:376 (1962).

66. F. Hoffmeister and G. Kroneberg, in Methods of Drug Evaluation (P. Mantegazza and F. Piccinini, eds.). Amsterdam: North-Holland Publ., 1966, p. 270.

67. E. Genonese, N. Bolego Zonta, P. A. Napoli, and R. Tammiso, Boll. Soc. Ital. Biol. Sper. 43:1719 (1967).

68. R. S. Grewal, Brit. J. Pharmacol. 7:433 (1952).

69. L. Paalzow, Acta Pharmacol. Suecica 6:207 (1969).

70. C. Vander Wende and S. Margolin, Fed. Proc. Fed. Amer. Soc. Exp. Biol. 15:494 (1956).

71. L. C. Hendershot and J. Forsaith, J. Pharmacol. Exp. Ther. 125:237 (1959).

72. R. I. Taber, D. D. Greenhouse, J. K. Rendell, and S. Irwin, J. Pharmacol. Exp. Ther. 169:29 (1969).

73. R. Okun, S. C. Liddon, and L. Lasagna, J. Pharmacol. Exp. Ther. 139:107 (1963).

74. C. Braun, F. Guzman, E. W. Horton, R. K. S. Lim, and C. D. Potter, J. Physiol. (London) 155:13 (1961).

75. D. Botha, F. O. Müller, F. G. M. Krueger, H. Melnitzky, L. Vermaak, and L. Louw, Eur. J. Pharmacol. 6:312 (1969).

76. G. D. Dickerson, R. J. Engle, F. Guzman, D. W. Rodgers, and R. K. S. Lim, Life Sci. 4:2063 (1965).

77. D. Armstrong, R. M. L. Dry, C. A. Keele, and J. W. Markham, J. Physiol. (London) 115:59P (1951).

78. D. Armstrong, R. M. L. Dry, C. A. Keele, and J. W. Markham, J. Physiol. (London) 120:326 (1953).

79. W. O. Evans, Psychopharmacologia 2:318 (1961).

80. W. O. Evans, Psychopharmacologia 3:51 (1962).

81. B. Weiss and V. G. Laties, J. Pharmacol. Exp. Ther. 131:120 (1961).

82. H. E. Hill, R. E. Belleville, and A. Wikler, Proc. Soc. Exp. Biol. Med. 86:881 (1954).

83. B. F. Skinner, The Behavior of Organisms. New York: Appleton-Century, 1938.

84. H. E. Hill, R. E. Belleville, and A. Wikler, Arch. Neurol. Psychiat. 73:602 (1955).

85. H. E. Hill, R. E. Belleville, and A. Wikler, Arch. Neurol. Psychiat. 77:28 (1957).

Chapter 5

THE TAIL-FLICK TEST*

WILLIAM L. DEWEY and LOUIS S. HARRIS

Department of Pharmacology
Medical College of Virginia
Richmond, Virginia

I. INTRODUCTION

The tail-flick test was initially described by D'Amour and Smith in 1941 [1] and was modified by Bass and Vander Brook in 1952 [2]. This procedure was developed to ascertain whether compounds possessed narcotic analgesic activity in rats. Although the basic elements of the apparatus have not changed since the work of D'Amour and Smith, the sophistication of the apparatus has been improved. Also, a few significant changes have been made in the basic methodology. Initially, complete analgesia was detected when a dose of drug caused a burn on the tail prior to a tail twitch by

*The preparation of this manuscript was supported in part by USPHS Grants DA00326 and DA00490.

the rat. Today, a cutoff time is usually used. For instance, if a mouse does not respond within 10 sec and a rat within 20 sec when tested following the administration of the drug, this dose is considered to be 100% effective and the animal is removed from the apparatus. This cutoff time allows one to determine graded effects of doses less than those that produce 100% effect. Another advantage of this modification is that burning of the tail or other immediately noticeable pathological damage is not observed within these time limits. For years the tail-flick test was used solely to determine the narcotic agonist activity of a compound. Its versatility has been expanded in recent years. Today it is used widely as an indicator of narcotic antagonist activity as well. That is, this test can be used to determine the ability of a compound to antagonize the analgesic activity of morphine or another narcotic. There is good correlation between potency or duration of action of narcotic antagonists in the tail-flick test and their potency and duration of action as antagonists in man. Finally, the tail-flick procedure has been modified in a number of different ways and used in a number of studies designed to elucidate the mechanism of action of morphine and other narcotics. For instance, premedication of animals with drugs that alter the neurochemical balance in the brain alters the action of morphine and other analgesics in the tail-flick test [3,4]. In general, these drugs cause a similar alteration in the analgesic potency of morphine in man. In 1953, Winter et al. [5] examined the effect of morphine in the tail-flick test in studies using spinal rats. More recently, Mayer et al. [6] have shown that electrical stimulation of the brain produces an inhibition of the tail-flick reflex similar to that found after the administration of morphine.

II. DESCRIPTION OF THE METHOD

The rodent is confined, with the aid of a cloth towel or a plastic holder, on a wooden block so that it is relatively immobile. The use of cloth over the animal tends to be less stressful and helps keep the animal calm. Of course, one must be careful not to suffocate the animal or hold it so tightly that it cannot flick its tail. The animal's tail protrudes from the end of the towel and is placed in a slit on a wooden stage which contains a photocell beneath the slit. Approximately 12 in. above the slit and the photocell, a light source is mounted within a photographic type of reflector which centers the light on a specific area over the photocell (on the tail). This light is connected electrically to a start button and a clock. A press of the start button simultaneously turns on the light and starts the clock. When the noxious stimulus from the light (heat) becomes so great that it is bothersome to the animal, the rodent flicks its tail off the slit, and the light falling on the photocell shuts off the light and the clock. The intensity of the light is controlled by means of a rheostat built into the apparatus. The rheostat is set so that the majority of animals flick their tails between 2 and 4 sec after the initiation of the noxious stimulus. Once the rheostat is set, it is not changed during an experimental session. The investigator should record the rheostat setting of each experiment in his or her data book. The reaction time for tails of mice or rats, or for that matter humans who place their fingers on the stage, is quite similar and reproducible from one individual to another. The occasional abnormal rodent that does not respond within 2-4 sec during the control test period, is discarded and not used in the experiment. These animals are not very prevalent in normal albino mice and rats used in scientific laboratories (e.g., less than 1% in our laboratory). A photograph of the tail-flick apparatus used in our laboratory is presented in Fig. 1. Alternately, a tail-flick apparatus may contain a heated wire beneath the slit in the block of wood. The tail is placed in the notch (over the wire) and the operator steps on a foot switch that starts the flow of current through the high-resistance wire at the same time that he starts a stop watch. When the rodent flicks its tail from the heat of the wire, the watch is stopped and the latency recorded. This type of apparatus requires much more work by the operator and therefore leaves more opportunities for possible error.

Another modification of the tail-flick test that appears to be useful is to place the mouse in a plastic cylinder with its tail protruding out of one end of the cylinder. The experimenter pulls the tail taut over a wire coil as described above and determines the latency until the mouse pulls his tail. This technique, used by Dr. Richard Ruening of Ohio State University, almost completely eliminated the variability in either control latency or morphine-induced latency when an inbred strain of mice was used. Unfortunately, when random-bred Swiss Webster albino mice were used, this

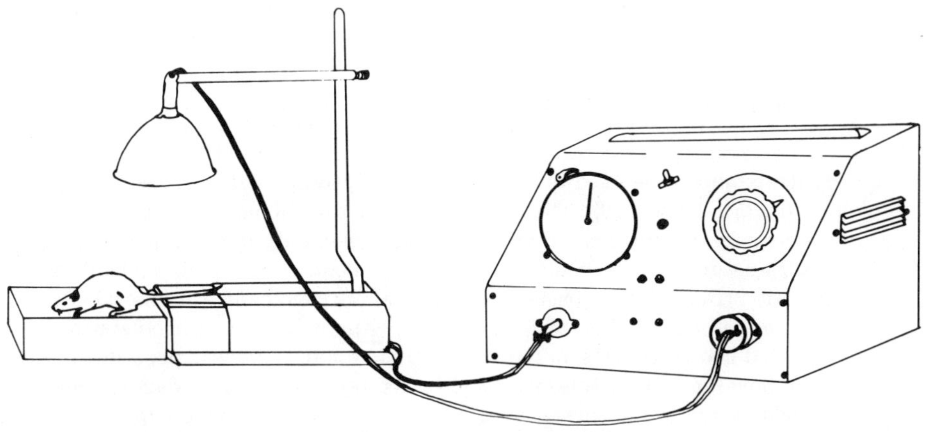

FIGURE 1. One type of tail-flick apparatus.

tail-pull method was as variable as the tail-flick procedures described above [7].

The tail-flick test affords one the option of obtaining either quantal or graded data. Some investigators determine the percentage of the animals tested that go to cutoff at each dose tested. These percentages are plotted vs dose on probability paper, the ED_{50} is read, and its 95% confidence limits are determined. Some investigators set an arbitrary increase in latency (for instance, a 4-sec increase) as a positive response and determine the percentage of the number of animals tested at a particular dose that reach this latency. Others have used a test reaction time greater than the control plus two or three times the standard error of the controls as a positive response. These data are then used as described above when the cutoff time was used as the indicator of a positive response. Many investigators, including these authors, prefer to use a graded response in the analysis of their data. In this method, one calculates the percent maximum possible response at each dose tested by use of the following formula, which has been published [8]:

$$\%\,\text{MPR} = \frac{\text{test latency - control latency}}{\text{cutoff - control latency}} \times 100$$

These percentages are handled as described above. Although these graded data do not lend themselves to the conventional statistical procedures used for comparisons of quantal data, one can determine differences between treatments with the analysis of variance and student's "t" test.

The antagonistic activity of a compound is obtained by giving a dose of the purported antagonist at a specifid period of time (usually 10 min prior) in relation to the injection of an active dose of morphine or another agonist. The percent antagonism is obtained by the use of the following formula.

$$\%\,\text{antagonism} = 100 - \left(\frac{\text{increased latency of morphine + antagonist}}{\text{increased latency of morphine + vehicle}} \times 100\right)$$

Rodents should be used only once in any of the analgesic procedures including the tail-flick test. The animals appear to associate the apparatus with the painful stimulus when they are used repeatedly in these procedures. This learning procedure causes a reduction in control and most probably in test reaction times. This phenomenon is not as troublesome in the tail-flick test as it is in the hot-plate technique. Another obvious problem in the repeated use of rodents in the tail-flick or other analgesic procedures is the rapid development of tolerance and cross-tolerance that occurs among compounds active in this procedure. One can miss an active compound because it was tested in rodents that had previously been given one or another of the analgesics. A final reason why repeated use of rodents in the tail-flick test is not a wise decision is the possibility that although one cannot detect gross pathological damage after one test exposure, there may be damage to sensory neurons or nerve endings. Such pathological damage which does occur during the testing of a highly active dose of a narcotic would obscure the duration of action of this effect if the tests were being run over and over again in the same animals. It is quite possible that the duration of action appears to be extended for many hours when the increased latency observed on subsequent testings is due to the inability of the rodent to flick its tail because of pathological damage and not to prolonged analgesic activity. One should inject a number of different groups of rodents with the compound and test a different group at each time period to determine duration of action of an analgesic agent in the tail-flick test.

Similarly, rodents should be used only once when one is determining the duration of action of a narcotic antagonist in the tail-flick test. The possibility exists that the rodent used over and over again would become tolerant to repeated administrations of morphine or another narcotic used as the agonist. This tolerance would give a false positive extended duration of action for the antagonist. Conversely, if a previous injection of an agonist had caused pathological damage, an active antagonist would appear to be inactive because the animal would not be able to flick its tail. Obviously, control groups could be run simultaneously in an attempt to minimize the problems described when animals are used repeatedly in the tail-flick test. The best testing procedure would be to use a different group of mice for each dose and time tested.

III. DISCUSSION

A large number of related screening procedures have been used in laboratory animals to assess the analgesic potency of compounds. There is a marked similarity in the basic procedure used in each of these screening tests. Animals are exposed to a brief noxious stimulus, and the normal reaction time is recorded as a control. The animal is then medicated with the drug and reexposed to the same noxious stimulus at a definite period of time following the administration of the drug. An increase in test reaction time over control reaction time is used as an index of the antinociceptive or "analgesic" activity of that dose of drug. As a group, these tests are relatively easy to perform, rapid, reproducible, and inexpensive, and most are predictable, within certain limits, of analgesic activity in man. The choice of one of these tests over the others may be based on any of a number of points, such as the experience of the investigator or the equipment available. Several authors have compared a number of these procedures from one point of view or another [9-11]. Since only a brief description is included here, the reader who is interested in more detailed comparisons among these tests is referred to these reviews.

The predictability of the tail-flick test for analgesic activity in man was demonstrated by Archer and his colleagues in 1964 [12]. They reported that the correlation coefficient for the potency of a series of narcotic analgesics in the rat tail-flick test and their potency as analgesics in man was 0.93. These workers also showed that there was an excellent correlation (0.93) between potency in the rat tail-flick test and potency in the mouse hot-plate test. These results indicate that these two procedures are very good and equal in predicting the efficacy of narcotic analgesic activity of a compound in man. The tail-flick test takes considerably less time to carry out than the hot-plate test, thereby presenting one advantage over this method. Another advantage of the tail-flick test over the hot-plate technique is the added selectivity of the tail-flick test, as described later in this chapter. We have used mice extensively in the tail-flick test in our laboratory and found that the relative potency of compounds in this test is practically the same when either mice or rats are the experimental animal. The correlation of the potency of a long series of narcotic analgesics and narcotic antagonists is exceptionally good between these two species in this procedure. The financial saving obtained when using mice instead of rats may make this a preferred species in this test procedure.

The tail-flick test is quite sensitive in that it can differentiate clearly between narcotic analgesics and weak analgesics such as aspirin and other drugs of this type. These drugs are not active in the tail-flick test at doses below those in the toxic range. Considerable question was raised as to the validity of the tail-flick test in predicting analgesic activity of strong analgesics in man upon the discovery of the narcotic antagonist analgesic pentazocine and its analogs in the early 1960s [8]. These compounds, like aspirin, are not active in the tail-flick test. However, pentazocine, cyclazocine, and other narcotic antagonist analgesics resemble morphine and other narcotics in that they relieve strong pain in man. For the first time, there existed a compound which was active in relieving strong pain in man and was not active in the rodent tail-flick test. Some years later, Gray [13] showed that if one lowered the stimulus in the rat tail-flick test, that indeed certain narcotic antagonists were active in this procedure. Gray decreased the intensity of the stimulus so that the control reaction times were somewhere between 7 and 10 sec rather than between 2 and 4 sec as was used prior to that time. When the noxious stimulus was set at this level, the narcotic antagonist analgesics did show good activity. There was one exception to a good relation between potency in the modified tail-flick test and potency in man with the narcotic antagonist analgesics. This exception was nalorphine, which was relatively inactive in Gray's procedure, but is as potent as morphine in relieving pain in man [14]. We have recently shown [15] that the narcotic antagonist analgesics pentazocine, nalorphine, and cyclazocine are active in the tail-flick procedure when a strong stimulus is used, providing that the animals are tested at short time intervals after the administration of the drug. These drugs were active in the tail-flick test at 1 and 5 min after either an intravenous or intraperitoneal injection. Interestingly, morphine and other narcotic analgesics were not active in the tail-flick test at these short intervals; instead, they appear to antagonize activity in the tail-flick and other tests of narcotic agonist activity soon after their intraperitoneal injection.

The tail-flick test is not as sensitive as some of the other tests which are used for narcotic analgesic screening. For instance, in our laboratories, the ED_{50} for morphine in the tail-flick test is approximately 6-8 mg/kg in mice or rats [3]. The ED_{50} for morphine obtained in the mouse hot-plate test in our laboratory is approximately 5 mg/kg and less than 1 mg/kg in the phenylquinone writhing test [3]. These data suggest that the tail-flick test may be the least sensitive of the three tests in detecting the activity of narcotic analgesics. This order of sensitivity among the three tests is also true for other narcotics. There is a poor correlation between potency in the acetic acid, acetylcholine, or phenylquinone writhing test and potency in relieving pain in man for narcotic analgesics and other compounds. A number of compounds that are inactive as analgesics in man show up as false positives in the writhing test. Although the correlation between activity in the hot-plate test and the activity in man is better than in the writhing test, a number of tranquilizers and other central nervous system depressants show up as false positives in the hot-plate test.

It has been proposed that activity of a compound to the noxious stimulus in the tail-flick test is due solely to an inhibition of a spinal reflex and has little relation to the effects of the compound in the brain. The proposal suggests that since this is a reflex, a compound need inhibit either conduction along the afferent axon, the monosynapse in the spinal cord, or conduction in the efferent somatic neuron in order to increase latency. Local anesthetics are not active at reasonable doses in this procedure unless injected into the tail. This decreases the probability that the mechanism of action of the analgesics is on conduction in either the afferent or efferent neurons. In addition, the narcotic analgesics, such as morphine, which are active in the tail-flick test at reasonable doses, do not block conduction in isolated neurons at comparable doses. It has been shown that if one transects the spinal cord of mice, and then exposes them to the noxious stimulus of the tail-flick procedure, the mice will still flick their tails. If one then administers morphine at doses up to and including 120 mg/kg, the reflex is not completely blocked [16]. Morphine is able to produce a 30% decrease in the response latency in the spinal mice. These data suggest that although the spinal reflex indeed is a factor in the tail-flick test, there is some supraspinal influence that is blocked by morphine in nonspinal animals and cannot be blocked by the narcotic in spinal mice. Therefore, the contention that activity in the tail-flick test is not representative of the effect of the drug in higher centers of the central nervous system appears to be unfounded. The work of Mayer et al. [6] has repeatedly shown that electrical stimulation in the paracentricular gray areas of the brain cause an increase in the latency of the tail-flick test. In addition, it has been shown that the intraventricular injection of morphine causes an increase in tail-flick latency. These results support our hypothesis that supraspinal mechanisms are involved in the actions of narcotics in the tail-flick procedure.

ACKNOWLEDGMENTS

The authors thank Dr. Mario Aceto for his helpful, constructive criticisms of a previous version of this manuscript.

REFERENCES

1. F. E. D'Amour and D. L. Smith, A method for determining loss of pain sensation. J. Pharmacol. Exp. Ther. 72:74-79 (1941).
2. W. B. Bass and M. J. Vander Brook, A note on an improved method of analgestic evaluation. J. Amer. Pharm. Ass. Sci. Ed. 41:569 (1952).
3. W. L. Dewey, L. S. Harris, J. F. Howes, and J. A. Nuite, The effect of various neurochemical modulators on the activity of morphine and the narcotic antagonists in the tail-flick and phenylquinone tests. J. Pharmacol. Exp. Ther. 175:435-442 (1970).
4. L. S. Harris, W. L. Dewey, J. F. Howes, J. S. Kennedy, and H. Pars, Narcotic-antagonist analgesics, interactions with cholinergic systems. J. Pharmacol. Exp. Ther. 169:17-22 (1969).
5. C. A. Winter and L. Flataker, The effect of cortisone, desoxycorticosterone and adrenocorticotrophic hormone on the responses of animals to analgesic drugs. J. Pharmacol. Exp. Ther. 103:93-105 (1951).
6. D. J. Mayer, T. Wolfle, H. Akil, B. Carder, and J. C. Liebeskind, Analgesia from electrical stimulation in the brainstem of the rat. Science 174:1351-1354 (1971).
7. R. Ruening, personal communication.
8. L. S. Harris and A. K. Puison, Some narcotic antagonists in the benzomorphan series. J. Pharmacol. Exp. Ther. 143:141-148 (1964).
9. F. R. Domer, Techniques for evaluation of analgesics. In Animal Experiments in Pharmacological Analysis. Springfield, Ill.: Thomas, 1971, pp. 275-318.

10. R. I. Taber, Predictive value of analgesic assays in mice and rats. In Narcotic Antagonists (M. C. Braude, L. S. Harris, E. L. May, J. P. Smith, and J. Villarreal, eds.). New York: Raven Press, 1973, pp. 191-212.

11. R. Banziger, Animal techniques for evaluating narcotic and non-narcotic analgesics. In Pharmacologic Techniques in Drug Evaluations (J. H. Modine and P. E. Siegler, eds.). Chicago: Yearbook Publ., 1964, pp. 392-396.

12. S. Archer, L. S. Harris, N. F. Albertson, B. F. Tullar, and A. K. Pierson, Narcotic antagonists as analgesics. Advan. Chem. Ser. 45: 162-169 (1964).

13. W. D. Gray, A. C. Osterberg, and T. J. Scuto, Measurement of the analgesic efficacy and potency of pentazocine by the D'Amour and Smith method. J. Pharmacol. Exp. Ther. 172:154-162 (1970).

14. A. S. Keats and J. Telfar, Nalorphine, a potent analgesic in man. J. Pharmacol. Exp. Ther. 117:190-196 (1956).

15. W. L. Dewey and L. S. Harris, Antinociceptive activity of the narcotic antagonist analgesics and antagonistic activity of narcotic analgesics in rodents. J. Pharmacol. Exp. Ther. 179:652-659 (1971).

16. W. L. Dewey, J. W. Synder, L. S. Harris, and J. F. Howes, The effect of narcotics and narcotic antagonists on the tail-flick response in spinal mice. J. Pharm. Pharmacol. 21:548-550 (1969).

Chapter 6

DETERMINATION OF ACTIONS OF NARCOTIC ANALGESICS AND THEIR ANTAGONISTS ON ELECTRICALLY STIMULATED GUINEA PIG ILEUM

SEYMOUR EHRENPREIS

New York State Research Institute
for Neurochemistry and Drug Addiction
Ward's Island, New York

I. INTRODUCTION

The guinea pig ileum has long been used as a tool for the study of narcotic analgesics and their antagonists, mainly in laboratories outside the United States [1-3]. The importance of this preparation in this country has only lately been recognized [4-6] and accordingly it is hoped that this chapter will stimulate additional research efforts with this unique and valuable pharmacological tool.

The ileum is composed mainly of two types of smooth muscle, longitudinal and circular. The tissue also contains a well-defined neural network, Auerbach's plexus, which arises from the vagus nerve. This consists of ganglia in close proximity to, or within, the muscle, preganglionic, and postganglionic fibers. When the tissue is impaled on external electrodes and current is passed, acetylcholine (ACh) is liberated from postganglionic nerves, causing muscle contraction. The smooth musculature itself is minimally excited by the applied current. Although preganglionic nerve stimulation with resultant liberation of ACh at ganglionic sites is another possible origin of impulses to the muscle, the evidence would appear to rule this pathway out as being involved with stimulation of the muscle. Thus, muscle contractions are only minimally affected when stimulation is carried out in the presence of fairly high concentrations of ganglionic blocking agents (hexamethonium, chlorisondamine) [5]. It is considered that the postganglionic fibers are selectively activated by the transmural shock.

When opiates are added to the bathing fluid surrounding a quiescent ileum, essentially no effect is noted. There is no sign of contraction or relaxation of the tissue; there is little if any effect of even high concentrations of the drugs on contractions produced by ACh, serotonin, bradykinin, or other smooth muscle stimulants. Thus, the opiates do not interact with muscle receptors or other muscular elements. On the other hand, the opiates are very potent in blocking contractions induced by electrical stimulation. The mechanism of this block has been well worked out and involves inhibition of release by the drugs of neuronal ACh [1-3]. This is a consequence of combination of the drugs with an opiate receptor located in the postganglionic nerves. The site of action is considered to be restricted to the terminals of these nerves. However, other sites are possible, e.g., within these nerve axons; in addition, many other drugs block electrically induced contractions by mechanisms that may or may not be similar to the opiates. It would be of some importance to review the sites with which a drug could interact to produce a block of contractions and to indicate how it is possible to distinguish among various mechanisms when the end point is essentially the same, namely inhibition of contraction. The following is a list of most of the readily recognized sites that could be involved in drug effects in the ileum:

1. The postganglionic nerve axon
2. Postsynaptic receptors, mainly ACh
3. Nonopiate receptors in nerve terminals
4. Extrajunctional "receptors" in conducting membrane of muscle
5. Extrajunctional sites within the muscle fiber (e.g., at the sarcoplasmic reticulum)

The means for determining whether one or more of these sites is involved are as follows:

1. An axonal site of blockade is difficult to differentiate from a purely terminal site: The net effect of blockade at either site would be to reduce ACh output, and since the ultimate measure is muscle contraction arising from ACh released by postganglionic nerve activity, either action would cause a block of contractions. At the present time there are no available methods for directly measuring neuronal activity in Auerbach's plexus. Such neurons are particularly vulnerable to action by many drugs since they are very fine and unmyelinated; indeed, Ritchie and Armett have shown that many drugs not considered to have local anesthetic activity can readily affect electrical properties of the desheathed vagus of the rabbit [7], neurons which may well resemble those in Auerbach's plexus. On the other hand, the concentrations required for these effects are higher by several orders of magnitude than those used to affect contractions in the ileum. In addition, the axonal blocking potency of morphine and other opiates is very low [8,9] and thus, at least by inference, it may be assumed that morphine and most opiates do not exert effects on conducting membranes of nerve axons. Furthermore, a recent study has shown that the axonal "receptor" lacks the stereospecificity for interaction with opiates [9]. Alternatively, if a drug shows fairly good nerve blocking activity, i.e., high local anesthetic potency, it would be a reasonable assumption that at least part of the block of contractions of the ileum would arise from axonal sites of action.

A mechanism of block of contractions by morphine and other opiates has been suggested which might explain why morphine action is confined to the nerve terminal: It and other opiates act by blocking the coupling of excitation to ACh release by inhibiting the activity of prostaglandin, the proposed modulator of ACh release [10]. The details of this proposal are beyond the scope of this presentation.

2. Postsynaptic ACh receptors: Drugs combining with and blocking ACh receptors would, of course, inhibit electrically induced contractions. The prime example of this type of drug is atropine. This site of action is readily distinguished from purely neuronal sites by examining the effect of exogenous ACh: If the dose-response curve to ACh is shifted to the right by

the drug at the time when block of contractions occurs, then receptor inhibition may be involved. However, other extrajunctional sites may also be affected (see below). A dose-dependent parallel shift in the curve would be indicative of a competition for ACh receptor sites, whereas if the shift is nonparallel other sites are probably involved. Another method for distinguishing between these two situations is to use KCl or $BaCl_2$ contractions, as discussed below. Other ways include effect of cholinesterase inhibitors or tetanic stimulation, although both of these would also affect block by a presynaptic action. Thus, if ACh concentration in the vicinity of the receptor is enhanced, displacement of the antagonist, at least temporarily (in the case of tetanic stimulation), could result in recovery of transmission. Both procedures can reverse atropine block. On the other hand, even at a time of complete morphine block of transmission, inhibition of ACh release is not complete (maximum perhaps 80%) and thus both cholinesterase inhibitors, as well as tetanic stimulation, can reverse morphine block. In other words, even use of these procedures cannot completely distinguish between purely neuronal and postjunctional site of action.

3. Nonopiate receptors in nerve terminals: Many drugs that have little affinity for either ACh receptors or axonal sites can block electrically induced contractions by a mechanism that appears to resemble that of the opiates, i.e., inhibition of release of ACh. However, it is clear that the nerve-terminal receptors for such drugs are not the opiate receptors since their block is not reversed by naloxone or by PGE [10].

4, 5. Extrajunctional sites: Perhaps the best way to test the involvement of such sites is to use a nonreceptor smooth muscle stimulant such as KCl or $BaCl_2$. Inhibition of their contractions by a drug at a time when it blocks electrically induced contractions would strongly suggest that the site of such block is neither neuronal or at the ACh receptor site.

II. DESCRIPTION OF THE METHOD

A. Detailed Procedure for Setting Up the Ileum and Longitudinal Muscle

The guinea pig should weigh between 200 and 300 g, although ilea obtained from animals much smaller or larger are quite satisfactory; however, the longitudinal muscle preparation (see below) cannot be easily made from very small guinea pigs. The animal is sacrificed by decapitation and the peritoneal cavity is carefully opened starting with a small incision in the midline that is widened with the fingers. The ileum is cut about 10 cm from the caecum with another cut being made some 30-40 cm from that point. The contents of the intestine are expelled by flushing with warm Tyrode's solution, the residual fluid being forced out by gentle "milking" of the tissue. Following this, we make a knot near the end of the tissue distal to the caecum since we start our experiments with the part closest to the caecum. The ileum is stored in Tyrode's solution; there is no need to oxygenate the solution to maintain viability.

It should be noted that the entire small intestine (ileum, jejunum, and duodenum) can be used to study drug effects on electrically induced contractions; it is generally considered that portions of the tract closest to the caecum are most sensitive to opiates.

If desired, the ileum can be kept for 1 or 2 days in buffer at 4°C without significant loss of sensitivity to electrical stimulation even without oxygenation; thereafter the tissue deteriorates markedly.

Ilea of several other species including mouse, rat, chicken, and gerbil, treated in the same manner as the guinea pig, respond very poorly to electrical stimulation and thus are not well suited for the study of these drugs.

No special precautions need be taken for preparing ilea from guinea pigs addicted to morphine by repeated injection of the drug.

We store the tissue that is not being used at the moment in the refrigerator at 4°C. This greatly reduces the amount of material leaching out of the tissue, possibly due to enzymatic degradation, as is observed when the tissue is kept at room temperature. A piece of tissue kept at low temperature for several hours requires longer equilibration at 37°C before reasonably good contractions are obtained.

The longitudinal muscle is set up as described by Rang [11]. A glass rod is inserted in a piece of ileum approximately 10 cm in length. Using a cotton swab, the tissue is brushed gently from both ends of the tissue beginning at the midline until almost all of the surface musculature has been bunched together. A piece of thread is tied to one end. The muscle bundle is then loosened from the underlying musculature by means of a forceps and mounted in the bath as described for the whole ileum. The only difference in the two preparations is that the tissue rests on the electrode rather than being impaled by it (see below).

B. Apparatus

Figure 1 shows the electrode setup used in this laboratory. It consists of a Plexiglas tube about 10 cm in length through which two insulated wires pass. These emerge at the base of the tube; at the other end are two connectors for banana plugs. A piece of ileum, approximately 3 cm long, is impaled in the two prongs as shown in Fig. 1; a piece of cotton is threaded through the other end of the tissue and attached to the force transducer.

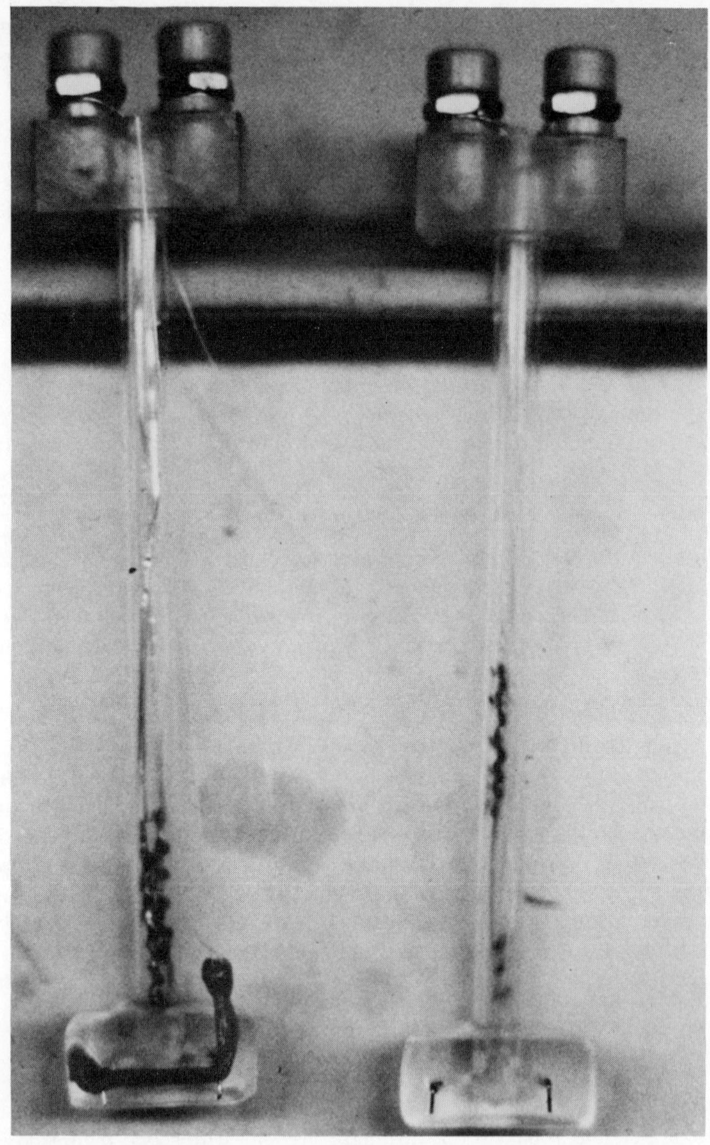

FIGURE 1. Electrode holders for stimulating guinea pig ileum.

The entire assembly is placed in a 50-ml organ bath at 37°C containing Tyrode's solution gassed with 95% O_2, 5% CO_2. The apparatus is connected to the stimulator and, after 20-30 min equilibration, 0.5 g tension is applied to the tissue. At this time the tissue should respond to electrical stimulation using the parameters set forth below. The contraction height at a sensitivity of 1 on the Grass model 79 polygraph should be 1.5-2.5 cm. If this is not achieved, the bath fluid should be changed and the tissue permitted to rest for an additional 10-20 min. Usually, rest will result in significantly greater contraction height, the maximum generally being achieved about 30-45 min after the tissue is placed in the organ bath. Regular contractions can be obtained for 4-5 hr from a single piece of tissue.

If the contraction is very weak, a brief tetanic stimulation (20 Hz, 10-30 sec) may suffice to begin fairly large contractions which will be sustained for long periods of time.

C. Stimulus Parameters

To determine the parameters for stimulating the tissue, one can vary current duration or voltage. We prefer current duration at constant voltage of 60 V. At this voltage, a current duration of 0.4 msec gives about 75-80% of maximum contraction height, which is achieved at a current duration of about 2 msec. These same parameters are used for the longitudinal muscle.

The stimulation rate differs for both preparations, being 0.2 Hz for whole ileum and 0.1 Hz for longitudinal muscle. Under these conditions both preparations will show fairly regular contraction heights over a period of 4 hr or more. However, it frequently happens that if a tissue is permitted to rest for an hour or so during the day, subsequent contraction heights show improvement.

At times it may be of interest to determine how a particular drug effect is altered by increased output of ACh. This can be achieved by use of tetanic stimulation of brief duration. The parameters we use are 20 Hz, 1 min for whole ileum and 10-20 Hz, 30 sec for longitudinal muscle. Under these conditions a normal tissue will respond fully to the control stimulus conditions within a few minutes after cessation of tetanic stimulation.

D. Duration-Response Relationships

We have recently found that the usual method of using a single set of stimulus parameters may not reveal subtle drug effects. Accordingly, we now examine the complete druation-response relationship before and after adding the drug. This procedure is carried out as follows:

Once tissue equilibrium is established under standard stimulation conditions (0.4 msec duration, 60 V), the current duration is dropped to threshold value, generally 0.03-0.04 msec. Contractions are recorded for 0.5-1 min, following which the current duration is increased to the point where contraction height becomes somewhat larger. This procedure is repeated until the maximum contraction height is obtained. The midpoint of the curve is calculated from a plot of the data (contraction height vs current duration) and compared with that determined in the presence of the drug.

This procedure has two distinct advantages over the single parameter method. First, there are examples of drugs which may affect to a minimum extent the contraction height elicited at high current intensity, yet may significantly alter the shape of the duration-response curve. Alternatively, the drug may greatly depress contraction height under standard conditions, this being submaximum, yet if current strength is increased it could be determined whether, indeed, the particular effect is exerted under all conditions of stimulation. Second, this eliminates the use of arbitrary parameters for the calculation of affinity of opiates to the tissue receptor. The blocking action of these drugs is particularly sensitive to changes in stimulation parameters, rendering calculation of potency meaningless except under the particular stated conditions. However, field strength also depends on bath size, volume of solution, etc. The duration-response relationship may obviate this problem provided the data can be treated in a meaningful manner.

One obvious drawback in the case of the duration-response curve determination is that it is somewhat time-consuming. In addition, there is evidence that opiate drug action is progressive [5] and that during the time of determination of the duration-response curve the effectiveness of the drug may increase. This could be tested by determining the duration-response curve a second time without washout of the drug.

The longitudinal muscle preparation responds in most respects identically to the whole ileum. This is true from both a quantitative as well as qualitative standpoint. One advantage of the longitudinal muscle is the general avoidance of spontaneous activity that sometimes becomes quite apparent in the case of whole ileum. One distinct difference between longitudinal muscle and whole ileum is that if the ileum is maintained in the cold for a period of 24 hr or so it is difficult, if not impossible, to have a viable longitudinal muscle preparation from such a stored tissue.

E. Determination of Opiate Potency

In this laboratory the cumulative dose-response (Fig. 2) is used to determine affinity of opiates for their receptor(s) [5]. The entire procedure requires only about 5 min and has a number of advantages over the individual dose method.

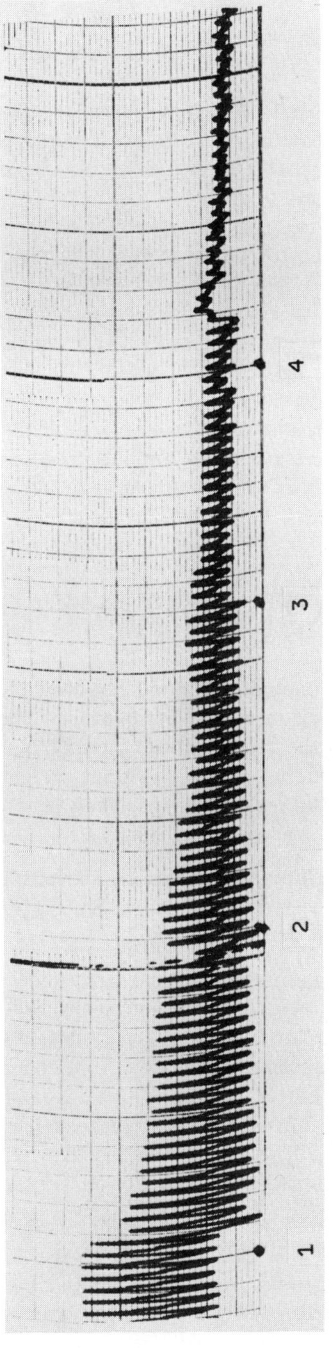

FIGURE 2. Cumulative dose-response curve for morphine. Current duration 0.4 msec, 40 V; stimulation rate 0.2 Hz; bath volume 50 ml; temperature 37°C. Morphine concentrations: 1, 4 ng/ml; 2, 8 ng/ml; 3, 16 ng/ml; 4, 32 ng/ml [5].

Paton [1] and Harris et al. [4] have shown that the ileum develops tolerance in vitro rather rapidly to morphine and other opiates. This may be due to the slow rate of exit of the drug from the tissue [12] or to some alteration in receptor configuration. In any event, very long washout periods are suggested, perhaps 30 min or more, in order for successive equal doses to give the same degree of block. In order to obtain the 4-5 points to construct the dose-response curve, 2-3 hr would be required, thus precluding use of the tissue for other studies. In the cumulative method, the data for the complete curve are obtained very rapidly and the same washout period (30 min) suffices to restore the tissue to control conditions. To be on the safe side, Harris and Dewey [4] replace the ileum after each determination of ED_{50} for a particular opiate. However, it should be noted that there may be considerable variability in the potency of an opiate between adjacent pieces of tissue on the same ileum; thus, it may not be possible to accurately compare results when one piece serves as a control for drug effects on the second. Our procedure is to use each piece of tissue as its own control.

III. NARCOTIC ANTAGONISTS: POTENCY, TYPE, AND DURATION OF ACTION

Narcotic antagonists such as naloxone, nalorphine, levallorphan, etc., readily antagonize the block produced by opiates. This action is exerted against all opiates, from the most potent, etorphine, to those which are relatively weak, e.g., codeine and meperidine. The method for determining affinity of antagonists to the opiate receptor has been developed by Kosterlitz and co-workers [13].

When tested against a series of opiates, the affinity of naloxone for the receptor was almost identical in each case, strongly suggesting that only a single type of opiate receptor is involved.

As is well known from animal studies, antagonists fall into two classes: pure and dual acting, i.e., having both antagonist and agonist action. A similar relationship holds for the ileum [13]. The pure antagonist naloxone fails to influence transmission even at very high concentrations whereas the other antagonists can block transmission if the concentration is raised somewhat above that showing reversal of opiate action. Because of its purely antagonistic action, it is recommended that naloxone be used for studies involving agonist-antagonist interactions in the ileum.

Duration of action of antagonists can be carried out as follows: The opiate is added to the bath at a concentration giving 50-80% inhibition. After a suitable period of wash, the tissue is exposed to the antagonist and then to the agonist. The effect of the agonist should be blocked. The tissue is then washed and the agonist added at the same concentration and the procedure repeated until complete recovery is the initial response is noted. Using this procedure, Kosterlitz et al. [13] showed that, as in the whole animal, the duration of action of naloxone can be quite short, the half-time for recovery being about 10 min. Of course, rate of recovery depends on concentration of the antagonist; Ehrenpreis et al. [5] showed that if the concentration of naloxone is quite high (initial naloxone/morphine ratio about 6/1) the duration of naloxone action is extended over several hours. These observations are quite consistent with observations concerning duration of naloxone action in a number of animals. In further agreement with in vivo results, the duration of antagonist action of cyclazocine proved to much greater than that of naloxone [5].*

IV. DEMONSTRATION OF TOLERANCE TO OPIATES

A. Induction of Tolerance

In vitro tolerance to morphine and other opiates was first reported by Paton [1] and later by Harris et al. [4]. Tolerance develops rapidly even when ilea from normal guinea pigs are used and is demonstrated by adding the same dose of drug repeatedly without washout. Inhibition of contractions gradually diminishes and eventually the added drug loses its effectiveness completely. No systematic study has been carried out to correlate this type of in vitro tolerance with tolerance production in animals.

Goldstein and Schulz [14] showed that following implantation of morphine pellets, ilea removed from such guinea pigs showed in vitro tolerance to morphine. Thus, the dose-response curve to morphine was progressively shifted to the right as the time of implantation increased, reaching a maximum degree of tolerance in 3-6 days. Ehrenpreis et al. [5] and Fennessy et al. [15] failed to demonstrate significant tolerance in vitro using ilea from guinea pigs injected several times daily with morphine for 7-10 days. One possible explanation for this discrepancy is that the dose of morphine in the latter experiments was insufficient to bring on tolerance. Nevertheless, guinea pigs so treated did show tolerance to <u>injected</u> morphine (see below). Another possibility is the method for determining the effectiveness of morphine, i.e., the method in which the dose-response curve was carried out. We noted that if the ileum from an addicted guinea pig is exposed to small doses of morphine (amounts giving 25-30% inhibition

*In contrast to reports by Kosterlitz et al. [13], we could not demonstrate significant antagonistic action of cyclazocine in the guinea pig ileum.

of contractions), then indeed a greater degree of tolerance was obtained than in control ilea. However, if a fairly large dose was given, e.g., 20-40 ng/ml, then the usual effectiveness was observed. Thus, the tolerance which is observed is of a complex nature, being manifested mainly at low doses of opiate.

Ehrenpreis et al. [5] were able to clearly show tolerance of the ileum to injected morphine. The experiment involved injection of a very large dose of the drug (500-700 mg/kg) into a control and addicted guinea pig (50 mg/kg/day for 7-10 days). Two hours later the ilea were removed, washed thoroughly, and set up for monitoring electrical stimulation. Figure 3 shows that whereas in the control ileum transmission was completely blocked, the ileum from the addicted animal contracted readily when shocked. This procedure could be used to ascertain whether or not a given drug produces tolerance in vivo. The fact that the ileum develops tolerance suggests that this phenomenon can occur by local adaptation of a peripheral tissue and is not confined to CNS sites. A possible mechanism for development of such tolerance has been suggested [5].

B. Withdrawal Syndrome in the Ileum

Withdrawal from opiates, in particular when precipitated by narcotic antagonists, is characterized by excitation; there is some suggestion that a sudden outpouring of ACh may account in part for the symptoms observed [16]. A similar type of excitation of the ileum can be demonstrated if naloxone is added in vitro to tissue removed from an addicted guinea pig. This is manifested as a contraction of the tissue (Fig. 4); naloxone has no effect on tissue from a control animal. Evidence has been obtained that this contraction results from the release of ACh by the added naloxone [5]. Thus, the guinea pig ileum as a model for the systematic actions of opiates and antagonists includes not only potency of such drugs but their ability to produce tolerance and demonstrate a type of withdrawal. The importance of these findings to the understanding of the mechanism of analgesia and addiction is self-evident.

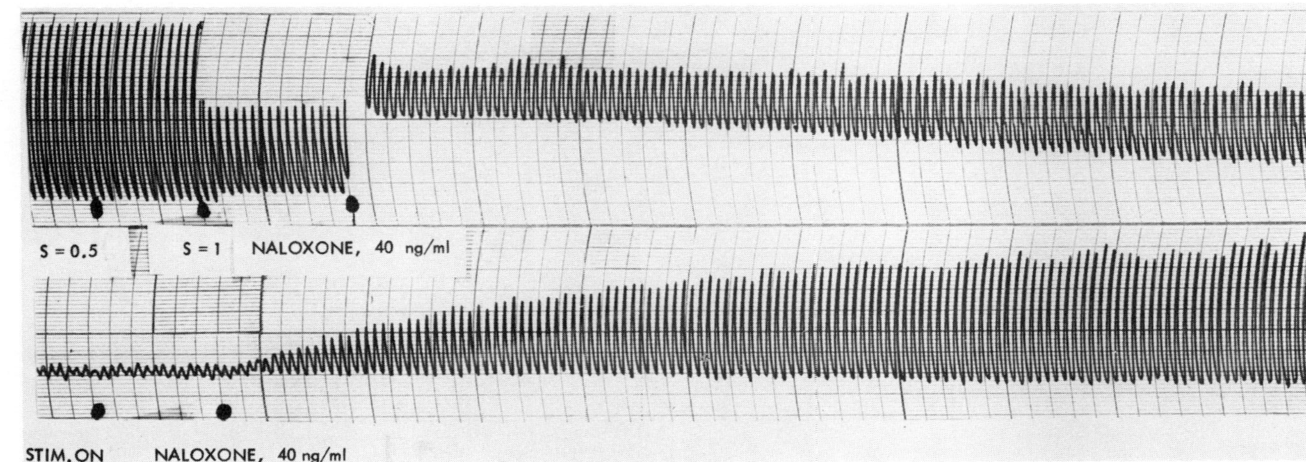

FIGURE 3. Effect of injecting large dose of morphine (600 mg/kg) into normal and addicted guinea pig: responsiveness of the ileum after injection [5]. Upper trace: addicted guinea pig. Note that contraction height is so great sensitivity had to be reduced. Following naloxone a large contracture is noted, this being a characteristic of the response of the ileum from an addicted animal to this drug (see Sec. IV, B). Lower trace: normal guinea pig ileum stimulated in the usual way. Note complete lack of responsiveness. Naloxone produces an immediate improvement in contraction height but no contracture.

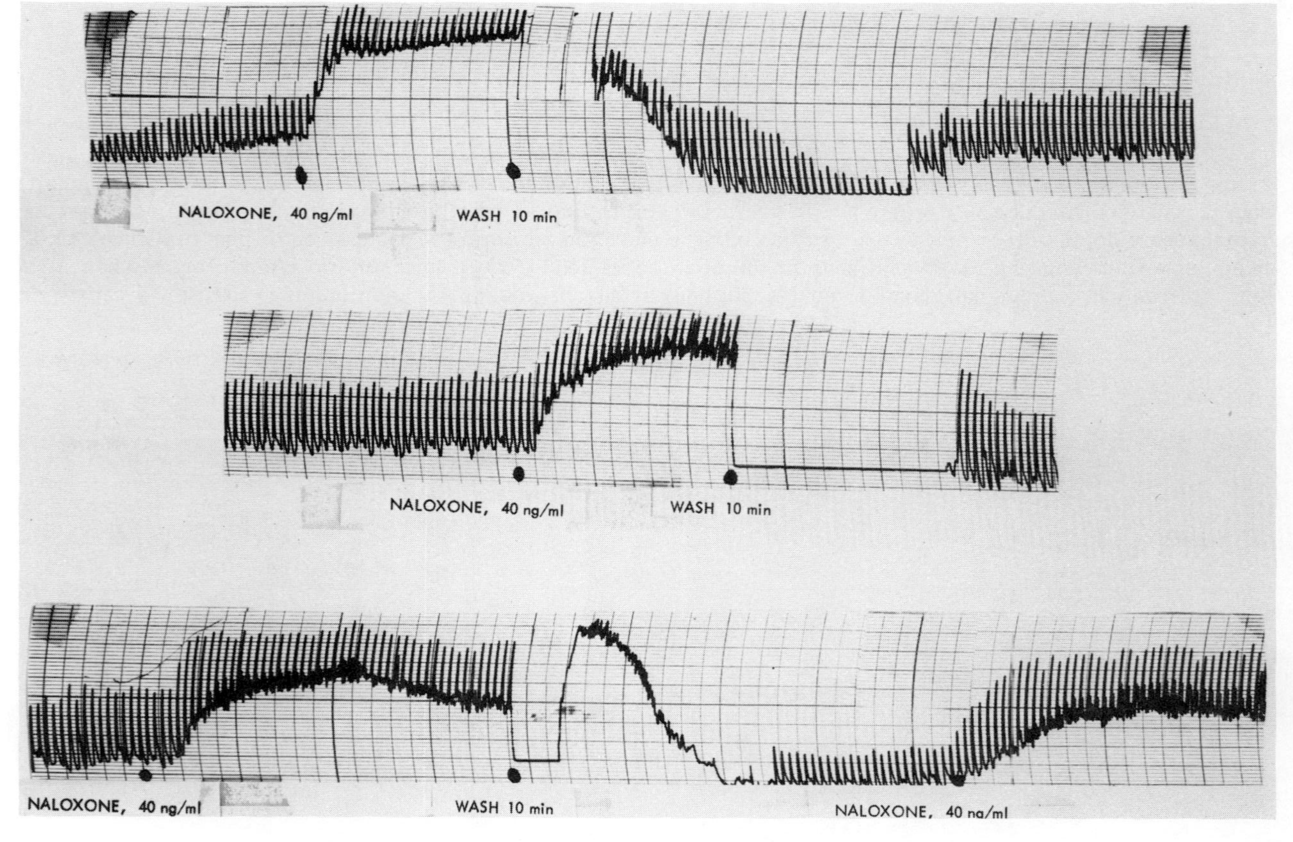

FIGURE 4. Naloxone contracture in ileum from addicted guinea pig. Note that this contracture can be elicited several times after washout, although the height of each contracture diminishes progressively [5].

REFERENCES

1. W. D. M. Paton, Brit. J. Pharmacol. 11:119 (1957).
2. W. Schaumann, Brit. J. Pharmacol. 12:115 (1957).
3. E. A. Gyang and H. W. Kosterlitz, Brit. J. Pharmacol. 27:514 (1966).
4. L. S. Harris, W. L. Dewey, J. F. Howes, J. S. Kennedy, and H. Pars, J. Pharmacol. Exp. Ther. 169:17 (1969).
5. S. Ehrenpreis, I. Light, and G. H. Schonbuch, in Drug Addiction: Experimental Pharmacology (J. M. Singh, L. H. Miller, and H. Lal, eds.). Mt. Kisco, N.Y.: Futura, 1972, p. 319.
6. A. Goldstein and R. Schulz, Brit. J. Pharmacol. 48:655 (1973).
7. J. M. Ritchie and C. J. Armett, Ann. N.Y. Acad. Sci. 167:504 (1967).
8. D. T. Frazier, K. Muryama, N. J. Abbott, and T. Narahashi, Proc. Soc. Exp. Biol. Med. 139:434 (1972).
9. P. Seeman, M. Chau-Wong, and S. Moygen, Can. J. Physiol. Pharmacol. 50:1181 (1972).
10. S. Ehrenpreis, J. Greenberg, and S. Belman, Nature New Biol. 245: 280 (1973).
11. H. P. Rang, Brit. J. Pharmacol. 22:356 (1964).
12. G. H. Schonbuch and S. Ehrenpreis, Fed. Proc. Fed. Amer. Soc. Exp. Biol. 31:482 (1972).
13. H. W. Kosterlitz, J. A. H. Lord, and A. J. Watt, in Agonist and Antagonist Actions of Narcotic Analgesic Drugs (H. W. Kosterlitz, H. O. J. Collier, and J. E. Villerreal, eds.). London: University Park Press, 1973, p. 45.
14. A. Goldstein and R. Schulz, Brit. J. Pharmacol. 48:655 (1973).
15. M. R. Fennessy, R. L. H. Heimans, and M. J. Rand, Brit. J. Pharmacol. 37:436 (1969).
16. L. S. Harris and W. L. Dewey, in Agonist and Antagonist Actions of Narcotic Analgesic Drugs (H. W. Kosterlitz, H. O. J. Collier, and J. E. Villerreal, eds.). London: University Park Press, 1973, p. 198.

Chapter 7

THE CLINICAL EVALUATION OF ANALGESIC EFFECTIVENESS

STANLEY L. WALLENSTEIN and RAYMOND W. HOUDE

Analgesic Studies Section
The Sloan-Kettering Institute for Cancer Research
New York, New York

I. INTRODUCTION

The application of appropriately designed experiments with adequate controls to cope with the problems of variability inherent in the clinical situation is a relatively recent development in the history of clinical analgesic studies. In 1948, K. D. Keele recognized that meaningful quantitative information on pain could be obtained by asking the patient to report its severity and by recording the responses on a daily pain chart [1]. He found this useful in evaluating analgesics, although his studies were uncontrolled. Denton and Beecher [2] recognized the importance of controls in the clinical measurement of subjective responses and of pain in particular, and put forth basic principles of experimental design: the "double-unknowns" (double-blind) technique, the use of a placebo and a standard of reference along with the test drug, randomization of the order of administration of study drugs, "correlated" (crossover) data, and "mathematical" (statistical) validation to establish supposed differences of effect among agents. Although the experimental design was relatively sophisticated for that time, Beecher and his group used only a gross quantal measure of analgesia. Their criteria, comfort and "at least 50% relief of pain" on two successive observations (45 and 90 min) after drug administration, provided information in terms of percentage of patients reporting positive results. From this, they calculated the AD_{90} (the "analgesic dose" in 90% of the population) for morphine to be 7-9 mg/150 lb body wt. However, subsequent studies by the same investigators [3] indicated that this was not a universal or absolute value: The average positive response to even 10 mg morphine/150 lb body wt varied from 55 to 94%, depending on the patient group in which it was assayed.

A wide variety of quantal and quantitative scales have been employed with varying success and sensitivity as measures of analgesia. These include "presence or absence of comfort" [2], "complete relief of pain" [4], "better," "no change," or "worse" days [5], and various scales of pain intensity [6-9]. Less satisfactory have been so-called therapeutic indices, which confound analgesia with side effects [10], or so-called objective measures, which attempt to correlate pain severity with observed behavior [11].

Although the principles outlined by Beecher for the controlled clinical study of analgesic drugs have received wide acceptance, they have not been without controversy. Batterman and Grossman [12] questioned the validity of the double-blind technique when they were unable to distinguish between a placebo and an active agent in a "double-blindfold" study but were able to in an open trial. These investigators, however, failed to recognize that their double-blind study, conducted in an outpatient population, was merely an insensitive one.

More controversial have been the objections of Free and Peters [4] and Meier and his co-workers [13] to crossover studies. They and others [14] have contended that, in postoperative and postpartum pain, definite time trends in pain severity adversely influence the results in crossover studies. They have also pointed up the possibility of interaction between a later medication and one given prior to it. On the other hand, other investigators [15] have found no impressive difference between an analysis of the effects of all doses given and first-dose-only data. This issue has not been definitely resolved, and an appropriate methodological choice would appear at present to be an empirical one, for the determinants may vary considerably from one clinical situation to another.

Experimental drug assay designs common to the laboratory were utilized by the authors in clinical studies of analgesics in patients with pain due to cancer [7,16-19]. In these studies, the effects of both standard and test drugs are employed to calculate relative potency estimates and their confidence limits. The twin crossover assay, an incomplete block crossover design used in some laboratory assays [20], has also been successfully employed by us in the study of clinical analgesic agents [21]. This design requires that each patient received only two medications and thus allows clinical analgesic assays to be carried out in patients with relatively short-lasting postoperative pain without losing the added information that crossover studies provide.

The basic methodology of double-blind, crossover comparisons has also been extended to the concurrent evaluation of oral and parenteral agents, thus permitting direct comparisons of analgesics administered by different routes in the same patient population [21-23].

Clinical analgesic studies utilizing a discrete, single-administration schedule of test medications are easier to manage and control than studies involving the repeated or chronic administration of analgesics. The situational variability and lack of adequate control over outpatients generally results in less sensitive studies in this population than in hospitalized patients [24]. There remains a need for studies of long-term administration of narcotic and narcotic antagonist analgesics in order to evaluate tolerance, cross-tolerance, and cumulative or toxic effects properly.

II. THEORETICAL BACKGROUND

The patient with pain of pathological or surgical origin is the subject of choice for the definitive evaluation of analgesics in man. No experimental pain model has yet been developed that can predict with any reliability the analgesic actions of drugs in patients with pain due to disease or trauma. Furthermore, so-called objective indices of pain have been unable to reflect adequately what the patient feels. Thus, despite the relative inconvenience and variability found in the clinical situation, it is here that the ultimate evaluation of analgesic effectiveness must be made, and this evaluation must rely on the subjective reports of patients with existing pain.

Measurements of subjective responses such as pain and pain relief in the clinical situation are subject to a multiplicity of biases, both conscious and unconscious, which can color study results. Perhaps most apparent to the investigator are the differences that exist among patients, both *physically* in terms of their disease, pain, and ability to handle drugs and *psychologically* in terms of their interpretation of pain and its connotations, their expectations concerning drug effect, and their understanding of the objectives of the study. More subtle are the variations that may occur within the same patients from time to time. Pain is affected by the current physical and/or psychological state of the patient and may vary from day to day as well as with the time of day. Psychological interactions based on the effects of previous therapy may also influence the reported effect of the drug under study.

Pharmacological variables may themselves be causes of potential study bias. The absorption and distribution of a drug may vary from patient to patient. Untoward side effects and idiosyncratic responses can influence the reports of patients. Drugs may react differently in ambulatory than in nonambulatory patients and interactions may occur with previously administered drugs. Last, tolerance and physical dependence to some drugs, such as narcotics, can substantially influence an analgesic assay.

Perhaps the most elusive variables for the observer to pinpoint, but by no means the least important, are the ones that he himself brings to the clinical situation. He must impose a definition of objectives and a study design on the clinical situation that may color the type of results he obtains. In evaluating subjective responses, communication with the subject is essential. The amount of insight the investigator chooses to impart to the subject as to the objectives of the study and his success or failure in communicating his definition of pain and criteria for relief are significant variables that are often overlooked. Finally, the investigator should be aware that the conscious or unconscious biases that he may have toward certain drugs can be tacitly communicated to the patient and are very much a part of the clinical experimental situation.

It is, of course, impossible to eliminate all these variables in any single clinical study, but by the use of appropriate experimental controls, one can balance the distribution of variables over treatments, and appropriate statistical analyses can provide the investigator with a measure of confidence in the reliability and validity of his results.

III. METHODOLOGY

A. General Considerations

A variety of questions relevant to the clinical usefulness of an analgesic can be answered by appropriately designed analgesic studies in patients with pain. Is the investigational drug an analgesic? If so, what is its potency relative to a standard reference drug? What side effects occur after administration of the drug, and what is the relative side effect liability compared to the standard drug at equianalgesic doses? How does its effectiveness compare by different routes of administration? If the drug is of the narcotic class, it is particularly relevant to know the degree to which tolerance, or cross-tolerance, to its analgesic effects develops with repeated use, and whether or not drug interactions with other narcotic agonists or antagonists occur.

Of course, no single clinical experiment can answer all of these questions adequately. Individual experiments must be designed to settle particular issues and some special designs will be discussed here in detail. However, regardless of the particular experimental design, the principles of a well-controlled clinical study are generally applicable.

To avoid latent or overt bias, the treatments in the study should appear indistinguishable to both the patient subject and the observer. This double-blind technique can be achieved most efficiently by preparing all treatments to be identical in appearance and packaging them in individual, sequentially numbered envelopes that identify the study, patient, and drug according to a prearranged randomized code.

Standard and control medications serve a dual purpose in the clinical experiment. They are landmarks against which the responses to the test medication can be compared and its relative efficacy measured. In addition, they serve as internal study controls, measuring study sensitivity and the ability of the patients to discriminate between active and inactive drugs, or between graded doses of an active drug. The standard and control medications can be employed to carry out both of these functions adequately only when they are included in the experimental study design and administered to the patients under the same conditions and subject to the same chance occurrence of the experimental variables as the test medication or medications.

Although a patient's responses vary from time to time, it has been our experience that, within the course of a study, differences are greater from patient to patient than within the same patient at different times, and that this holds true even when evaluating pain of relatively short duration, such as postoperative pain. It is therefore our belief that, wherever practical, studies should be designed as crossover rather than noncrossover comparisons, so that responses to the study medications can be compared within the same patient, and so that the variability among patient groups receiving the various treatments under study can be measured and more adequately controlled. The possibility of pharmacological and/or psychological interaction with previously administered pain medication has been used as an argument against the crossover design. However, this situation generally pertains to even single-dose, noncrossover studies for very few eligible candidates for clinical studies are naive subjects in the sense that they have not had recent previous experience with analgesic medications. It is therefore essential that studies be designed with appropriate time intervals between medications and, in crossover comparisons, be balanced for order of administration of study drugs. Furthermore, if there is indeed interaction among study drugs, this can best be determined and measured in a well-designed crossover comparison.

The proposition that pain is a subjective phenomenon about which valid information can be obtained only in terms of subjective reports of patients with pain implies the necessity for the development of an adequate system for dialogue between patient and observer. This involves defining pain in terms meaningful to both the patient and observer for the purpose of collecting data that can be put in a form amenable to statistical analysis and testing. Graded responses of severity of pain or degree of relief of pain which can be rated on even a quasi-quantitative scale are in general more sensitive than quantal responses involving only reporting the presence or absence of pain. Although degrees of pain or amounts of relief represent a continuum of effect, these are subjective estimates that can be communicated meaningfully only in gross terms, and only relatively limited scales of pain and relief have been developed that provide clinically useful and meaningful measures of analgesic effect. It has been our experience that relief can conveniently and reasonably be categorized on a five-point scale as "none," "slight," "moderate," "lots," or "complete." Categories such as "none" or "complete" are easy to define, but intermediate categories require a clear specification and understanding between subject and observer.

Adequate communication is facilitated when the patient has a general understanding of the aims and objectives of the study. The use of the double-blind technique need not imply that the patient must be kept in total ignorance. Briefing the patient on what is being looked for and the form the investigation will take before he is assigned to the study will generally improve the quality of information obtained and, incidentally, can make for a more meaningful informed consent on the part of the patient.

B. Details of Methodology

The following is a description of the method and procedures employed by the authors in cancer patients at the Memorial Sloan-Kettering Cancer Center. These methods have proven reliable in assays of most of the commonly employed analgesic drugs that we have conducted in the course of the past two decades.

1. Patient Selection

Adult patients with pain are examined by the research team physician and are selected on the basis of an appraisal of the cause of pain, the appropriateness of treatment with analgesics in general and with the study drugs in particular, and the ability of the patients to communicate. They are informed by the physician that he is interested in learning what drug best controls their pains and that they will receive several drugs during the course of the study, some of which may be more effective than others. Properties of new investigational drugs are explained to the patient at this time. They are informed that they will be seen at hourly intervals by a nurse observer who will inquire about the severity of their pains, administer study medications when required, and ask them to estimate the degree of relief obtained from these medications. The scales for intensity of pain and degree of relief are explained to the patients, and they are asked to give their written consent to participate in the study.

Patients are excluded from participating in the studies when there is reason to doubt that their reports of pain are due to physical causes or can be validly assessed even when the cause may be apparent. This category consists of patients whose psychiatric, mental, or physical conditions may be expected to detract from their ability to estimate their degrees of pain, and patients incapable of communicating effectively with the nurse observer because of language or speech difficulties. Patients are also excluded when the investigator feels that the administration of the study drugs would be unduly hazardous to the patient and/or medically contraindicated, e.g., pregnant women, patients with a prior history of adverse or idiosyncratic reactions, or patients with advanced renal or hepatic disease. Unless studies are designed to evaluate the effects of test drugs in patients who are tolerant or physically dependent on narcotics, these patients too would not be selected. However, as most cancer patients with chronic pain are likely to have some evidence of pulmonary, hepatic, or renal disease and frequently have had some prior exposure to narcotics, a priori exclusion from the study is based on the investigator's judgment of whether these are of sufficient degree to compromise patient safety or to bias the results. In large measure this assessment is based on the patient's responses to previous analgesic medications administered in the hospital.

2. Collection of Data

Patients selected for study are seen at hourly intervals by a trained, full-time nurse observer, and are questioned about the severity of their pains, awakening them if they are asleep. Pain severity is scored on the four-point scale from none to severe as 0 to 3. If the patient requests medication for pain and has not received an analgesic drug for at least 3 hr and if pain is reported as moderate or severe, a study medication is given by the nurse observer. Observations are continued at hourly intervals for 6 hr or until pain has returned to the premedication level and another medication is administered. If medication for pain is required before the 6-hr period has expired, it is assumed that there is no analgesia from the study medication for the balance of the period. After administration of the study drug, the patients are also questioned hourly as to their estimates of degree of relief on a five-point scale from none to complete (0 to 4), whether or not their pains have been at least half relieved, and whether they consider the drug acceptable. The presence and severity of observed or volunteered side effects are also noted. The Sloan-Kettering Institute analgesic study form used to collect this information is illustrated in Fig. 1. The upper portion of the form is a worksheet for the observer to fill out when interviewing the patient. The various categories are coded as follows: Pain: 0 = none, 1 = slight, 2 = moderate, and 3 = severe. Relief: 0 = none, 1 = slight, 2 = moderate, 3 = lots, and 4 = complete. 50% Relief and Acceptability: 1 = yes and 2 = no; Pain Site: 0 = multiple, 1 = head, 2 = face, 3 = neck, 4 = chest, 5 = arms, 6 = abdomen, 7 = back, 8 = legs, and 9 = pelvis and perineum; Pain Character: 1 = circumscribed and sharp, 2 = dull, aching, and diffuse, 3 = radiating or shooting, 4 = crampy, 5 = pressing or tight, 6 = burning, 7 = throbbing, and 8 = other. The data are subsequently transposed to the appropriate boxes below. Each box corresponds to a column on computer punch cards and is numbered accordingly on the second of the three tear-off sheets. The top line of boxes is for study and patient identification; the next line identifies the test medication and the analgesic, if any, administered prior to it; analgesic data are recorded on the following two lines. Side effects are recorded below using an open-ended alphameric system and are punched on separate cards.

3. Study Design

Patients are assigned to the study according to a prearranged randomized design generated specifically for the study. Only one dose of study medication is given per day. All analgesic and sedative medication orders are under the control of the investigator while the patient is on the study.

The particular design employed reflects the objectives of the study and can conveniently be divided into three categories:

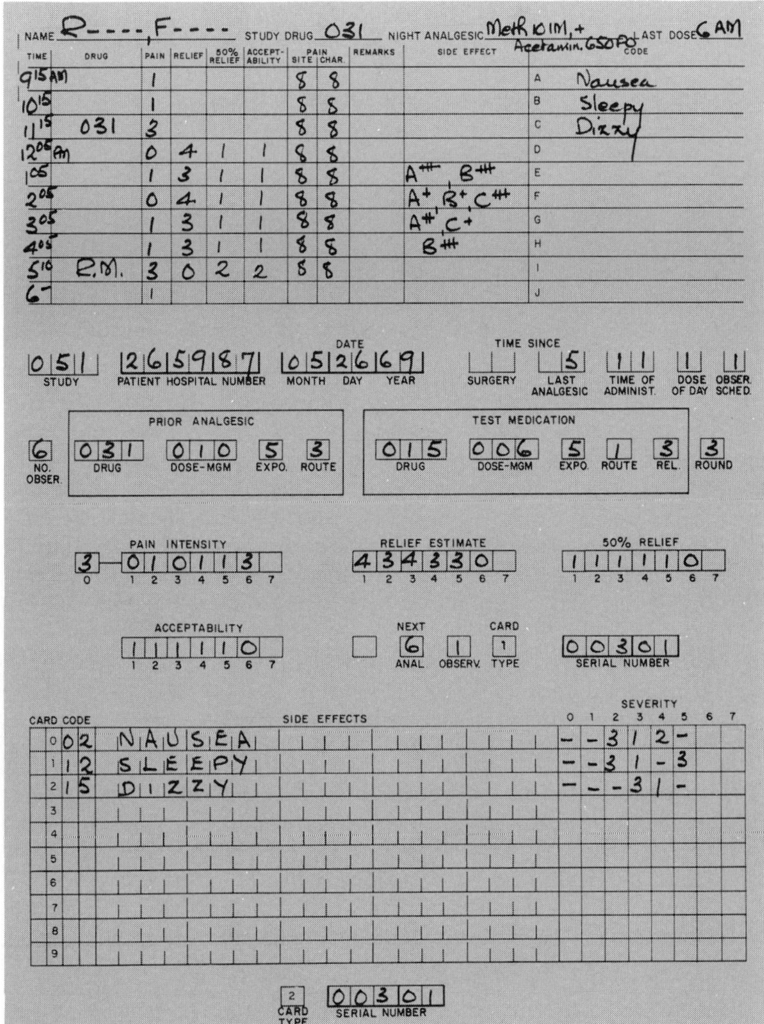

NAME R----, F---- STUDY DRUG 031 NIGHT ANALGESIC Meth 10 IM, + Acetamin. 650 PO LAST DOSE 6 AM

TIME	DRUG	PAIN	RELIEF	50% RELIEF	ACCEPT-ABILITY	PAIN SITE	PAIN CHAR.	REMARKS	SIDE EFFECT	CODE
9^{15} AM		1				8	8			A Nausea
10^{15}		1				8	8			B Sleepy
11^{15}	031	3				8	8			C Dizzy
12^{05} AM		0	4	1	1	8	8			D
1^{05}		1	3	1	1	8	8		A### B###	E
2^{05}		0	4	1	1	8	8		A+ B+ C###	F
3^{05}		1	3	1	1	8	8		A## C+	G
4^{05}		1	3	1	1	8	8		B###	H
5^{10}	P.M.	3	0	2	2	8	8			I
6-		1								J

STUDY 051 | PATIENT HOSPITAL NUMBER 2659871 | DATE: MONTH 05 DAY 26 YEAR 69 | TIME SINCE: SURGERY | LAST ANALGESIC 5 | TIME OF ADMINIST. 11 | DOSE OF DAY 1 | OBSER. SCHED. 1

NO. OBSER. 6

PRIOR ANALGESIC: DRUG 031 | DOSE-MGM 010 | EXPO. 5 | ROUTE 3

TEST MEDICATION: DRUG 015 | DOSE-MGM 006 | EXPO. 5 | ROUTE 1 | REL. 3 | ROUND 3

PAIN INTENSITY: 0: 3 | 1–7: 0 1 0 1 1 3

RELIEF ESTIMATE: 1–7: 4 3 4 3 3 0

50% RELIEF: 1–7: 1 1 1 1 1 0

ACCEPTABILITY: 1–7: 1 1 1 1 1 0

NEXT ANAL 6 | OBSERV. 1 | CARD TYPE 1 | SERIAL NUMBER 00301

CARD CODE		SIDE EFFECTS	SEVERITY 0	1	2	3	4	5	6	7
0	02	NAUSEA	–	–	3	1	2	–		
1	12	SLEEPY	–	–	3	1	–	3		
2	15	DIZZY	–	–	–	3	1	–		
3										
4										
5										
6										
7										
8										
9										

CARD TYPE 2 | SERIAL NUMBER 00301

FIGURE 1. The Sloan-Kettering Institute analgesic study form. A triplicate form for recording the patient's fluctuations in pain and analgesic responses to study medications, and for ready conversion of data to punch cards for computer analysis.

1. Studies to determine the presence or absence of analgesic effect may be simple, single-dose comparisons of the test drug with a standard and a control. This design depends on the ability of the investigator to select an appropriate dose of the test medication, and in reality asks the specific question, Is this particular dose of the test medication analgesic? More complicated designs may include graded doses of the test and/or standard drugs, or may include more than a single test drug. However, practical considerations would limit the number of study medications in crossover studies, and, indeed, it is usually more efficient to design a series of small experiments than to carry out a single, unwieldy, large study.
2. Studies of drug interaction may similarly be designed as a simple factorial experiment (a placebo, single doses of each of two drugs both alone and in combination) or may consist of more complicated designs including graded doses of either one or both of the drugs alone and in combination. The specifics of the design are, of course, dictated by the type of interaction under investigation. The analgesic effects of combinations of narcotics and salicylates, for example, may be simple and additive, while combinations of narcotics and narcotic antagonists may produce enhancement of, or interference with, analgesia depending on a variety of factors including the ratio of doses of narcotic to antagonist and the degree of tolerance or physical dependence.
3. Assays of relative potency are carried out to determine equianalgesic doses of the test medication and a commonly employed standard medication, such as morphine, in the usual therapeutic range of doses. These assays are particularly useful to the clinician in determining the appropriate dose of a test drug that may be substituted for a standard. In addition, estimates of side effect liability are most meaningful when obtained in the equianalgesic range of the two drugs.

A relative potency estimate requires the assumption that the test drug is acting as a diluent of the standard, i.e., that the dose-effect slopes of the two drugs are parallel, and this assumption should either be tested in the experiment or be independently verified. The classical relative potency assay supplies the investigator with graded dose information on the drugs under study and can be considered valid when the following conditions are met: (a) A positive slope for the study is obtained; (b) there is no significant difference in parallelism of the slopes of the two drugs; and (c) there is no significant difference in the effect levels obtained with the two drugs, so that extrapolation of the dose-effect curves is not required to obtain the relative potency estimate. This is best accomplished when the assay encompasses as wide a range of doses of the study drugs as possible. However, a variety of circumstances may limit the number of test medications that can reasonably be administered to any one patient in a crossover comparison. This assay may therefore be designed as a series of small, sequentially related experiments, each experiment including as few as two doses each of standard and test medication with the ratio of doses of test to standard being varied from experiment to experiment. The relative responses of the patients to the test and standard medications in the current experiment determine the ratio of doses to be employed in the subsequent experiment. This sequential decision-making process is continued throughout the assay and can be carried out after the results are obtained in a small group of patients in each experiment. In this way, a wide range of doses can be assayed, with the bulk of the data obtained in the equianalgesic effect range of the two drugs.

Certain types of clinical pain, however, may be so short-lived that it is not feasible to include even two doses of each drug in complete crossover studies. In the past, investigators utilizing such patients have felt constrained either to abandon obtaining slope estimates for both drugs, or to sacrifice the advantages inherent in crossover design. The problem, however, can be largely overcome by the employment of an incomplete block or twin crossover assay, a bioassay design that provides estimates of slope and relative efficacy in a crossover comparison in which each subject receives only two drug administrations [19,20]. In this assay, each patient receives the upper dose of one study drug and the lower dose of the other, on separate days. A group of four patients represents a crossover block balanced for drug, dose, and order (Table I). To maintain this balance, it is necessary to substitute patients for those who fail to complete the study. The assignment of patients is randomized within each crossover block. Randomization is accomplished by blind selection from a shuffled deck of cards of the twenty-four possible orders of administering four different

TABLE I

A Sample Block Design for a Twin Crossover Assay[a]

	Standard drug		Test drug	
Patient	Lower dose	Upper dose	Lower dose	Upper dose
A	1[b]			2
B		2	1	
C		1	2	
D	2			1

[a]Selected from an assay containing several randomized blocks.
[b]Numbers denote order of administration.

medications. Like the complete crossover assay, the twin crossover assay can readily be carried out as a series of sequentially related experiments. An appropriate end point for decision making here would be after every block of four patients. For example, if the sum of the total relief scores in the four patients were greater for the standard drug than for the test drug, a decision to employ higher doses of test drug would be made. Conversely, if the test drug scores were higher, the decision would be to employ lower doses. If the scores were equivalent, the ratio of doses would be kept the same.

Special applications of the various study designs mentioned above may be undertaken to answer specific questions: (a) Patients may be separated into groups according to the degree of presumed tolerance to narcotic drugs. This may be based simply on the amount of narcotics the patients are taking prior to being placed on study, or may be determined experimentally, for example, by the patients' responses to challenge doses of a narcotic antagonist. (b) When distinct divisions can readily be made according to type of pain (such as chronic or postoperative pain), the two patient populations may be studied separately so that the results in each group can be compared. (c) It may be of interest to compare drugs by different routes of administration, as in factorial studies involving combinations or parenteral narcotics and oral salicylates, or in relative potency assays of a single drug given by different routes, i.e., relative oral-intramuscular analgesic potency assays. Studies of this type are carried out on a double-blind basis by including appropriate dummy medications in coded envelopes so that the patient will receive medication by both routes whenever a study drug is required. For example, in an oral-parenteral study, the patient receives an oral placebo with his injection of drug, or a saline injection with his drug capsule or tablet.

C. Special Requirements

Analgesic studies such as these stand or fall on the accurate recording and interpretation of subjective reports of patients. This is not likely to be accomplished with any degree of reliability by the casual observations of a busy floor nurse. Generally it is best to employ a full-time observer, indoctrinated as to the pitfalls of preconceived bias, and trained to elicit the specific information desired. The observer should not be burdened with other major responsibilities that could detract from the appointed analgesic rounds. The observer should have more than a casual understanding of the rationale and objectives of investigation and, indeed, of the particular studies being carried out. A knowledge of the properties of the drugs under investigation is desirable in the clinical setting and is not inconsistent with the double-blind technique. A specially trained registered nurse who is adept at establishing good rapport with patients makes for the best possible observer.

Whether or not it is advisable to employ more than one observer for a single study is a matter that has been debated but not conclusively resolved. A second observer introduces an additional variable in a situation already loaded with potential sources of bias. Differences in patient-observer interaction may influence results and cannot be easily dismissed. Overnight observations, when the patient is usually asleep, contribute little to studies of this type and it would thus seem prudent, whenever possible, to limit observations to the working hours of a single observer.

The randomization, encoding, and packaging of study drugs may be carried out by an outside sponsor of the study, or may be done by a member of the analgesic study team who does not participate in the observation and interview of the patients on study. In either case, copies of the drug code should be kept on hand so that the code of a particular study medication can be readily broken in the case of a medical emergency.

Not all patients with pain are suitable subjects for any single study. Some may not be able to take drugs by a particular route, some may be appropriate candidates only for the milder analgesics, and some only for the stronger. Considering the not insignificant investment in time and effort in establishing an analgesic study group, it may be advisable to plan for different types of studies which can be run concurrently. Because of the diversity of patients in most clinical settings, this will make for most efficient use of the research team.

D. Sensitivity

The sensitivity of clinical analgesic studies is determined by the multiplicity of variables inherent in the clinical situation as well as by the verbal limitations in communicating subjective responses. Nevertheless, reproducible results are obtainable in adequately designed and controlled studies. Graded dose-effect responses are routinely achieved with drugs of the narcotic class, and significant differences between placebo and commonly employed doses of analgesics can also be expected.

In quantitative relative potency assays, λ, an index of precision, can be calculated in terms of the ratio of standard error to slope. This value (s/b) is independent of the units in which doses are measured and of the experimental design and the number of observations [25]. It is thus possible to compare the sensitivity of a variety of clinical assays, and even to compare the precision of the clinical assay with laboratory assays in animals. The smaller the value of λ, the greater the assay precision. In our experience, values for λ in the range of 0.4-0.6 are commonly obtained in relative potency assays of intramuscularly administered narcotics. In studies involving oral administration, λ is somewhat higher and probably reflects greater variability of drug absorption. Whether the study is a complete or a twin crossover design does not apparently affect the value of λ to any great extent. By way of comparison, Winder [26] has reported λ of 0.27 for laboratory assays of analgesics in guinea pigs and, indeed, one would expect more precise assays under laboratory conditions than in a clinical milieu.

When λ is known, it is possible to estimate the minimum number of subjects required for an assay with specified confidence limits. For calculating the number of subjects required for 95% confidence limits with a relative potency range of 2X, Gaddum gives the formula $170\lambda^2$ [25]. Thus, for $\lambda = 0.6$, a minimum of 61 subjects would be required. A comparable calculation for the minimum number of guinea pigs in the laboratory assay reported by Winder in which $\lambda = 0.27$ would be 12. Results in the clinical situation can thus be expressed in terms commonly employed in the laboratory and allow for direct comparisons if an appropriate number of subjects are employed.

E. Limitations

In the laboratory, the investigator usually has a wide variety of options for manipulation and control of his experimental design. In the clinic, the clinical situation itself most often dictates what can or cannot be done. The number of patients with pain available for study, the length of time that they are available, the type and severity of their pains, and the appropriateness of the treatments for the patients are all factors which, of necessity, must serve as significant determinants in the planning, design, and execution of clinical analgesic studies. When clinical studies are planned for a situation in which they have not been carried out before, it is wise to carry out a pilot study using noninvestigational, regularly employed analgesics. This can serve the dual purposes of validating the method by demonstrating that the study is capable of picking up differences between an active drug and placebo or between graded doses of a known analgesic, and also of alerting the investigator to any special situational problems that can best be solved before a commitment is made to an inappropriate experimental regimen.

IV. TYPES OF DATA OBTAINABLE

The information generated by the hourly patient interviews represent arbitrary categorizations of the patients' subjective responses. They differ from other clinical measures such as temperature or blood pressure in that they are not absolute values, even though we assign them numerical scores. We have no way of knowing whether "moderate" and "severe" pain, or "slight" or "some" relief, or any of the other categories employed mean the same thing from one patient to another. Even the quantal responses to questions such as "Is your pain at least half gone?" are not free from slippage [27] or differences in interpretation by different patients. Pain is notoriously difficult to define and quantify and it follows that analgesia is at least as difficult. Thus, an analgesic "score" has specific meaning only in terms of the experience of the particular patient from whom it was elicited. The relationship to the responses of other patients is neither clear-cut nor easily defined, although this becomes somewhat academic in crossover studies in which drugs are compared in the same patients. It is obvious that the validity of the response cannot be resolved in advance on an individual basis, but must be determined empirically from the study results themselves. If a group of patients is able to discriminate between a placebo and a standard analgesic, or between graded doses of an analgesic, and the observed differences are not likely to have been caused by chance, this can be accepted as evidence of the sensitivity of the method. If the study population cannot make these discriminations, the validity of the study is open to question. Thus, statistical evaluation of results becomes a vital aspect of the clinical analgesic assay. For quantitative data, analysis of variance may be carried out with patients, treatments, and replications (when patients receive more than one round of study medications) serving as the sources of variation. Although analgesic data may be skewed, differences in responses to drugs tend to be normally distributed in crossover studies, so that deviations from normality have been found not to affect the analysis significantly.

Problems of normality of distribution can be circumvented by weighting or transforming the data so that they will either approach normality or become distribution-free. The ridit transformation formulated by Bross [27] is a nonparametric transformation developed especially for use with subjective measurement scales. Based on an empirically identified distribution within the study (such as the responses to a dose of standard drug) rather than on a theoretical normal distribution, the ridit is distribution-free and extends from 0 to 1 with the mean of the identified distribution at 0.5. It is a property of ridits that, when examining the same effect in different studies, agreement will be good regardless of differences in the original scales. The ridit is therefore particularly useful in equating scales among different studies, or even those of different investigators, so that results can be directly compared [28]. Ridit scores can be subjected to the same statistical tests as can the raw scores.

In relative potency assays, the mean squares of the orthogonal treatments components for common slope, differences in parallelism between the individual drug slopes, and differences in the effect levels of the standard and test drugs are computed and tested for significance. A valid assay will have a significant common slope, insignificant deviations from parallelism, and insignificant differences in effect between the study drugs. Standard methods for the calculation of relative potency and appropriate confidence limits have been discussed by Gaddum [25]. A detailed application of these statistical techniques to a clinical analgesic assay has been presented by Seed et al. [7].

The criteria for the twin crossover assay are somewhat different than those for the complete crossover in that the test for parallelism of the drug slopes is not a crossover comparison and thus can be confounded by individual differences [29]. Since intersubject differences do not bias the estimate of relative potency in this assay, the contrast for parallelism is not an appropriate assessment of validity. Discussion of the twin crossover assays and detailed descriptions of their analysis are reported by Finney [20] and Rerup [30].

Hourly observations of the patients provide quantitative data for the calculation of dose-effect and time-effect curves in terms of either peak drug effect (the highest score obtained during the first three hours after drug administration), or total effect (an estimate of the area under the time-effect curve arrived at by totaling the hourly scores for 6 hr). These can be obtained either in terms of the patients' reported changes in severity of pain after administration of the test medication or in terms of their estimates of degree of relief.

Quantal data, in the form of whether or not the patient estimates that at least half his pain is relieved or whether or not he considers the drug acceptable at any particular hour, also provide useful clinical information. The estimate of acceptability is not a pure measure of analgesia, for it undoubtedly is influenced by other factors such as side effects. Differences in these two end points may be revealing in studies of certain drugs, such as the narcotic antagonists, where disquieting psychotomimetic effects may occur. Quantal measures such as these are distribution-free and can be analyzed by standard statistical techniques such as chi^2 or the Mosteller sign test [31]. However, they provide less information and are considerably less sensitive than quantitative data and serve mainly as complementary information.

These studies are not designed primarily for the evaluation of drug side effects and information on them must be considered as only supplementary to the data on analgesia. Patients are not questioned in detail regarding possible side effects, nor are laboratory tests performed except in special circumstances. Those side effects that are recorded are either obvious to the observer or volunteered by the patient, and may be the result of their disease rather than the drug. Nevertheless, dose-related drug effects can be and are picked up in this fashion and provide additional information on the potential therapeutic roles of the drugs under study. Side effects can be unpredictable, particularly with new or investigational drugs, and it is advisable that the procedure for recording them be open-ended so that significant side effects will not be lost in a miscellaneous category. To be most meaningful, all comparisons of drugs in terms of side reactions should be carried out in terms of equianalgesic doses.

V. COMPARISON OF VARIOUS PROCEDURES

The ultimate test of any experiment is of course whether or not the results are reproducible. Criteria for measuring pain and analgesia vary from one investigator to another so that absolute analgesic scores, e.g., percent relieved, AD_{90}, etc., cannot be meaningfully compared. Nevertheless, well-designed experiments have provided information on the relative effects of analgesics which have been found to be reproducible in a wide variety of painful states and clinical conditions [32]. Our estimates of the relative potency of methadone and morphine in parallel independent assays in patients with postoperative pain and patients with chronic pain have been virtually indistinguishable. Moreover, in studies employing identical methodology and end points, but working independently at separate institutions, Eddy and Lee [33] arrived at an almost identical estimate of the relative potency of oxymorphone and morphine as we did earlier at Memorial Sloan-Kettering Cancer Center.

The therapeutic usefulness of any putative analgesic is the prime, but not the only, objective of the clinical analgesic assay. Appropriately controlled studies designed to define parameters of pharmacological effects can provide the medicinal chemist with clues helpful in developing analgesics whose spectrum of activity may be preferable to the currently used narcotic analgesics and may provide the pharmacologist with insights into the modes of action of analgesic drugs. Undoubtedly further refinements in methodology will be forthcoming as we learn more about how to manipulate psychological variables and how blood and other body fluid drug levels correlate with analgesic activity.

ACKNOWLEDGMENT

The authors wish to express their appreciation to Miss Julie Franchi for her assistance in the search of the literature and for her help in the preparation of this manuscript.

REFERENCES

1. K. D. Keele, Lancet 2:6 (1948).
2. J. E. Denton and H. K. Beecher, J. Amer. Med. Ass. 141:1051 (1949).
3. A. S. Keats, H. K. Beecher, and F. C. Mosteller, J. Appl. Physiol. 1:35 (1950).
4. S. M. Free, Jr., and F. Peters, J. Chronic Dis. 7:379 (1958).
5. R. W. Boyle, C. E. Solomonson, and J. R. Petersen, Ann. Intern. Med. 52:195 (1960).
6. A. J. Hewer, C. A. Keele, K. D. Keele, and P. W. Nathan, Lancet 256:431 (1949).
7. J. C. Seed, S. L. Wallenstein, R. W. Houde, and J. W. Bellville, Arch. Int. Pharmacodyn. Ther. 116:293 (1958).
8. L. Lasagna, Ann. N.Y. Acad. Sci. 86:28 (1960).
9. C. M. Gruber and A. Baptisti, Clin. Pharmacol. Ther. 4:172 (1963).
10. R. C. Batterman, G. J. Mouratoff and J. E. Kaufman, Curr. Ther. Res. Clin. Exp. 4:81 (1962).
11. E. C. Kast, Int. J. Neuropsychiat. 3:1 (1967).
12. R. C. Batterman and A. J. Grossman, J. Amer. Med. Ass. 159:1619 (1955).
13. P. Meier, S. M. Free, and G. L. Jackson, Biom. Bull. 14:330 (1958).
14. T. G. Kantor, A. Sunshine, E. Lasker, M. Meisner, and M. Hopper, Clin. Pharmacol. Ther. 7:447 (1966).
15. L. Lasagna and T. J. DeKornfeld, J. Pharmacol. Exp. Ther. 124:260 (1958).
16. W. T. Beaver, S. L. Wallenstein, R. W. Houde, and A. Rogers, Clin. Pharmacol. Ther. 7:740 (1966).
17. R. W. Houde, S. L. Wallenstein, J. W. Bellville, A. Rogers, and L. A. Escarraga, J. Pharmacol. Exp. Ther. 114:337 (1964).
18. W. T. Beaver, S. L. Wallenstein, R. W. Houde, and A. Rogers, Clin. Pharmacol. Ther. 7:436 (1966).
19. W. T. Beaver, S. L. Wallenstein, R. W. Houde, and A. Rogers, Clin. Pharmacol. Ther. 10:314 (1969).
20. D. J. Finney, Statistical Method in Biological Assay, Chap. 10. New York: Hafner, 1964.

21. S. L. Wallenstein, W. T. Beaver, and R. W. Houde, Pharmacologist 8:207 Abst (1966).

22. W. T. Beaver, S. L. Wallenstein, R. W. Houde, and A. Rogers, Clin. Pharmacol. Ther. 8:415 (1967).

23. W. T. Beaver, S. L. Wallenstein, R. W. Houde, and A. Rogers, Clin. Pharmacol. Ther. 9:582 (1968).

24. W. Modell and R. W. Houde, J. Amer. Med. Ass. 167:2190 (1958).

25. J. H. Gaddum, Pharmacol. Rev. 5:87 (1958).

26. C. V. Winder, Ann. N.Y. Acad. Sci. 52:838 (1950).

27. I. D. J. Bross, Biom. Bull. 14:18 (1958).

28. R. W. Houde, S. L. Wallenstein, and W. T. Beaver, in International Encyclopedia of Pharmacology and Therapeutics (L. Lasagna, ed.), Sec. 6 Vol. I, Chap. 5. New York: Pergamon, 1966.

29. C. Rerup, in Quantitative Methods in Pharmacology (H. deJonge, ed.). Amsterdam: North-Holland Publ., 1961, pp. 101-115.

30. C. Rerup, Acta Pharmacol. Toxicol. 17:390 (1960).

31. F. Mosteller, Biom. Bull. 8:220 (1952).

32. R. W. Houde, S. L. Wallenstein, and W. T. Beaver, in Analgetics (G. deStevens, ed.), Chap. 3. New York: Academic Press, 1965.

33. N. B. Eddy and L. E. Lee, J. Pharmacol. Exp. Ther. 125:116 (1959).

Part III

DETERMINATION OF BEHAVIORAL EFFECTS OF NARCOTICS

Chapter 8

MORPHINE-WITHDRAWAL AGGRESSION*

HARBANS LAL

Department of Pharmacology and Toxicology
Department of Psychology
University of Rhode Island
Kingston, Rhode Island

---

*The investigation described in this chapter was supported by research grants MH 18346 and MH 20115 from the National Institute of Mental Health, Public Health Service.

I. INTRODUCTION

Aggression-related behaviors are among the most consistent symptoms observed during narcotic withdrawal in the rat and several other animal species. They are present during both acute and protracted withdrawal. Moreover, the withdrawal aggression is somewhat specific to narcotic withdrawal. It is seen after withdrawal from morphine, methadone, or fentanyl. It is not seen during withdrawal from prolonged ingestion of amphetamine, phenobarbital, or ethanol given in drinking water [1].

The study of aggression in relation to narcotic dependence bears an additional research interest when we consider the fact that among the CNS effects, aggression is the only withdrawal symptom of which the psysiological mechanism is somewhat understood. By virtue of this fact, the study on aggression not only is related to the mechanisms of narcotic addiction but also provides a tool to investigate the neurobiology of aggression.

This chapter describes the methods of studying morphine-withdrawal aggression and summarizes the information known about the underlying mechanisms. The discussion is limited to morphine withdrawal, although aggression from methadone withdrawal [2] and fentanyl withdrawal (unpublished data) has been reported. The rat has been used for most studies on morphine-withdrawal aggression. However, morphine-withdrawal aggression has been seen in mice [3], guinea pigs [4], and monkeys [5].

II. METHODS

A. Methods to Produce Morphine Dependence

There are several procedures known to produce morphine dependence in rodents. A number of them have been described elsewhere in this book (see Chapters 10-15). A typical procedure used routinely in our laboratory consists of three injections of morphine per day in increasing doses. The injection schedule for a typical experiment is illustrated in Table I.

TABLE I

Schedule of Morphine Sulfate Injections to Produce Morphine Dependence in Rats

Day of injection	Dose/injection[a] (mg/kg)	Total dose (mg/kg)
1	15	45
2	30	90
3	45	135
4	60	180
5	75	225
6	90	270
7	105	315
8	120	360
9	135	405[b]
10-13	135	405

[a]Given three times a day equally spaced between 7 a.m. and 11 p.m.

[b]A maintenance dose for at least 5 days or as long as it is necessary to maintain dependence.

We obtain male hooded rats of Long-Evans strain, weighing about 250 g, from Charles River Farms. After a period of 5-7 days of acclimation, we distribute them in individual cages and inject them with morphine sulfate solution every 8 hr around the clock (7 a.m., 3 p.m., 11 p.m.), 7 days a week. Once the maintenance dose of 405 mg/kg/day is reached by gradual increase of doses, the rats are maintained at this dose for at least 5 days before withdrawal (see Table I for details).

At withdrawal (24-48 hr after last injection), the morphine-dependent rats show severe signs of withdrawal. These include hypothermia, loss of body weight, body shakes, piloerection, writhing, ptosis, and anorexia. They are described in detail in Chapters 12-14.

B. Stereotaxic Brain Lesions

Under ether anesthesia, electrolytic brain lesions are made with a monopolar stainless-steel electrode with a noninsulated tip. The electrode is placed into the brain with a stereotaxic instrument. The coordinates for the placement of electrodes can be found in any stereotaxic atlas available. For illustration [6], in order to make lesions in the nigrostriatal bundle the electrode is placed 1.5 mm posterior to the bregma, 2 mm lateral to the midline suture, and 8.5 mm below the surface of the cranium [7]. To cause complete destruction, a current of 2 mA is passed through the electrode for 30 sec.

C. Measurement of Aggressive Responses

To measure aggression we place three or four rats together in an observation chamber [8,9]. Then we reset the recording counters to zero and begin to record the aggressive responses. Digital counters can be obtained from any of the manufacturers of electronic equipment for behavioral experiments. We have been using the counters obtained from LHV Electronics (BRS/LHV Model DC-904). Typically, we observe these rats for 60 min, taking 10-min counts of aggressive responses (see below). However, the duration of observation may vary according to the objective of the experiment. The aggression can be continuously observed in the same group of rats for many hours or days. Usually there is no lethality in the first hour. An illustration of 10-min counts of aggressive responses is given in a paper by Lal et al. [9]. We measure aggression as three discrete responses as given below.

1. Rearing

Rearing is defined as total number of seconds for which at least two of the rats in a group are found standing on their hind legs facing each other in an aggressive posture but during which no attacks or bitings are emitted. When the rats are found in this posture, which is illustrated in Fig. 1, the experimenter depresses a switch and keeps it depressed as long as the rearing position is maintained. The switch closure is recorded on a running time meter (Model RT 904/412-01, BRS/LVE) that accumulates the duration, in seconds, for which rearing posture is maintained.

2. Vocalization

The number of discrete vocalizations is recorded by a voice-operated relay (Audio Threshold Detector Relay, Model no. 761-A, supplied by Scientific Prototype Mfg. Co.), modified to detect a frequency range of 2400-4000 Hz. The relay closures are recorded as digital counts on electromechanical counters. Vocalization of a typical group of rats, once recorded on a magnetic tape, can be subsequently used to periodically calibrate the sensitivity characteristics of the detection and recording devices. A cumulative record of vocalization is illustrated in Fig. 2.

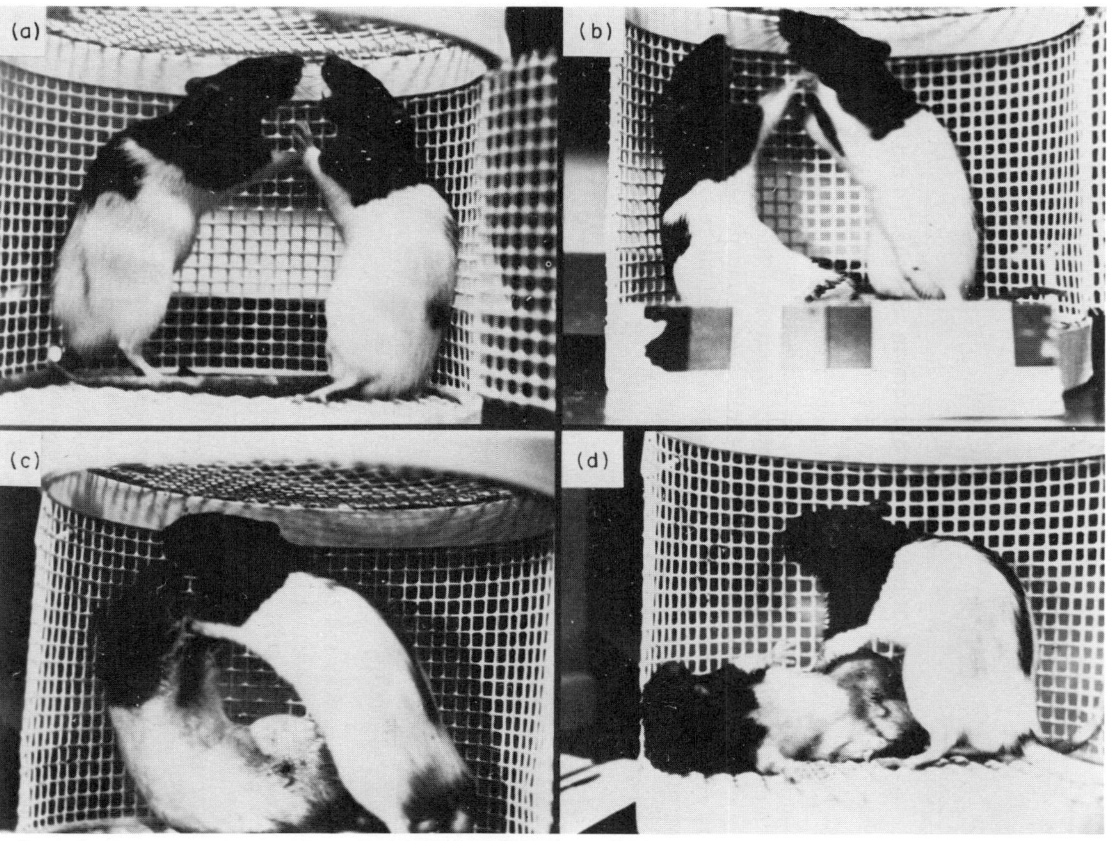

FIGURE 1. Rats in various postures of aggressive behaviors. Rearing is shown in panel (a), and various acts of attack/bite are shown in panels (b), (c), and (d). (Courtesy of G. McKenzie.)

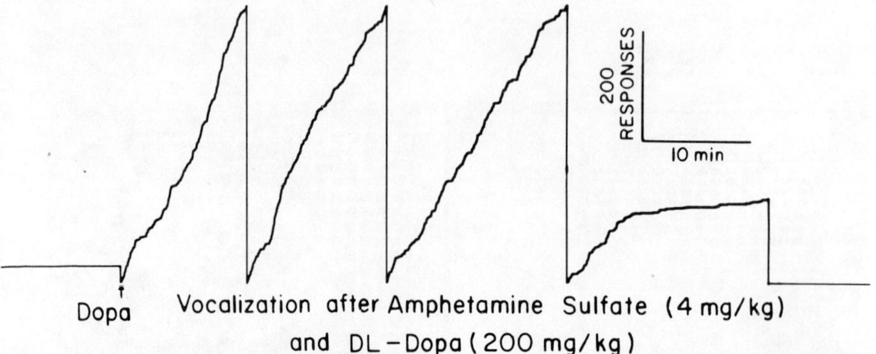

FIGURE 2. Cumulative recording of vocalization associated with drug-induced aggression. The cumulative record here illustrates the elicitation of intense vocalization after dopa administration in animals pretreated with amphetamine. Similar vocalization is recorded in morphine-withdrawn rats grouped together. Each vocal response moved the recording pen upward.

3. Attacks/Bites

The number of attacks and/or bites as observed by the experimenter is recorded on digital counters. When the experimenter detects an actual attack by one rat on another, or if a biting movement takes place, he depresses a switch to register this event on an electromechanical digital counter as a discrete event. One must realize that attack/bites are subjective measures and high variability is obtained.

All recording and counting devices are reset to zero every 10 min to obtain counts at 10-min intervals, usually through a print-counter (BRS/LVE Model POC-112).

D. Pain-Induced Aggression

Rats are placed in pairs on a metal grid connected to a shock generator-scrambler (BRS/LVE Model SGS-003). After approximately 1 min the shocker is turned on for 0.5 sec. The scrambler changes the polarity of each grid 56 times per second to prevent the rat from selecting two grids of the same polarity in order to avoid paw shock. The occurrences of vocalization, rearing, and attack/bite are recorded by the experimenter as discrete responses to each shock. Vocalization can be recorded automatically through a voice-operated relay as described above. We use eleven graded shock intensities varying from 0.2 to 4.0 mA. Five trials are given at each shock intensity and 15-60 sec are allowed between each shock. The data are plotted as the frequency of occurrence of each response against each shock intensity (see Lal et al. [8] for detailed procedure and illustration of typical results).

III. CHARACTERISTICS OF MORPHINE-WITHDRAWAL AGGRESSION

A. General Considerations

Morphine-withdrawal aggression can be observed either during precipitated withdrawal that is produced by an antagonist or during a withdrawal caused by cessation of the maintenance dose of the narcotic drug. It consists of rearing, vocalization, attacks, and biting directed toward other animals as well as toward the experimenter's hand when it is introduced into the cage. The biting results in oozing of blood and one sees blood smeared on the walls and the bottom of the cage, as well as on the body surface of the fighting animals.

As is obvious, the aggressive responses are seen when the addicted subjects are grouped during withdrawal. Intense aggression during withdrawal in higher animals has gone virtually unnoticed because higher animals are rarely housed in colony cages during abstinence. Seevers and Deneau [5], who have extensive experience working with primates in which rage can readily be recognized, reported the occurrence of vocalization, aggressive postures, and difficulty in handling individually housed rhesus monkeys during abstinence.

In rats, aggressive reactions are difficult to recognize unless they are manifested against each other in a group situation. Therefore, one must pair withdrawn rats or house them in groups to objectively observe aggression. Morphine-withdrawal aggression is definitely social in nature as no attack or biting is directed toward an anesthetized rat or toy rat made of synthetic material or a mouse placed in the cage.

It is customary to aggregate rats into groups of three or four for the study of aggression. Although two rats aggregated together usually show considerable aggression, the aggression may not be continuous since one of two rats may become exhausted and too weak to fight back and will withdraw from the contest, so that the other rat will stop attacking. The presence of a third rat in the cage ensures the continuation of hostilities in that case.

B. Aggression During Precipitated Withdrawal

Usually one can cause withdrawal symptoms to occur by administering small doses of narcotic antagonists. However, a dose of nalorphine as high as 20 mg/kg [10] or a dose of naloxone as high as 8 mg/kg* failed to reliably cause aggression in the addicted rats. There was aggression in some groups but not in others. However, when the antagonist-treated rats are challenged with small doses of amphetamine or apomorphine, intense aggression always results.

C. Aggression After Withholding of Morphine

As soon as morphine-withdrawn rats are placed together, aggressive responses begin. No provocation other than social confrontation is necessary to provoke aggression. Depending on the degree of addiction prior to withdrawal, aggressive episodes last for various intervals of time. The rats fight for several minutes, then stop fighting for a few minutes and start fighting again. This pattern of activity may continue for several hours and for several days if the fighting animals are not separated and housed in socially isolated conditions. After the withdrawn rats are aggregated for the first time, the aggression is continuous for approximately 2 hr. After that time, periods of inactivity begin to appear and these periods are lengthened as the time goes by. For the most consistent measurement of aggression, the first 2 hr of observation is recommended.

The time course for morphine-withdrawal aggression does not perfectly coincide with the intensity of other withdrawal symptoms. In the rat, most autonomic and somatic symptoms of morphine withdrawal are seen 24 hr after the last morphine injection. The intensity of symptoms is markedly reduced by 72 hr. Morphine-withdrawal aggression, on the other hand, is minimal at 24 hr after the last morphine injection and reaches its maximum by 72 hr of withdrawal [9]. After that period, when most other withdrawal symptoms are at their lowest level, the withdrawal aggression remains quite intense and marked. It can be observed in great intensity even 30 days after the last morphine administration [11,12]. To date, withdrawal periods longer than 30 days have not been studied.

Spontaneous aggression, once initiated, may continue in an episodic manner for several days. However, one observes lethality under these circumstances only occasionally, although marked injuries are always observed.

---

*G. Gianutos, R. B. Drawbaugh, M. D. Hynes, and H. Lal, unpublished data, 1974.

D. Pain-Induced Aggression and Morphine Withdrawal

Paw shock has been known to normally elicit aggression in all rats. However, during narcotic withdrawal the shock threshold to cause aggression is markedly reduced [1]. We previously reported that chloramphetamine effectively blocks shock-induced aggression in normal rats [13]. When this drug is administered to the morphine-withdrawn rats, it significantly reduces shock-induced aggression [14]. These data are illustrated in Fig. 3.

IV. AGGRESSION-INDUCING DRUGS IN MORPHINE-WITHDRAWN RATS

It has been found that morphine-withdrawal aggression can be enhanced markedly by certain drugs. Dihydroxyphenylalanine (L-dopa), amphetamines, methylphenidate, or apomorphine, when given in small doses to the morphine-withdrawn rats, transform their usual aggressive responses into the most violent aggression ever recorded in the rat. Amphetamine, L-dopa, or methylphenidate does not cause clear-cut aggression in normal animals, in any dosage, although rage-like reactions have been reported with these drugs. In order to cause aggression in normal animals, a large dose of apomorphine [15] or a combination of L-dopa and amphetamine, both given in large doses [16], is usually required. However, several times smaller doses of these drugs cause marked potentiation of aggression in morphine-withdrawn rats. These doses are completely ineffective in causing aggression in nondependent rats. The effect of apomorphine on withdrawal aggression is illustrated in Fig. 4. The effect of several aggression-inducing drugs in morphine-dependent rats undergoing acute withdrawal is illustrated in Table II. As is evident from the data shown in this table, all of these drugs increase the rate of aggressive responses several-fold. Both levo and dextro forms of amphetamine are effective in enhancing morphine-withdrawal aggression [9]. These effects of selected drugs are reliable and are easily reversible.

The effects of apomorphine rarely last beyond 2 hr after injection of the drug in morphine-withdrawn rats. The effect of a single dose of amphetamine in enhancing morphine-withdrawal aggression has been recorded for as long as 24 hr and can be very easily seen until 8 hr after the single dose. Usually the sensitization of morphine-withdrawal aggression caused by these drugs lasts longer than the other commonly measured effects of the same drugs.

Aggression-inducing drugs generally enhance the intensity of morphine-withdrawal aggression to a very high level. If the morphine-withdrawn rats after treatment with these drugs are left together for long enough periods, nearly one-forth of them are killed in fighting or die of exhaustion. This is particularly true of the use of relatively longer acting drugs, such as amphetamines, which enhance morphine-withdrawal aggression.

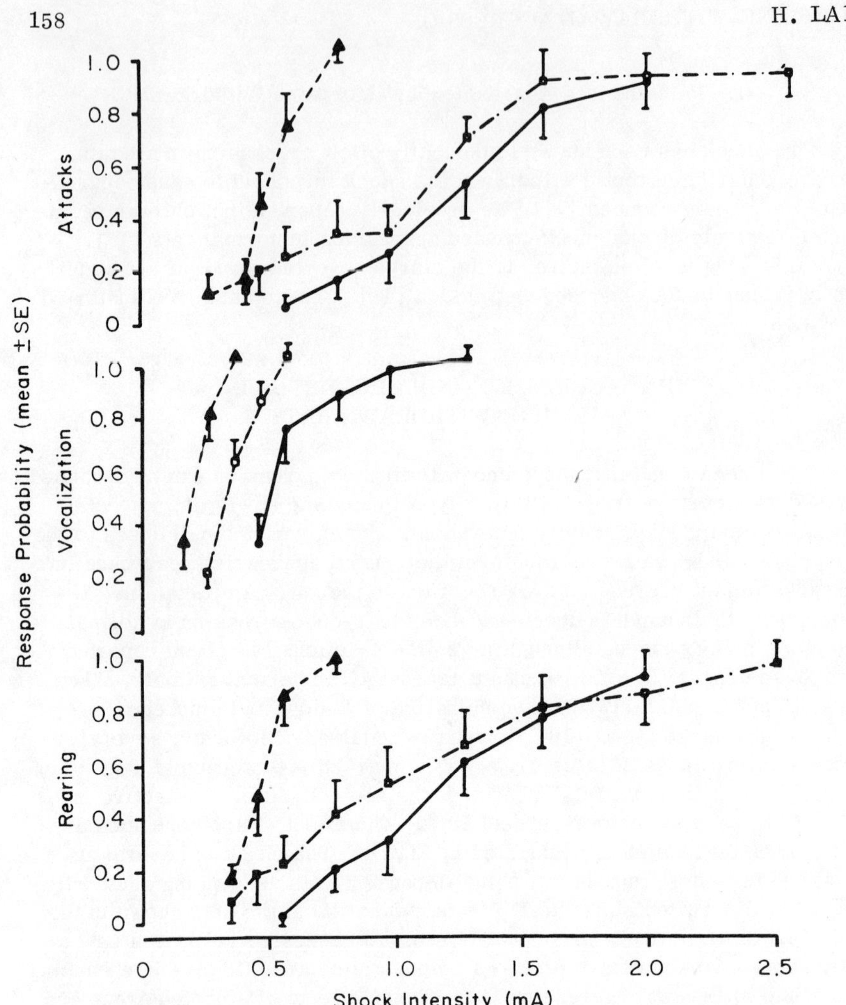

FIGURE 3. Effect of morphine withdrawal and chloramphetamine on shock-elicited aggression. Morphine withdrawal enhanced sensitivity to paw shock, while chloramphetamine reversed the effect of morphine withdrawal. Key: •, control; ▲, morphine withdrawal (72 hr); □, morphine withdrawal (72 hr) plus p-chloramphetamine (3 mg/kg). (Adopted from Lal et al. [14].)

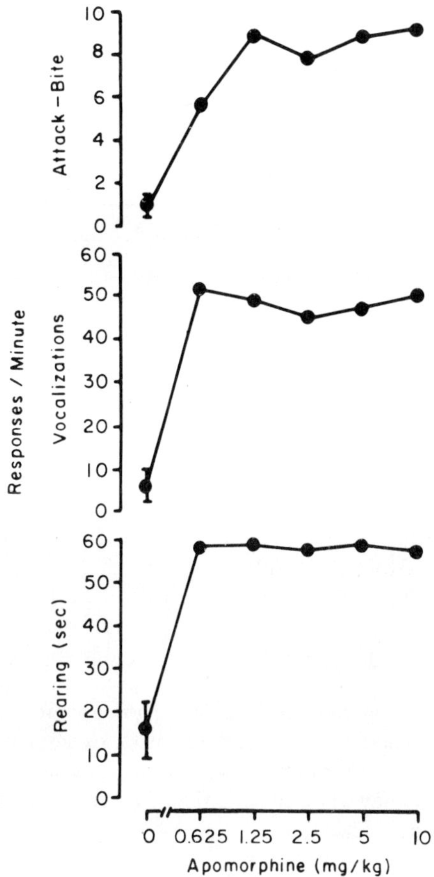

FIGURE 4. Effect of apomorphine treatment on morphine-withdrawal aggression. There was no aggression in the morphine-naive rats with any of the apomorphine doses employed. Doses higher than those shown in the graph produced some aggression responses in naive rats. (Adopted from Lal and Puri [10].)

V. PROTRACTED ABSTINENCE AND AGGRESSION

In narcotic-dependent subjects there are many physiological measures that require several months following withdrawal to return to normal. Martin and Sloan [18] proposed the term protracted abstinence syndrome to describe those characteristics of narcotic dependence. Since the early

TABLE II

Effect of Various Drugs on Morphine-Withdrawal Aggression

Pretreatment drug[a]	Dose[b] (mg/kg)	N[c]	Morphine-withdrawal[d] aggression[e] (responses/min, mean ± SE) Attack/bites	Vocalizations	Rearing
None		4	0.53 ± 0.089	3.32 ± 0.46	4.93 ± 1.45
L-Dopa	50	1	1.34	37.56	27.67
DL-Dopa	200	3	1.52 ± 0.17	21.34 ± 1.45	28.40 ± 3.54
Amphetamine	2	3	4.25 ± 0.18	36.59 ± 2.76	50.24 ± 1.82
Apomorphine	1.25	7	7.01 ± 0.80	33.07 ± 3.47	53.81 ± 2.88
Haloperidol	0.63	1	0.08	0.22	0.28

[a] All drugs were administered immediately before grouping of the rats for aggression except haloperidol, which was given 2 hr before testing.

[b] In the pilot projects, determined to be a dose with maximum effect.

[c] Number of groups of rats. Each group contained four addicted rats.

[d] 72-hr withdrawal from a maintenance dose (400 mg/kg/day) of morphine.

[e] Aggression was measured for 1 hr in dopa-, apomorphine-, or haloperidol-treated rats. There were no attack/bites or rearing in the dependent rats not withdrawn from morphine or the normal rats not made dependent on morphine. They showed less than 0.2 vocalization/min. (Adopted from Puri and Lal [17].)

work of the Lexington group, several other symptoms associated with the protracted abstinence have been described. Withdrawal aggression is the most intense symptom of all those reported to date.

Once made morphine dependent, rats spontaneously show intense aggression upon grouping even 30 days after complete abstinence from morphine [11,12]. The aggression seen after 30 days of abstinence is only slightly less intense than that seen after 3 days of abstinence and is much more marked than the aggression seen after 24 hr of abstinence.

Aggression associated with protracted abstinence is blocked by low doses of morphine [12]. It is markedly enhanced by small doses of apomorphine given just before grouping of the abstinent rats (Table III).

TABLE III

Effect of Apomorphine and Brain Lesions on Morphine-Withdrawal Aggression[a,b]

Treatment[c]	No. of rats tested	Aggressive responses/hr (mean ± SE)		
		Attacks/bites	Rearing (sec)	Vocalization
Isolated controls				
No drug	24	1 ± 0.3	52 ± 48	4 ± 2
Apomorphine[d]	16	0	9 ± 9	14 ± 3
72-hr morphine withdrawal				
No drug	12	26 ± 5.8	3599 ± 1	2191 ± 271
30-day morphine withdrawal				
No drug	36	23 ± 9	1513 ± 280	828 ± 260
Morphine[e]	8	0	0	
Apomorphine[d]	20	56 ± 10	3017 ± 138	1961 ± 155
MFB lesion[f]	12	33 ± 5.2	1423 ± 298	753 ± 59
NSB lesion[f]	28	1 ± 0.8	39 ± 39	18 ± 6
NSB lesion[f] plus apomorphine[d]	16	42 ± 21.5	625 ± 267	528 ± 222

[a]Adopted from Gianutsos et al. [12].

[b]For testing, these rats were distributed into groups of four. Responses from these groups were used to calculate mean and standard error.

[c]MFB, medial forebrain bundle; NSB, nigrostriatal bundle.

[d]1.25 mg/kg.

[e]10 mg/kg 30 min prior to testing.

[f]Lesions were produced 24 hr before testing; MFB denotes medial forebrain bundle and NSB, nigrostriatal bundle.

VI. BRAIN LESIONS AND MORPHINE-WITHDRAWAL AGGRESSION

Brain lesions have been extensively used to localize the site of action of drugs as well as the neuroanatomical sites of discrete behaviors. On the basis of their proven usefulness in the past, brain lesions were employed in the investigation of morphine-withdrawal aggression. These studies have been centered around the lesioning of the nigrostriatal bundle and medial forebrain bundle. The nigrostriatal bundle is the major nerve trunk that carries nerve fibers from dopaminergic brain cells in the substantia nigra to brain areas in the striatum. The medial forebrain bundle is the major nerve trunk carrying nerve fibers mostly from serotonin-containing nerve cells and some from noradrenergic nerve cells.

As is illustrated in Table III, lesioning of the nigrostriatal bundle was found to completely eliminate aggression in narcotic-abstinent rats [11,12]. Similar lesioning of the medial forebrain bundle is without any effect on that aggression [12].

Brain lesioning per se may cause general debilitation which may attenuate behaviors. Moreover, lesioning of the nigrostriatal bundle may injure motor systems that influence the animal's ability to show aggression-related motor responses. These factors confounded with the brain lesioning must be taken into account before one can arrive at specific conclusions from such studies.

Lesioning of the medial forebrain bundle did not block aggression (Table III). This shows that a possible debilitation associated with the stress of the lesioning procedure is not sufficient to reduce the intensity of aggressive behaviors. The dependent rats with nigrostriatal lesions produced during withdrawal did not show any aggression. However, these rats are capable of full expression of aggressive response because they show intense aggression when given small doses of apomorphine [11,12]. Therefore, the antiaggression effect of nigrostriatal lesioning is not an artifact of injury to motor systems but is specific to the blockade of morphine-withdrawal aggression.

VII. DRUGS THAT ACT AGAINST MORPHINE-WITHDRAWAL AGGRESSION

Spontaneous aggression in withdrawn rats can be markedly reduced or completely eliminated by a number of drugs. As expected, morphine and methadone are potent narcotics with antiaggression potency. A dose of 10-20 mg/kg in either case is effective in abstinent rats even though the rats have been made tolerant to these drugs during addiction [12,17]. However, development of tolerance to narcotic drugs is seen with respect to their antiaggression potency when used repeatedly in withdrawn rats. Antiaggression action of morphine may not be due only to narcotic substitution: Morphine has been shown to be antiaggressive in nonaddicted rats that were provoked to aggression by paw shocks (Fig. 5).

Among the nonnarcotic drugs effective as antiaggression agents in abstinent rats, only a few have been investigated. Haloperidol and α-methyl-p-tyrosine (MPT) have been found to be active in this respect. Haloperidol,

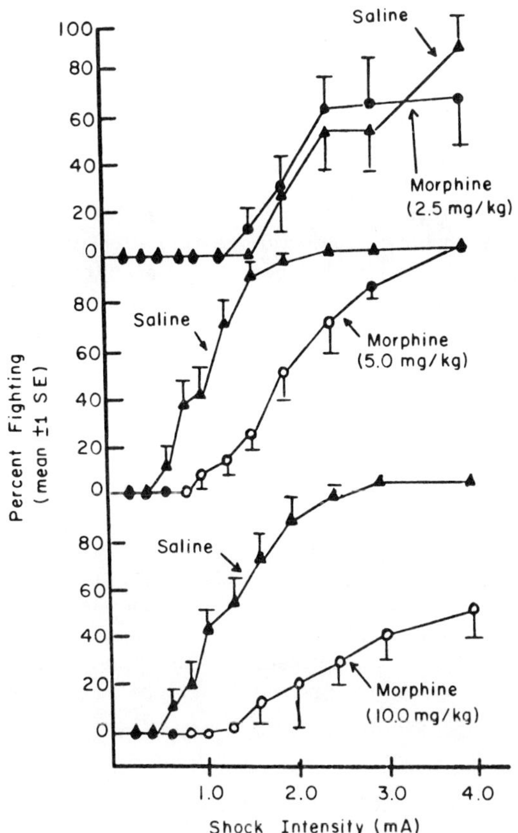

FIGURE 5. Effect of morphine injected intraperitoneally on aggression elicited by paw shock in naive rats.

a potent neuroleptic, is very effective against aggressive responses in rats undergoing morphine withdrawal (Table II). Even if the effect is measured immediately after drug administration, when the drug has not had sufficient time to act, complete blockade of aggression is obtained with a usual pharmacological dose of haloperidol [17]. If an appropriate period is allowed for the drug to act maximally, smaller doses show marked antiaggression potency. Recently, effectiveness of haloperidol in markedly reducing agitation seen during acute detoxification [21,22] or long-term heroin abstinence [23] was confirmed in human addicts. Chlorpromazine antagonizes morphine-withdrawal aggression only in high doses.*

*S. K. Puri and H. Lal, unpublished data, 1971.

Another drug not yet available for human use, but found effective against aggression during morphine withdrawal, is MPT. Given in a dose of 200 mg/kg 4 hr before the rats are allowed to confront each other, MPT effectively blocks narcotic-withdrawal aggression. Use of this drug, however, is limited to experimental animals because of its potential side effects when used in the high doses required for therapeutic effects.

The four drugs discussed above as being effective against spontaneous aggression during morphine withdrawal are also effective when used in abstinent rats in which aggression has been potentiated by other drugs. All of these drugs are effective in the same doses as described above. The effectiveness of methadone is illustrated in Fig. 6. It is effective in small doses when given for the first time, but the development of tolerance is seen when used subsequently. A time course of effectiveness for haloperidol is shown in Fig. 7, and dose-response is shown in Fig. 8. In the above experiments the response of haloperidol was measured immediately after its administration. Usually, 2 hr should be allowed for the optimum effect of haloperidol to occur.

Data obtained from the study with MPT in addicted rats are illustrated in Fig. 9. This drug blocked aggression in withdrawn rats treated with saline or dextroamphetamine. However, the potency of apomorphine in enhancing morphine-withdrawal aggression was not affected. This was taken to suggest that MPT pretreatment does not reduce the effectiveness of direct stimulation of dopamine receptors (see below) in causing aggression [17].

VIII. MECHANISMS

It is only recently that the aggressive behaviors associated with morphine withdrawal were first reported in experimental animals [24]. Therefore, there is insufficient information to evolve a precise mechanism underlying that aggressive syndrome. A working hypothesis, however, has been proposed. Based on a number of observations enumerated below, it was proposed that the aggressive syndrome in narcotic abstinence is associated with the hyperactivity of dopamine receptors that were rendered supersensitive during the addicting process [10,17,20,25-27]. The evidence in favor of this hypothesis can be briefly described as follows.

1. Dopamine stimulation caused by a number of drugs results in aggressive behavior in the experimental animal (dopa plus amphetamine [16,28], dopa plus Pargyline [29], or apomorphine given alone [15]. All of these drugs are known to directly or indirectly produce dopamine-receptor stimulation. On the other hand,

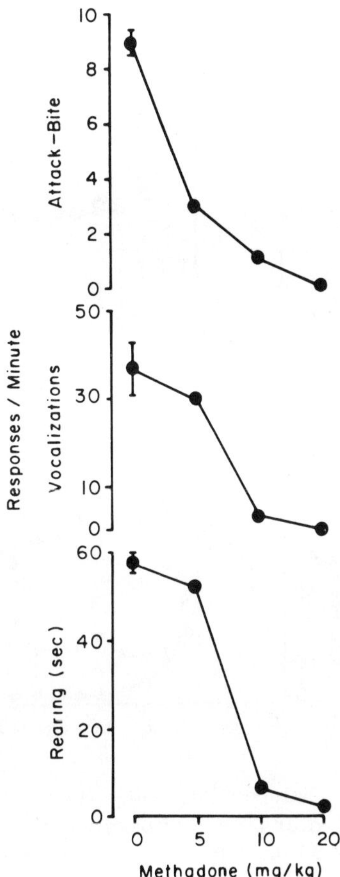

FIGURE 6. Effect of methadone on morphine-withdrawal aggression. Apomorphine hydrochloride (1.25 mg/kg) was injected to potentiate morphine-withdrawal aggression. Following the 20-min measurement of aggression (data not given), no drug (seven groups) or methadone (one group with each dose) was injected and the resulting effect on aggression was measured for 60 min. Each group contained four rats. (Adopted from Puri and Lal [17].)

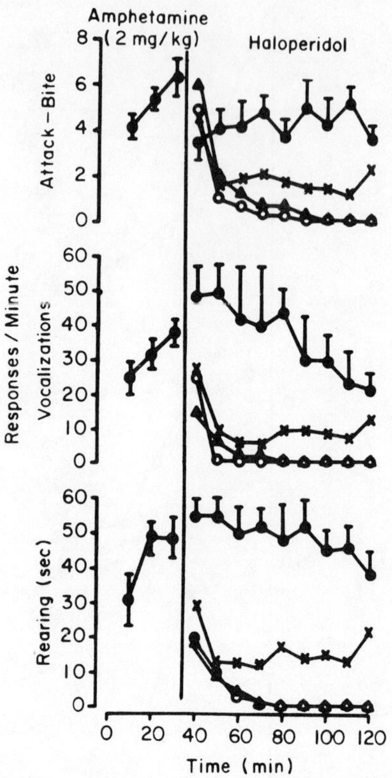

FIGURE 7. Effect of haloperidol on morphine-withdrawal aggression. Haloperidol was injected after 30 min of baseline measurement (x, 1.25 mg/kg haloperidol; Δ, 1.25 mg/kg; ○, 2.5 mg/kg; •, 0). (Adopted from Lal and Puri [10].)

dopamine-receptor-blocking drugs, such as haloperidol or morphine, block drug-induced aggression [9,17].

2. It is well known that pharmacological blockade of postsynaptic receptor sites causes supersensitivity of those receptors to their specific neurotransmitters such as acetylcholine, norepinephine, and dopamine [12,13,30-34]. Narcotic drugs such as morphine [19,35] and methadone [36] are known to inhibit dopamine receptors in the central nervous system. Therefore, continuous use of these drugs is likely to cause disuse supersensitivity of the dopamine receptors. In fact, evidence to this effect has already been reported [8,10,12,17,27].

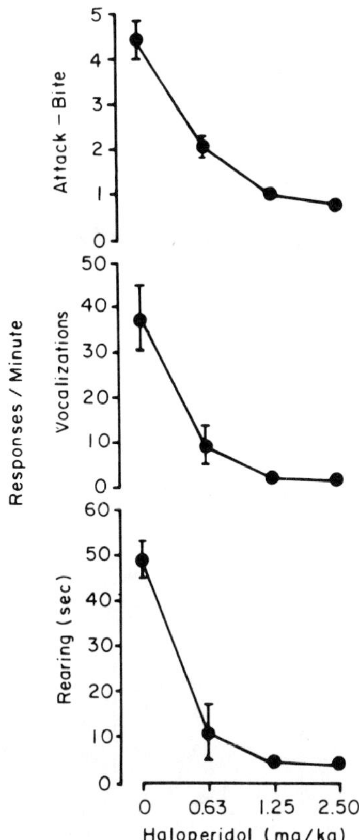

FIGURE 8. Effect of haloperidol on morphine-withdrawal aggression. Amphetamine (2 mg/kg ip) was injected to potentiate the withdrawal aggression. Following the measurement of aggression for 20 min (data not given), no drug (three groups) or haloperidol (two groups with 0.63 mg/kg dose and one group each with subsequent doses) was injected and the resulting aggression was measured for 60 min. Each group contained four rats. (Adopted from Puri and Lal [17].)

3. In morphine-dependent rats, otherwise ineffective doses of dopamine-receptor-stimulating drugs (dopa, amphetamine, apomorphine) intensify the withdrawal aggression markedly. This aggression is blocked by dopamine-blocking drugs such as haloperidol, MPT, methadone, or morphine [17]. Moreover, inactivation of presynaptic dopamine nerve endings by lesioning of the nigrostriatal nerve trunk also abolishes the aggression in morphine-withdrawn rats [11,12].

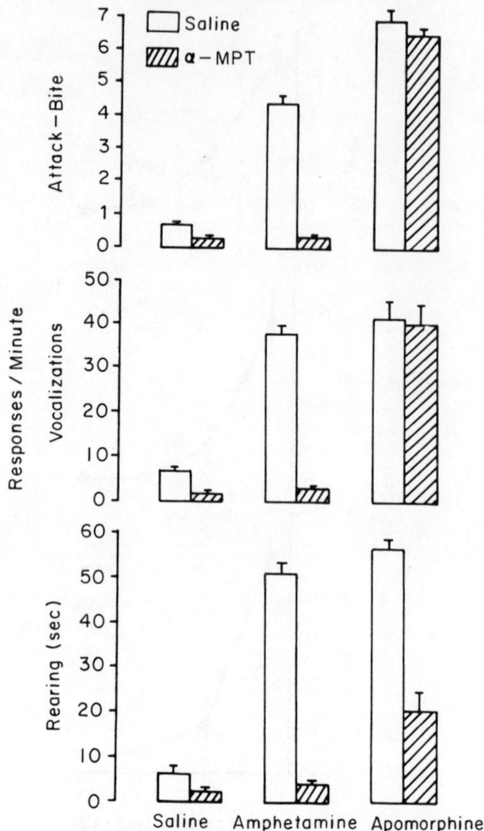

FIGURE 9. Effect of α-methyl-p-tyrosine (α-MPT) (200 mg/kg ip, 4 hr pretreatment) on morphine-withdrawal aggression in rats treated with saline (1 ml/kg, four groups), d-amphetamine sulfate (2 mg/kg, three groups), or apomorphine hydrochloride (1.25 mg/kg, seven groups). Each bar represents mean for that group with standard error. Each group contained four rats. (Adopted from Puri and Lal [17].)

ACKNOWLEDGMENTS

The drugs used in this study were supplied free of charge by their manufacturers. Richard Drawbaugh, Martin Hynes, Gerald Gianutsos, John O'Brien, Arthur Pitterman, Surendra Puri, and Chejerla R. Reddy conducted experiments and provided technical assistance. Mrs. Lucie Johnson provided secretarial assistance in preparing the manuscript.

REFERENCES

1. S. K. Puri and H. Lal, Reduced threshold to pain-induced aggression specifically related to morphine-dependence. Psychopharmacologia 35:237-242 (1974).

2. M. D. Singh and J. M. Singh, Methadone-induced aggressive behavior. Toxicol. Appl. Pharmacol. 25:452 (1973).

3. A. Weissman, Jumping in mice elicited by α-napthyloxyacetic acid (NOAA). J. Pharmacol. Exp. Ther. 184:11-17 (1973).

4. A. Goldstein and R. Schulz, Morphine-tolerant longitudinal muscle strip from guinea pig ileum. Brit. J. Pharmacol. 48:655-666 (1973).

5. M. H. Seevers and G. A. Deneau, Physiological aspects of tolerance and physical dependence. In Physiological Pharmacology (W. S. Root and F. G. Hofmann, eds.), Vol. 1. New York: Academic Press, 1963, pp. 565-640.

6. J. A. Harvey, A. Heller, R. Y. Moore, H. F. Hunt, and L. J. Roth, Effect of central nervous system lesions on brain serotonin. J. Pharmacol. Exp. Ther. 144:24-36 (1964).

7. G. A. Oltsman and J. A. Harvey, LH syndrome and brain catecholamine levels after lesions of the nigrostriatal bundle. Physiol. Behav. 8:69-78 (1972).

8. H. Lal, J. J. DeFeo, and P. Thut, Effect of amphetamine on pain-induced aggression. Commun. Behav. Biol. 1:333-336 (1968).

9. H. Lal, J. O'Brien, and S. K. Puri, Morphine withdrawal aggression: Sensitization by amphetamines. Psychopharmacologia 22:217-223 (1971).

10. H. Lal and S. K. Puri, Morphine withdrawal aggression: Role of dopaminergic stimulation. In Drug Addiction: Experimental Pharmacology (J. M. Singh, L. H. Miller, and H. Lal, eds.), Vol. 1. Mt. Kisco, New York: Futura, 1972, pp. 300-310.

11. G. Gianutsos, M. D. Hynes, R. B. Drawbauch, and H. Lal, Morphine withdrawal aggression during protracted abstinence: Role of latent dopaminergic supersensitivity. Pharmacologist 15:348 (1973).

12. G. Gianutsos, M. D. Hynes, S. K. Puri, R. B. Drawbaugh, and H. Lal, Effect of apomorphine and nigrostriatal lesions on aggression and striatal dopamine turnover during morphine withdrawal: Evidence for dopaminergic supersensitivity in protracted abstinence. Psychopharmacologia 34:37-44 (1974).

13. H. Lal, J. J. DeFeo, and P. Thut, Prevention of pain-induced aggression by parachloroamphetamine. Biol. Psychiat. 2:205-206 (1970).

14. H. Lal, S. K. Puri, R. B. Drawbaugh, and C. Reddy, Morphine withdrawal syndrome in mice and rats: Partial blockade by p-chloroamphetamine. Fed. Proc. Fed. Amer. Soc. Exp. Biol. 33:487 (1974).

15. G. M. McKenzie, Apomorphine-induced aggression in the rat. Brain Res. 34:323-330 (1971).

16. H. Lal, J. O'Brien, A. Pitterman, G. Gianutsos, and C. Reddy, Aggression after amphetamine and dihydroxyphenylalanine. Fed. Proc. Fed. Amer. Soc. Exp. Biol. 31:529 (1972).

17. S. K. Puri and H. Lal, Effect of dopaminergic stimulation or blockade on morphine-withdrawal aggression. Psychopharmacologia 32:113-120 (1973).

18. W. R. Martin and J. W. Sloan, The pathophysiology of morphine dependence and its treatment with opioid antagonists. Pharmakopsychiat. Neuro-Psychopharmacol. 1:260-270 (1968).

19. S. K. Puri and H. Lal, Effect of morphine, haloperidol, apomorphine and benztropine on dopamine turnover in rat corpus striatum: Evidence showing morphine induced reduction in CNS dopaminergic activity. Fed. Proc. Fed. Amer. Soc. Exp. Biol. 32:758 (1973).

20. S. K. Puri and H. Lal, Effect of apomorphine, benztropine or morphine on striatal dopamine turnover: Evidence of latent supersensitivity of dopaminergic receptors in morphine dependent rats. Pharmacologist 13:247 (1973).

21. Y. Karkalas and H. Lal, Haloperidol in the treatment of opioid addiction. Clin. Toxicol. 5:59 (1972).

22. J. Karkalas and H. Lal, A comparison of haloperidol with methadone in blocking heroin-withdrawal symptoms. Int. Pharmacopsychiat. 8:248-251 (1973).

23. J. J. Friedman and G. LeCompte, Detoxification and maintenance of heroin addicts with haloperidol in an outpatient population. Paper presented at Second International Symposium on Drug Addiction, New Orleans, March 1973.

24. S. C. Boshka, H. M. Weisman, and D. H. Thor, A technique for inducing aggression in rats utilizing morphine withdrawal. Psychol. Rec. 16:541-543 (1966).

25. H. Lal, S. K. Puri, and Y. Karkalas, Blockade of opioid withdrawal symptoms by haloperidol in rats and humans. Pharmacologist 13:263 (1971).

26. S. K. Puri, J. O'Brien, and H. Lal, Potentiation of morphine withdrawal aggression by d-amphetamine, dopa, or apomorphine. Pharmacologist 13:280 (1971).

27. S. K. Puri and H. Lal, Tolerance to the behavioral and neurochemical effects of haloperidol and morphine in rats chronically treated with morphine or haloperidol. Nauyn-Schmeidebergs Arch. Pharmakol. 282:155-170 (1974).

28. H. Lal, B. Nesson, and N. Smith, Amphetamine induced aggression in mice pretreated with dihydroxyphenylalanine (DOPA) and/or reserpine. Biol. Psychiat. 2:299-301 (1970).

29. A. Randrup and I. Munkvard, Pharmacological studies on the mechanisms underlying two forms of behavioral excitation: stereotyped hyperactivity and "rage." Ann. N.Y. Acad. Sci. 159:928-938 (1969).

30. A. L. Boura and A. F. Green, Adrenergic neuron blocking agents. Annu. Rev. Pharmacol. 5:183-212 (1965).

31. N. Emmelin, Supersensitivity following pharmacological denervation. Pharmacol. Rev. 13:17-37 (1961).

32. S. K. Sharpless, Reorganization of function in the nervous system: use and disuse. Annu. Rev. Pharmacol. 26:357-388 (1964).

33. V. Trendelenburg, Supersensitivity and subsensitivity to sympathomimetic amines. Pharmacol. Rev. 15:225-276 (1963).

34. G. Gianutsos, R. B. Drawbaugh, M. D. Hynes, and H. Lal, Behavioral evidence for dopaminergic supersensitivity after chronic haloperidol. Life Sci. 14:887-898 (1974).

35. S. K. Puri, C. Reddy and H. Lal, Blockade of central dopaminergic receptors by morphine: Effect of haloperidol, apomorphine, or benztropine. Res. Commun. Chem. Pathol. Pharmacol. 5:389-401 (1973).

36. M. A. Sasame, J. Perez-Cruet, G. DiChiaro, A. Tagliamonte, P. Tagliamonte, and G. L. Gessa, Evidence that methadone blocks dopamine receptors in the brain. J. Neurochem. 19:1953-1957 (1972).

Chapter 9

THE IMPLICATION AND SIGNIFICANCE OF EEG AND SLEEP-AWAKE ACTIVITY IN THE STUDY OF EXPERIMENTAL DRUG DEPENDENCE ON MORPHINE*

NAIM KHAZAN

Department of Pharmacology and Therapeutics
University of Cincinnati Medical Center
Department of Pharmacology
Merrell-National Laboratories
Cincinnati, Ohio+

---

*Supported by National Institute of Mental Health Grants MH-16693, MH-34429, MH-23386, DA00461, and DA01050.

+Present address: Department of Pharmacology and Toxicology, University of Maryland School of Pharmacy, Baltimore, Maryland.

I. INTRODUCTION

A. Literature Survey

The discovery of electrical potentials of the brain is thought to have been made by Caton [1], who in 1875 presented the results of his research with rabbits and monkeys to the British Medical Association in Edinburgh. Half a century later, in 1929, in Jena, Austria, Berger discovered human brain waves [2] and, hence, is recognized as the father of electroencephalography. From these momentus findings arose modern electroencephalography, the recording of oscillations in the potential differences between two points in the brain.

Different states of awareness, such as full consciousness, drowsiness, or sleep, bring about prominent changes in the electroencephalogram (EEG). Moruzzi and Magoun [3] discovered that high-frequency stimulation of the brain stem recticular formation or presentation of alerting stimuli produced EEG tracings with fast frequency and low amplitude, referred to as EEG activation or desynchronization. On the other hand, the behavioral state of drowsiness or sleep was associated with a low-frequency, high-amplitude EEG referred to as EEG deactivation or synchronization.

Carefully controlled EEG and electromyogram (EMG) recordings, collected from animals prepared with acute or chronic electrodes, have provided useful information about the action of drugs with central nervous system (CNS) activity. Correlation between changes in the EEG and behavior and in sleep-awake activity occurring spontaneously or after drug administration has been reported. Central stimulants, in general, induce EEG activation associated with arousal behavior. Electroencephalogram deactivation is induced by CNS depressants, and here also a correlation between the behavioral depression and the EEG synchrony has been shown [4-11]. Wikler [12] found that such association between the EEG and the behavioral changes was lost, however, after treatment with morphine, N-allylnormorphine, or atropine. In this state of "dissociation," the EEG of an atropine-treated dog failed to change in the direction of activation or desynchrony during behavioral wakefulness or even excitation. Rinaldi and Himwich [13] showed that intravenous (iv) administration of atropine to rabbits evoked EEG patterns typical of sleep and, moreover, inhibited all EEG alerting responses either to physiological stimuli or to direct stimulation of the midbrain.

During the awake state, low-voltage, high-frequency EEG activity and EEG desynchrony associated with active EMG tracings prevail. The EEG synchrony, high-voltage, slow-wave recordings with low EMG activity are termed slow wave sleep (SWS). In the rat, rapid eye movement (REM) sleep is a state of sleep distinguished by a desynchronized, low-voltage, fast-frequency EEG similar to that seen in the awake state but accompanied by conjugate eye movements, twitches of the vibrissae, ears, and digits, irregular respiration, and loss of body muscular tone. This stage of sleep has also been called paradoxical sleep (PS), rhombencephalic sleep, deep sleep, activated sleep, and dreaming sleep or "D-state" sleep [14-17]. Although the phenomenon of REM sleep was discovered recently [18], there is already a wealth of literature dealing with the pharmacological manipulation of this sleep state by psychoactive drugs (for review, see Kay [19]).

During my association in 1962-1963 with C. H. Sawyer and his colleagues in the Department of Anatomy and the Brain Research Institute, University of California, Los Angeles, we explored several physiological and pharmacological aspects of REM sleep. From continuous EEG recordings collected at slow chart speed from unrestrained, freely moving rabbits prepared with chronically implanted cortical and subcortical electrodes, we studied the phenomenon of REM sleep deprivation [20]. Spontaneous episodes of REM sleep were plentiful in rabbits adapted to the experimental surroundings, but REM sleep episodes were almost completely inhibited when continuous "white" background noise was introduced into the animal's cage. However, this noise did not prevent occurrence of SWS. When the white noise was terminated, a large increase in REM sleep time (REM rebound) occurred. Further studies of drug effects on REM sleep in these rabbits revealed that LSD-25, pentobarbital, morphine, and chlorpromazine inhibited REM sleep, whereas phenobarbital, diphenhydramine, and ethanol had less effect [21]. We also studied averaged evoked potentials collected during REM sleep episodes and found them to be similar to those obtained during the arousal state of behavior [22]. In this study, the effects of several psychotropic drugs on the evoked potential during REM sleep state were assessed and reported. These included amphetamine, LSD-25, atropine, reserpine, morphine, chlorpromazine, and barbiturates.

B. Theoretical Background

By 1963, numerous facets of the pharmacology of narcotics had been explored, using the rat as the experimental animal [23-33]. The operant behavior experiments in which the rat, by pressing a lever switch, self-administers morphine at will via a chronically indwelling iv cannula were first used in 1962 by James R. Weeks [34] of the Upjohn Company, Kalamazoo, Michigan. Such rats maintained a dependent state for as long as 3 months. Intrigued with the possibility of applying the technique of chronic electrode implantation to monitor EEG and sleep-awake activity in morphine-dependent rats and the likelihood of gaining vast information in this field, I joined Dr. Weeks' efforts in 1963. Collaborative efforts to integrate these two approaches were achieved, and our addiction studies were begun a decade ago. The results of these and subsequent studies conducted during the past 12 years, with the collaboration of J. R. Weeks, L. Schroeder, P. Brown, J. Masur, B. Colasanti, P. Nash, and recently T. Roehrs and J. Moreton, are presented in this chapter. The applicability of this experimental model to the study of opiate dependence [35] and other addictive and psychotropic agents is presented and discussed.

II. DESCRIPTION OF THE METHOD

A. Chronic EEG and EMG Electrode Implantation

Adult female Sprague-Dawley rats (250-300 g) are used. Implantation of chronic electrodes for the recording of the EEG and EMG is performed after an intraperitoneal (ip) injection of pentobarbital (35 mg/kg) or ketamine HCl (150 mg/kg), the anesthesia being supplemented by ether when necessary. The rat is mounted on a stereotaxic frame. Left and right ear bars are inserted into the ear canal in a manner permitting the skull to pivot freely about the axis of the ear canal, with minimal lateral movement of the skull. The incisor bar and hose clamp are then adjusted and gently, but securely, tightened.

Taking care not to cut the underlying bone, one makes a midline incision with a scalpel blade, and the periosteum is dissected bluntly from the skull with scissors. The incision may be held open by hemostatic forceps. Next, the periosteum or bone covering is scraped from the top of the skull with a dull scalpel.

For the preparation of the EMG electrode, cut a 9.0-cm length of Teflon-coated wire, and place a knot 1.5 cm from one end. Remove the insulation from the longer section of the wire by applying a soldering iron to the Teflon near the knot, effecting a break in the insulation. Then, strip the 7.5-cm insulation with the fingernail. Strip the tip of the insulated 1.5-cm wire, and tin the end of the insulated wire after it is etched with concentrated phosphoric acid. To implant these EMG electrodes, expose the left and right temporalis muscles and thread one of these electrodes through a surgical needle and suture deeply into the temporalis muscle in a "Z" fashion. Enter the temporalis muscle at the anterior dorsal aspect and exit at the posterior ventral aspect.

Five holes are drilled into the skull: two holes, 3 mm posterior and 2 mm lateral; two holes, 2 mm anterior and 2 mm lateral; and a fifth hole, 5 mm posterior and 2 mm lateral to the bregma and sagittal sutures, respectively (Fig. 1a). Four stainless-steel screws, to which electrode wires were soldered earlier, are threaded into the first four holes of the skull, above the frontal and parietal areas of the cortices for subsequent bipolar EEG recordings. The fifth (anchor) screw is threaded into the remaining hole to supply additional support for the chronic preparation (Fig. 1b). Wire leads from the EEG and EMG electrodes are then soldered to a small Amphenol connector and fixed in place with acrylic (Fig. 1c and 1d), after which approximately 1 week of postoperative recovery is permitted.

B. Intravenous Cannula Construction and Implantation

Weeks' technique for preparation and implantation of the iv cannula in the rat [36] was followed and found to be very satisfactory. Since this or a similar technique has been described elsewhere in this book, I have chosen to avoid repetition (see Chapter 1).

C. Experimental Setup

Rats are maintained in special individual cages that serve as their home cage throughout the experiment and permit drug administration and continuous recording of EEG and EMG. The majority of results of the chronic experimentations are obtained under lighting conditions that provide a timer-regulated dark period from 10 p.m. to 6 a.m. To permit free

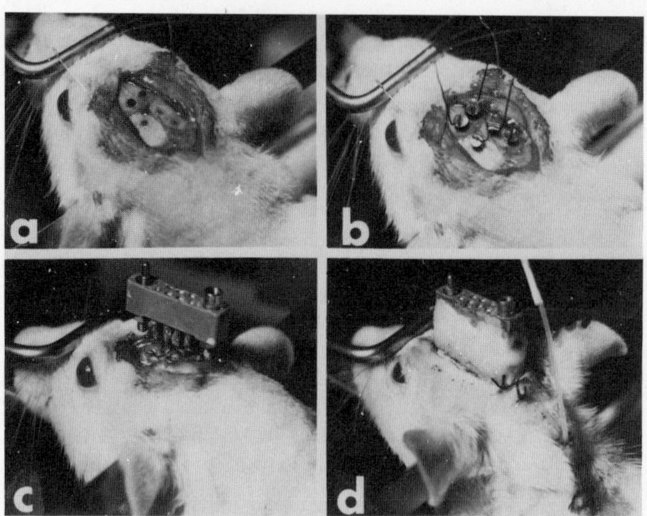

FIGURE 1. Illustration of the holes drilled into the skull of the rat in the designated locations (see text). The EEG and EMG electrodes are positioned and soldered to an Amphenol connector. Dental cement is then used to fix electrodes and connector in place.

movement of the rat, each cage is equipped with a cable connector having concentric pools of mercury as noise-free sliding contacts (Fig. 2). A modified 10-channel Grass, Model 7, polygraph, with five event markers added, is used for simultaneous recording of the EEG, EMG, lever-pressing activity, and drug injections of five rats. Responses and reinforcements are also recorded at slow paper speed on an Esterline-Angus event recorder. Lehigh Valley Electronic solid-state components are used for timing and delivery of automatic or self-administered injections of the narcotic.

For quantification of the mean EEG voltage output, the EEG voltage integrator (Model 23, Coldspring Instrument Corp.) is used. The operation of the integrators is based on the continuous cumulative measurement of the area under successive waves, both positive and negative [38]. The resulting output is a series of pulses, the rate of which is directly proportional to the EEG "energy content" or voltage output. These pulses are recorded on one of the channels of the polygraph. The method used in the quantification of the EEG voltage is a modified form of that suggested by Munoz and

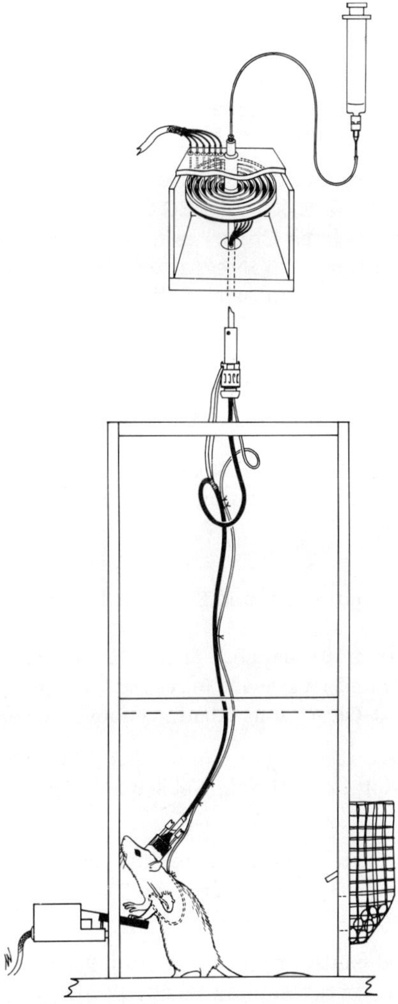

FIGURE 2. The home cage of a rat chronically implanted with cortical and myographic electrodes and with a silicone rubber cannula. Notice the modified Sutton and Miller mercury contacts built around the swivel to allow the rat free movement without twisting the cable [37]. (Reprinted with modification from Khazan [11], p. 182, by courtesy of Raven Press, New York.)

Goldstein [39] and Goldstein et al. [40,41] in which episodes corresponding to the behavioral states of sleep, REM sleep, and wakefulness are selected from the EEG recordings, and 30-sec intervals are sampled representing maximal synchrony in the case of sleep and maximal desynchrony in the case of REM sleep and wakefulness.

For examination of qualitative and quantitative changes in the major frequency components of the EEG, an EEG frequency analyzer (San ei, Type EA-201, Medical Systems Corp.) is used. This instrument consists of matched band-pass filters with integrators, the output of which is a spectrogram of the relative magnitude of the EEG activity present in five frequency bands: 2-4, 4-8, 8-13, 13-20, and 20-30 Hz, over a 10-sec integration period. For the quantification of these frequency bands of the EEG, a procedure similar to that of Martin and Eades [42] is followed. Spectrograms are evaluated within 1-min intervals of episodes of sleep, REM sleep, and wakefulness. Two sets of five cages connected to the EEG recorder, an event recorder, an oscilloscope, EEG voltage integrator and frequency analyzer, and solid state trigger mechanism for injection are used (Fig. 3).

D. Equipment and Supplies Required

1. Polygraph. Modified 10-channel, Model 7, to consist of five EEG and five EMG channels and five event markers. Supplier: Grass Instrument Company, 101 Old Colony Road, Quincy, Massachusetts 02169.

2. EEG frequency analyzer. Type San ei, EA-201. Supplier: Medical Systems Corporation, 230 Middle Neck Road, Great Neck, New York 10021.

3. EEG voltage output integrator. Model 23. Supplier: Coldspring Instrument Corporation, 800 W. Jericho Turnpike, Huntington, New York 11743.

4. Lehigh Valley solid-state programming components. To include solid-state power supply, programming leads, predetermining counter (5 digit), multirange timers, and counter panel, for the control of automatic and self-injections. Former supplier: Lehigh Valley Electronics, Inc., P. O. Box 125, Fogelsville, Pennsylvania 18051. Present supplier: Tech Serve, Inc., BRS/LVE, 5301 Holland Drive, Beltsville, Maryland 20705.

5. Event recorder. A unit to record lever-pressing activities and injections at a low chart speed, Model A620T (no. 188397) and chart paper (no. 37020-C). Supplier: Esterline-Angus, Division of Esterline Corporation, Box 24000, Indianapolis, Indiana 46224.

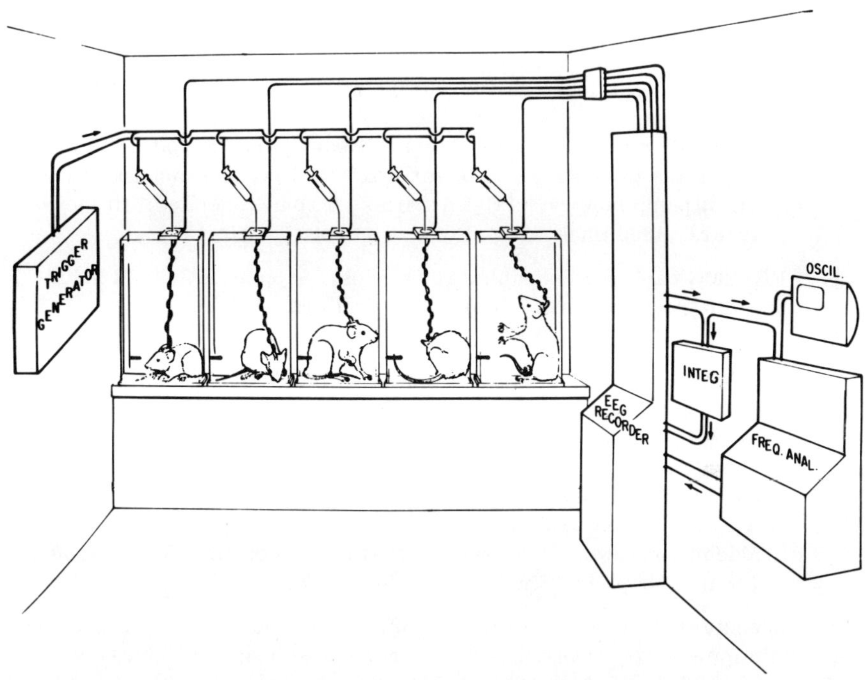

FIGURE 3. Diagram showing the experimental design employed in our drug addiction studies. The EEG and EMG tracings are collected continuously during control, addiction, and abstinence states. (Reprinted with modification from Khazan [35], p. 161, by courtesy of Symposia Specialists, Miami, Florida.)

6. Swivels. Custom built, mercury pool, six-conductor with feed-through cannula. Supplier: Technical Concepts, Inc., 84 W. 238th Street, Bronx, New York 10463.

7. Cannulas.
   a. Silastic medical-grade tubing. Dow Corning, 0.012 in. i.d., 0.025 in. o.d. Supplier: Crocker-Fels Company, 990 Dalton Street, Cincinnati, Ohio 45203.
   b. Polyethylene tubing. Intramedic, PE 10 and PE 20. Supplier: Crocker-Fels Company.
   c. Shrinkable tubing, FIT-221, 3/64 in. Supplier: Terminal Hudson Electronics, Inc., 236 West 17th Street, New York, New York.
   d. Bridges for cannula system. Stainless-steel hypodermic needles. Supplier: Small Parts, Inc., 6901 N.E. 3rd Avenue, Miami, Florida 33138.

8. Injection system.
   a. Syringes. Yale infusion, Luer-lok, 10 cc (catalogue no. 02-0010) and 20 cc (catalogue no. 02-0014). Supplier: Becton, Dickinson and Company. Rutherford, New Jersey 07070.
   b. Harvard portable infusion pumps. Model 1100. Supplier: Harvard Apparatus Company, 150 Dover Road, Millis, Massachusetts 02054.
   c. Hurst pump motors. PC-DA series, 6 rpm. Supplied: Hughes-Peters, 4865 Duck Creek Road, Cincinnati, Ohio 45227.

9. EEG-EMG cable. Flexicable, 200 series. Supplier: Caltron Industries, 2015 Second Street, Berkeley, California 94710.

10. Electrodes.
    a. Cortical electrode. Stainless-steel wire, Teflon coated, 0.010 in. (catalogue no. 316). Supplier: Medwire, 421 S. Columbus, Mt. Vernon, New York.
    b. Muscle electrode. Stainless-steel wire, Teflon coated (catalogue no. AS6325). Supplier: Cooner Wire Company, 9439 Turline Avenue, Chatsworth, California 91311.
    c. Machine screws. Stainless-steel screws, no. MX080-2F, 0-80 x 1/8 in. Supplier: Small Parts, Inc.

11. Connectors. Microminiature MM-22, female (no. MM7-22-SGDS) and male (no. MM7-22PGDSK). Supplier: Weststates Electronics Corporation, 20151 Bahama Street, Chatsworth, California 91311.

12. Cement adhesive. Eastman 910 adhesive. Supplier: Any photography supply store.

13. Stereotaxic instrument. Supplier: David Kopf Instruments, 7324 Elmo Street, Box 636, Tujunga, California 91042.

14. High-speed dental drill. Supplier: Any dental supply store. Use no. 3 carbide bit available from S. S. White, Philadelphia, Pennsylvania, or local vendor.

15. Soldering iron, gun, and tips. Supplier: Any hardware store.

E. Sensitivity

In conjunction with the drug self-administration technique, we found the continuous recording of the EEG and EMG to be invaluable in a finer assessment of the course of the addiction cycle, which includes the development of tolerance, physical dependence, drug-seeking behavior, and immediate and protracted abstinence. The changes observed in the EEG and EMG and in the sleep-awake pattern were most characteristic during any of the above states. The results of our EEG and behavioral approach to the study of postaddicts provided further evidence of long-term central effects detectable for extended periods after termination of the dependence state in these rats. Moreover, with the use of this experimental EEG model, the characteristics of a "pure" narcotic antagonist were easily delineated.

F. Pitfalls

The experimenter is alerted to some precautionary measures regarding the preparation of the experimental setup and the collection and interpretation of the data.

The adaptation of the technique previously described in this text for the preparation and implantation of the EEG and EMG electrodes is not at all laborious. Such methodology is being used by many laboratories involved in the study of the sleep-awake cycle in experimental animals. The same is true with regard to the preparation and implantation of chronic iv cannulas. With a successful preparation, the rat can be used for a period of up to 1 year.

The ability to visually detect and evaluate the normal pattern of the EEG of the rat during the sleep-awake cycle and to distinguish between real changes in the EEG and possible artifact can be acquired with experience. It is also essential that one become acquainted with the normal EEG and EMG recordings at different chart speeds before the introduction of drugs. As a beneficial exercise, study the circadian rhythm with regard to sleep-awake patterns of activity in these rats.

It is desirable to acquire the aid of an electronic engineer or qualified technician to assist in the installation and maintenance of the equipment. To ensure adequate EEG and EMG recordings, mercury pools should be cleaned periodically, once every 4-6 weeks. At the same time, to eliminate the oxidized layer, the mercury should be filtered or changed.

III. TYPE OF DATA OBTAINABLE

A. Studies in Naive Rats

1. Effects of Single Injections of Morphine on EEG and Overt Behavior

The rat shifts frequently among the three behavioral states of sleep, REM sleep, and wakefulness. Figures 4-6 show EEG and EMG tracings during these behavioral states, before drug treatment.

Morphine injections are followed by the appearance of bursts of high-voltage activity in the EEG (Fig. 7), while the rat is behaviorally awake

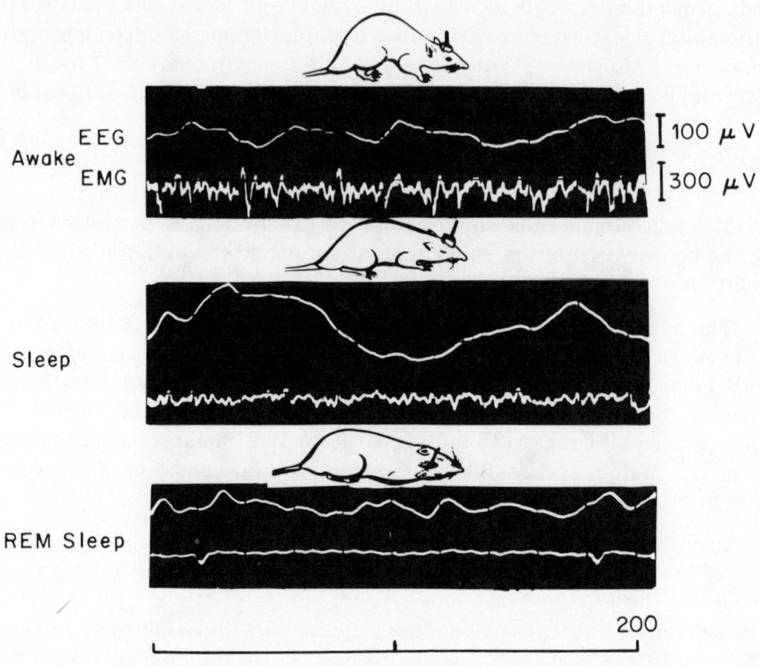

FIGURE 4. Comparison of the oscilloscope tracings of the EEG and EMG during the three stages of normal sleep-awake cycle in the rat. Note the high voltage, low frequency of the EEG and the quiet EMG during sleep. Also note the awake-like pattern of EEG with the highly suppressed EMG activity during REM sleep.

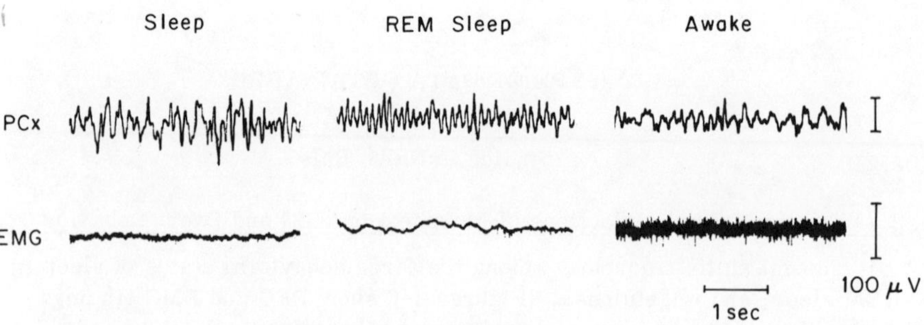

FIGURE 5. EEG and EMG tracings at a low chart speed. Note the contrast between the recordings collected during the three stages. (PCx denotes posterior cortex.) (Reprinted with modification from Khazan [11], p. 197, by courtesy of Raven Press, New York.)

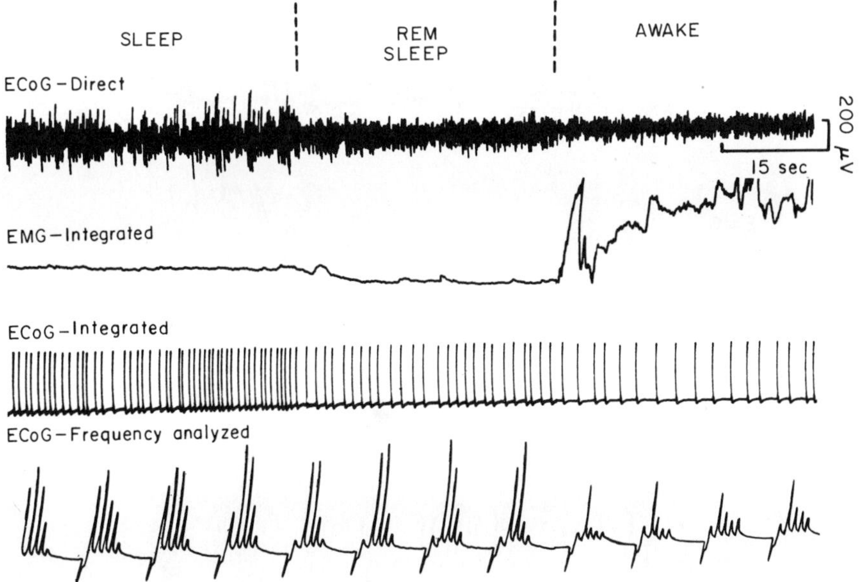

FIGURE 6. Comparison of the cortical EEG (ECoG) and the temporalis EMG during states of the sleep-awake cycle in the normal rat. Note the awake-like EEG pattern with highly suppressed EMG activity during REM sleep. The integrated voltage output of the ECoG decreases in the transition from sleep to REM sleep and then to wakefulness. The frequency-analyzed spectrogram of the ECoG shows a definite decrease in the slow-wave components associated with the awake state. (Reprinted from Khazan and Colasanti [43], p. 493, by courtesy of Williams & Wilkens Co., Baltimore.)

with eyes open but is immobile and stuporous. These EEG bursts, when collected at a higher chart speed, their voltage integrated and frequency analyzed, reveal the presence of high-voltage, low-frequency components; thus, the term EEG "slow bursts" [43,44], as depicted in Fig. 8. Our findings with the use of this animal model have replicated and extended the earlier observations of morphine-induced slow-wave activity in the rat, dog, rabbit, monkey, and man [45-50] (for review, see Isbell and Fraser [51] and Wikler [52]).

Control recordings of the EEG and EMG of the rat were collected over a period of 2 hr. A 10 mg/kg challenge dose of morphine or an equivalent volume of saline was then administered ip and polygraphic and behavioral

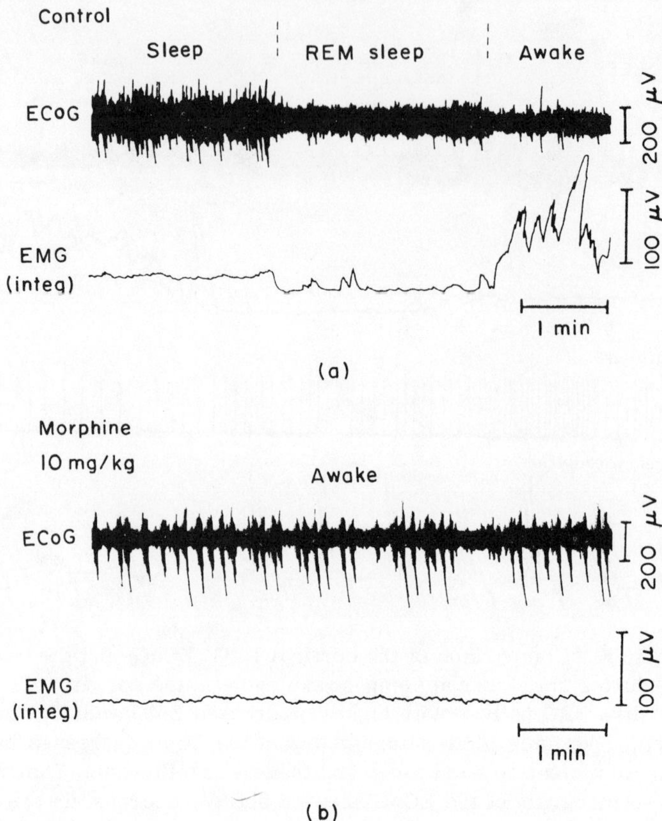

FIGURE 7. (a) EEG and EMG tracings of the sleep-awake cycle in the rat collected during the control period. (b) In contrast, tracings collected 15 min after the administration of morphine, 10 mg/kg ip. The EEG shows bursts of high-voltage activity while the rat is behaviorally awake, immobile, and stuporous. SWS and REM sleep are suppressed (see Khazan et al. [44]). (Reprinted from Colasanti and Khazan [45], p. 465, by courtesy of Pergamon Press, Elmsford, New York.)

correlates were obtained over an additional period of 3-4 hr; this period extended to the appearance of the first EEG, EMG, and behavioral sleep. It was found that a morphine injection of 10 mg/kg in the naive rat was followed by a biphasic pattern of behavioral depression and subsequent stimulation. During the initial depressed phase, which extended for 60-90 min and was associated with behavioral stupor, the EEG tracings showed

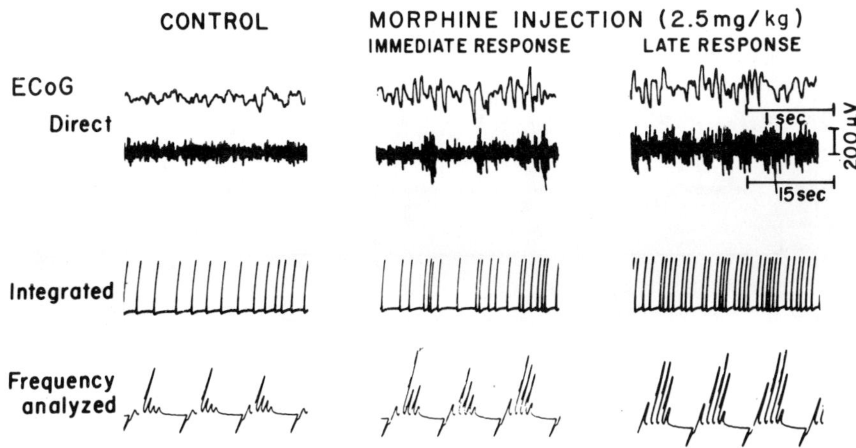

FIGURE 8. Effect of a single injection of morphine, 2.5 mg/kg iv on the ECoG of a control rat. High-voltage EEG slow bursts appeared almost immediately after the injection, and within half an hour a sleeplike EEG pattern was observed to coincide with awake behavior. These high-voltage slow-wave EEG bursts are reflected as changes from the baseline of the integrated and frequency-analyzed ECoG. (Reprinted from Khazan and Colasanti [43], p. 494, by courtesy of Williams & Wilkens Co., Baltimore.)

high-voltage slow bursts. During the phase of stimulation and behavioral arousal, lasting an additional 60-90 min, the EEG revealed desynchronized awake tracings; only a few short episodes of behavioral stupor with EEG slow bursts intervened in this period. This phase was characterized by increased locomotor activity, stereotyped behavior, and episodes of startle reactions [53]. The biphasic response to morphine of the naive rat is shown schematically in Fig. 9.

2. Effects of Single ip Injections of Morphine-like Agonists, Antagonist-Analgesics, or a Pure Antagonist on EEG and Overt Behavior

In order to determine whether the induction of EEG slow bursts is a property of the narcotic analgesics in general rather than a unique action of morphine, the EEG and behavioral correlates of the morphine-like narcotics codeine, methadone, and meperidine were examined. All three agents were found to induce high-voltage EEG slow bursts at dose levels equivalent to their relative analgesic potencies, with methadone the most potent and codeine the least potent. The appearance of EEG slow bursts was accompanied by immobility and stuporous behavior of the rat, as in

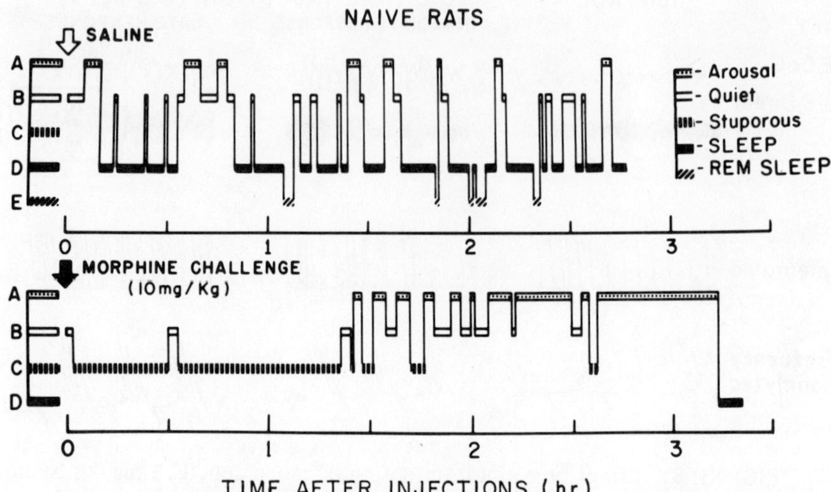

FIGURE 9. Diagrams showing the normal alternation of the states of the sleep-awake cycle in the naive rat after saline injection in contrast to the response to a 10 mg/kg morphine challenge. Note after morphine challenge the biphasic pattern of CNS depression, manifested as behavioral stupor, followed by stimulation and behavioral arousal. (Reprinted from Khazan and Colasanti [53], p. 60, by courtesy of Springer-Verlag, New York.)

the case of morphine. Similarly, the administration of the narcotic antagonist-analgesics nalorphine, pentazocine, or cyclazocine induced high-voltage slow activity in the EEG. Accompanying these EEG slow waves was behavioral stupor of the rat during wakefulness, as in the case of the narcotic analgesics. The narcotic antagonist naloxone, however, was devoid of this effect, and EEG and behavior of naloxone-treated rats appeared to be normal within 15 min after its administration.

The interaction between morphine and narcotic antagonists on the EEG was also studied [54]. Administration of nalorphine 5 min before the injection of 10 mg/kg morphine reduced the duration of the EEG and behavioral effects of morphine. The dose of 2.5 mg/kg of nalorphine appeared to shorten predominantly the initial phase of EEG and behavioral stupor occurring after morphine administration. The dose of 1.25 mg/kg of nalorphine, on the other hand, chiefly reduced the second phase, i.e., that of EEG and behavioral arousal. In contrast to nalorphine, a 2 mg/kg dose of naloxone administered 5 min before the 10 mg/kg dose of morphine completely antagonized both phases of the morphine response, and EEG and behavioral sleep occurred within 15 min after the morphine injection. This was followed by regular alternations of the behavioral states of sleep, REM sleep, and wakefulness as seen during the control period [55].

Thus, our animal model has permitted us to demonstrate that the induction of high-voltage slow activity in the EEG during behavioral stupor of the rat occurs after the administration of the narcotic analgesics. The narcotic antagonists nalorphine, pentazocine, and cyclazocine were also found to affect the EEG, inducing slow bursts and EEG synchrony in association with behavioral stupor. Naloxone, however, was devoid of such activity. This dual feature of the EEG synchrony and behavioral immobility and stupor, followed by behavioral arousal, therefore appeared to be an agonistic property characteristic of the narcotic analgesics as well as the antagonist-analgesics. The complete absence of such agonistic activity by naloxone further supported the pharmacodynamic profile of this compound as a "pure" narcotic antagonist.

Also, when the duration of high-voltage EEG slow activity was used as the dependent variable, a dose-response relationship could be determined for the various narcotic analgesics and antagonist-analgesics. As shown in Fig. 10, methadone was the most potent in this respect and was followed in decreasing order by morphine, codeine, and meperidine. Of the narcotic antagonist-analgesics, cyclazocine was the most potent, whereas pentazocine was the least potent.

3. Role of Brain Amines in the EEG Effects of Morphine

Morphine injections of 10 mg/kg given ip to rats pretreated with p-chlorophenylalanine (PCPA), which blocks the synthesis of serotonin (5-HT) by inhibition of trytophan hydroxylase [56], were followed by an almost complete abolition of the initial period of EEG and behavioral stupor, which was succeeded by a marked prolongation of the period of EEG and behavioral arousal. Administration of 5-hydroxytryptophan (5-HTP), the immediate precursor of 5-HT, 30 min before the morphine injection reversed this effect of PCPA [45], as is shown in Fig. 11. The antagonism of the response to morphine in rats treated with PCPA and reversal of this antagonism by injection of 5-HTP suggested that brain 5-HT may mediate production of the initial EEG and behavioral depression after morphine administration. These findings are in direct agreement with the work of Eidelberg and Schwartz [57], who demonstrated the absence of the initial phase of depression of spontaneous locomotor activity induced by morphine in rats pretreated with PCPA. Similar effects of both PCPA and median raphé lesions in rats treated with morphine have been reported [58,59].

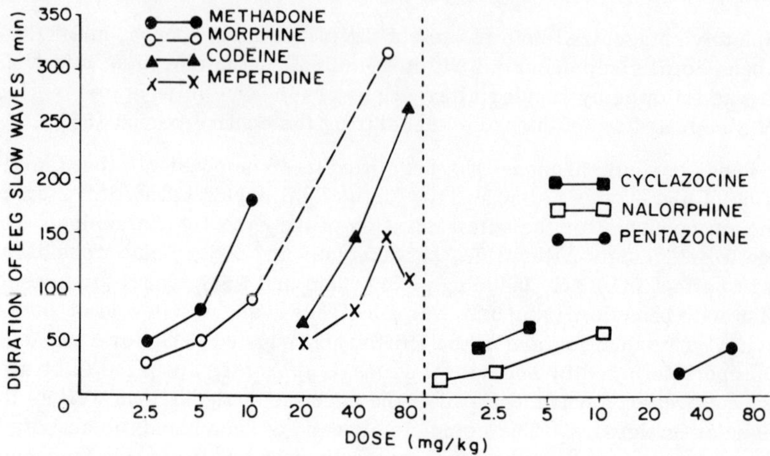

FIGURE 10. Duration of EEG synchrony induced by narcotic analgesics (left) and antagonist-analgesics (right) at the specified doses. Each point represents the mean value for three to five rats. Note the similarities in the slopes of the dose-response curves within each group of drugs. (Reprinted from Colasanti and Khazan [55], p. 622, by courtesy of Pergamon Press, Elmsford, New York.)

Morphine injections given to rats pretreated with α-methyl-p-tyrosine (AMPT), which blocks synthesis of catecholamines by inhibition of tyrosine hydroxylase [60], resulted in a slight but significant reduction of the initial period of stuporous behavior in association with EEG slow bursts. The duration of the secondary phase of EEG and behavioral arousal, however, was unaffected [44]. The antagonism by PCPA of the biphasic response to morphine was partially reduced by concomitant pretreatment of the rats with AMPT. Thus, it appeared that the availability of 5-HT and catecholamines plays a joint role in the mediation of the immediate morphine EEG and behavioral effects. The role of serotonin in the development of physical dependence on morphine is disputed [61-64].

Several studies have shown that morphine impairs the release of acetylcholine (ACh) at the peripheral [65-67] and central [68-71] cholinergic synapses. It has been suggested that the hypoactivity and stuporous phase induced by morphine is related to its inhibition of central ACh release [72].

B. Studies in Rats Made Physically Dependent on Morphine

A complete cycle of addiction to iv morphine in the rat comprises three stages: control period, induction of dependence on morphine by

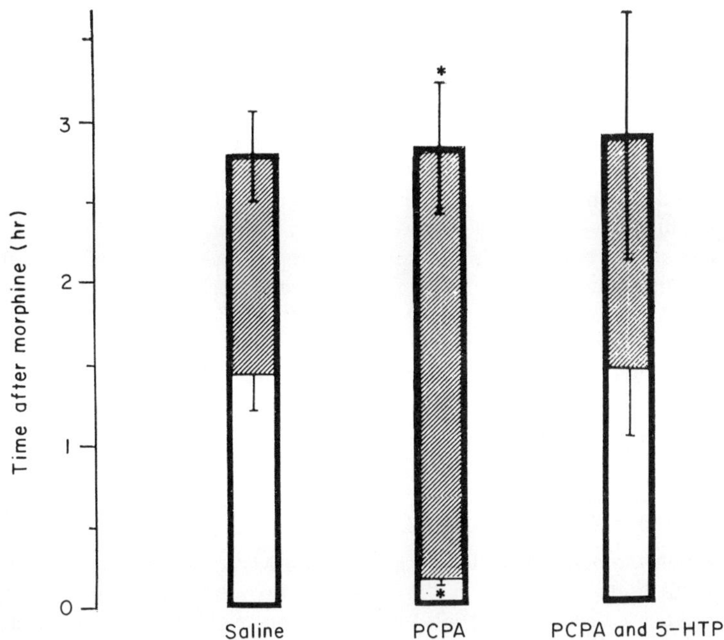

FIGURE 11. Effects of 10 mg/kg injection of morphine in rats pretreated with PCPA or PCPA plus 5-HTP. A biphasic pattern of response was produced in the saline control rats, consisting of an initial period of behavioral depression associated with the appearance of high-voltage EEG slow bursts (unshaded) and a secondary phase of EEG and behavioral stimulation (shaded). The initial period of EEG and behavioral depression was almost completely abolished by pretreatment with PCPA (100 mg/kg per 24 hr for 3 days), an effect that was reversed by 5-HTP, 75 mg/kg, administered 30 min prior to the morphine injection (asterisk signifies $P < 0.01$). (Reprinted from Colasanti and Khazan [45], p. 466, by courtesy of Pergamon Press, Elmsford, New York.)

automatic injections and by self-administration, and abstinence [44,73]. The control stage allows the rat to adjust to the experimental setup. Morphine sulfate is then injected automatically every hour at an initial dose of 2 mg/kg during the 24 hr of the first day. The dose is gradually increased in geometric progression over successive days to 3.1, 4.7, 7.1, 11.1, 17.0, 26.1, and 40.0 mg/kg/hr. More recently [43], a shorter treatment regimen was adopted whereby the initial dose of morphine is 1.25 mg/kg given hourly for 24 hr and is then increased on successive days to 2.5, 5.0, 10,0, and 20.0 mg/kg/hr. The final dose of 20 mg/kg/hr is maintained for 2 days. The volume of injections varies from 0.05 to 0.3 ml, depending on the dose. These dose schedules induce a state of morphine dependence in the rat, and the behavioral manifestations of the abstinence syndrome become evident when the injections are discontinued. During the self-maintained dependent state, in which previously addicted rats self-administer morphine by pressing a lever switch for 10 mg/kg injections, the aspect of drug-seeking behavior is included. Under a fixed ratio (FR) schedule of reinforcement, morphine injections are given initially for each lever response. After responses become regular (2-3 days), the number of lever responses necessary for morphine injections is progressively increased, usually on successive days, from the initial FR 1 through FR 5, FR 10, and finally FR 20. The dependent state is terminated by abstinence, wherein morphine injections are either discontinued or replaced by injections of isotonic saline or 5% glucose.

1. Development of Tolerance to Morphine: EEG Correlates

During the control period, EEG and EMG tracings indicated less sleeping time at night and in the early morning hours than at other hours of the day as expected from the usually greater nocturnal activity of the rat. After initiation of hourly automatic injections of morphine, sleep was greatly reduced and REM sleep was virtually eliminated. High-voltage slow bursts appeared in the EEG of the awake state. By the third day of treatment, however, in spite of the increasing doses of morphine, the period covered by behavioral stupor and EEG slow bursts decreased, and the total amounts of sleep and REM sleep gradually approached normal values. These circumstances reflect the development of tolerance to the drug [44].

2. Dependence State and Drug-Seeking Behavior

During the next stage of addiction, the dependent state, in which the rat self-administers morphine by pressing a bar on an FR schedule, a state of wakefulness prevailed immediately after an injection, whereas prolonged episodes of sleep and REM sleep predominated in the period before the injection [44,74], as depicted in Fig. 12. EEG slow bursts appeared directly after the morphine injection (Fig. 13) and disappeared by the time of the next injection. (For patterns and factors affecting iv self-injection by morphine-dependent rats, see Weeks and Collins [75, 76].)

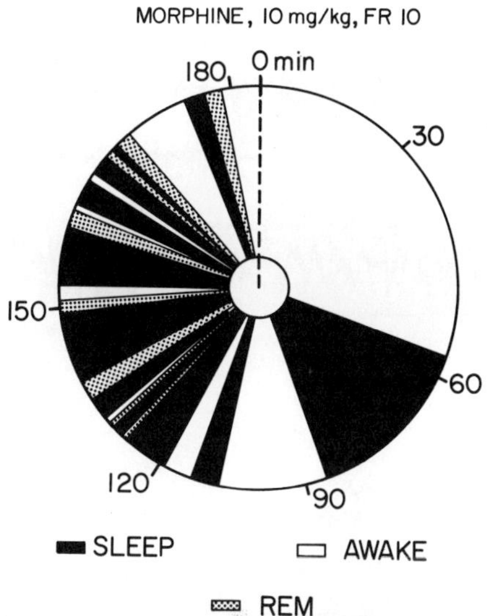

FIGURE 12. The distribution of sleep, REM sleep, and wakefulness during an interinjection interval of a morphine-dependent rat bar pressing for morphine self-injection. Note the dominant wakefulness after morphine injection and the sleep and REM sleep prior to the next injection. (Constructed from published data [44], by courtesy of Williams & Wilkens Co., Baltimore.)

C. The Abstinence Syndrome

1. Immediate EEG and Behavioral Changes

Upon withdrawal of morphine, sleep and long REM sleep episodes predominated in the first 4-6 hr. After this period, sleep progressively decreased until wakefulness and behavioral hyperirritability prevailed. This biphasic depressed and aroused pattern of behavior observed in rats reminded us of a description of clinical signs and symptoms of the abstinence syndrome [77]:

> The signs and symptoms ... begin to appear some six to twelve hours after the last dose of the narcotic, consisting initially of a vague awareness of the impending illness. The patient

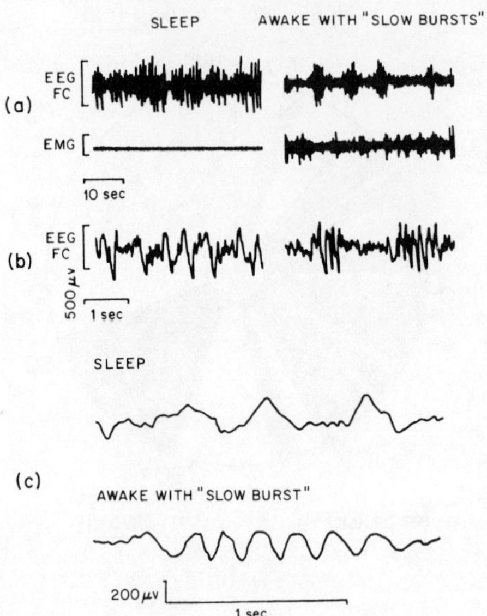

FIGURE 13. High-voltage 4- to 7-Hz slow bursts in the EEG from the rat frontal cortex (FC) during the behavioral awake state following a voluntary morphine injection and contrasted with the sleep states. Paper speeds are (a) 1.5, (b) 15, and (c) 60 mm/sec. (Reprinted from Khazan et al. [44], p. 526, by courtesy of Williams & Wilkens Co., Baltimore.)

> then begins to yawn, has tearing of the eyes (lacrimation), a stuffy or runny nose (rhinorrhea) and begins to sweat. He then may enter into a fitful disturbed sleep called the "sleepy yen." As the abstinence syndrome becomes more intense he is awakened and becomes restless,...and twitchings of various muscle groups become apparent.

The initial depressed stage of the abstinence syndrome in the rat with much sleep and REM sleep, followed by hyperirritability, may be compared to the initial "sleepy yen" stage and restlessness, respectively, as described in man. The typical withdrawal symptoms of tremor, piloerection, ptosis, and diarrhea accompanied the behavioral irritability. Frequent "wet dog shakes" as well as tail chasing and startle reactions also appeared with the beginning of this stage of hyperactivity. Sleep EEG tracings correlated with incidences of behavioral sleep in an awake posture which were followed occasionally by short REM sleep episodes. During this period, however, total sleep time decreased and no slow wave bursts appeared in the EEG tracings.

By continuously recording the EEG and EMG at a low chart speed, we observed that the EEG voltage output obtained from rats withdrawn from morphine was considerably lower than that during the foregoing states of control or morphine dependence [44]. Quantification of the EEG voltage output was therefore determined with the aid of an EEG voltage integrator. The results revealed that upon withdrawal, first a brief rise and then a progressive decline in the mean integrated voltage occurred in the sleep, REM sleep, and awake EEG of all the dependent rats. The decline in the mean EEG voltage output of the individual rats ranged from 35 to 70% of the control value for the sleep state and from 35 to 55% for the awake state. Maximal decline of the EEG voltage output of the rats as a group was reached toward the end of the first 8 hr of abstinence. The low-voltage output of the awake state EEG endured for 2-3 days [43,78]. The reduction of the voltage output of the abstinent rat is shown in Fig. 14.

Low-voltage EEG tracings have been frequently considered a correlate of either anxiety and psychic tension or lowered vigilance [79]. We noted no report describing a low EEG voltage output during abstinence from morphine or other narcotic analgesics in experimental animals or man. Decreases in voltage output of the EEG were shown, however, accompanying the behavioral stimulation and excitation seen after the administration of amphetamine [39] or LSD-25 [40]. Our findings of a decline in the EEG voltage output, concomitant with the development of hyperirritability of the rat during morphine abstinence, consequently lend further support to the generalization of Wikler [80] that EEG desynchronization occurs in association with anxiety, hallucination, fantasies, illusions, or tremor, regardless of the nature of the drug.

2. Protracted REM Sleep Rebound

In view of the clinical studies describing prolonged rebound in REM sleep time after the withdrawal of addictive agents such as narcotic analgesics [81] and barbiturates from man [82,83], experiments were undertaken to determine whether a rebound in REM time would likewise follow the withdrawal of morphine from dependent rats. Total REM time was determined for the rats by evaluation of the EEG and EMG recordings collected continuously at a low paper speed during the periods of control, induction of morphine dependence, and abstinence. Upon withdrawal of morphine, REM sleep time was significantly enhanced during the first 4-6

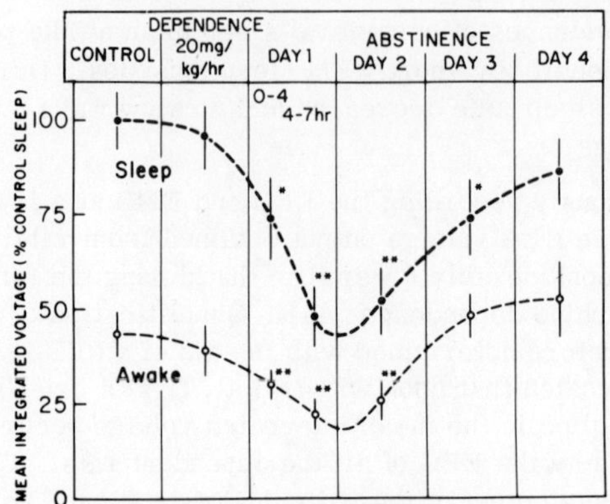

FIGURE 14. Time course of changes in the mean voltage output of the EEG during morphine abstinence. The means of the individual rats in each time period were pooled to obtain group means. The values for days 2, 3, and 4 are the means for the 8-hr period studied (single asterisk signifies $P < 0.01$; double asterisk, $P < 0.001$). (Reprinted from Khazan and Colasanti [43], p. 496, by courtesy of Williams and Wilkens Co., Baltimore.)

hr. The duration and the mean EEG voltage output of REM sleep episodes declined to minimal levels within the remainder of the first day of withdrawal. Both REM time and the integrated REM EEG voltage had returned to control values by the third day, after which a significant rebound occurred in both parameters. While the elevation of the REM EEG voltage output extended to the sixth or ninth day, the rebound in REM time remained evident up to the twelfth day of withdrawal studied (Figs. 15 and 16). These results, demonstrating a protracted REM rebound after morphine withdrawal in the experimental rat [84,85], were consistent with the clinical findings mentioned above.

Deprivation of REM sleep in experimental animals and in man is generally followed by a rebound in REM sleep time. After REM deprivation produced in the rabbit with the use of white masking noise, a rebound occurred in both the frequency and the duration of REM sleep episodes [20]. Likewise, REM sleep deprivation produced in man by selective awakenings at REM onset was followed by a rebound recovery which amounted to 65-75% of the REM time lost during deprivation [86]. Suppression of REM sleep also was found to follow the administration of many psychotropic drug

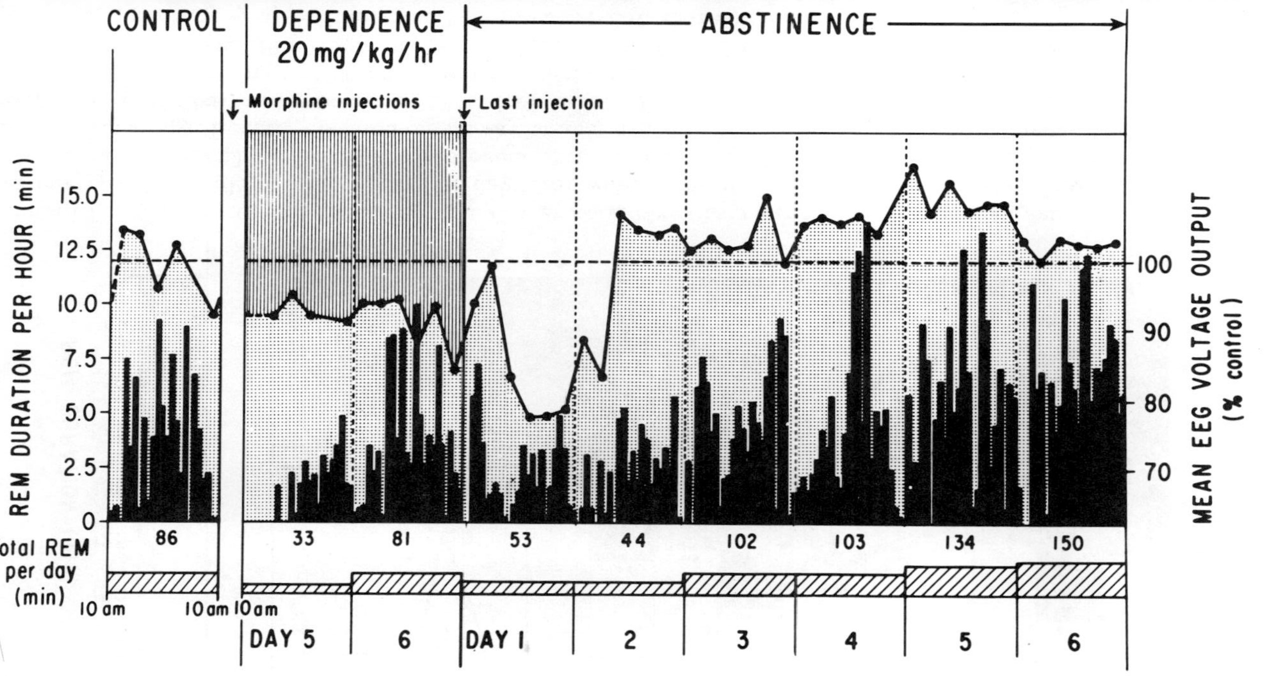

FIGURE 15. Duration and mean EEG voltage output of REM sleep for a representative rat during the periods of control, morphine dependence at 20 mg/kg/hr, and the abstinence state. REM sleep time is shown for 1-hr intervals (vertical bars), whereas the mean voltage output of the REM sleep EEG is depicted for intervals of 4 hr (points on the upper curve). Although REM time returned to the baseline values on the second day of morphine administration at the 20 mg/kg/hr dose, a marked suppression of REM sleep and a concomitant decline in the voltage output of the REM sleep EEG occurred within the first day of withdrawal. Note the rebound increases in both REM time and the REM EEG voltage output after the third day of morphine abstinence. (Reprinted from Khazan and Calosanti [84], p. 27, by courtesy of Williams and Wilkens Co., Baltimore.)

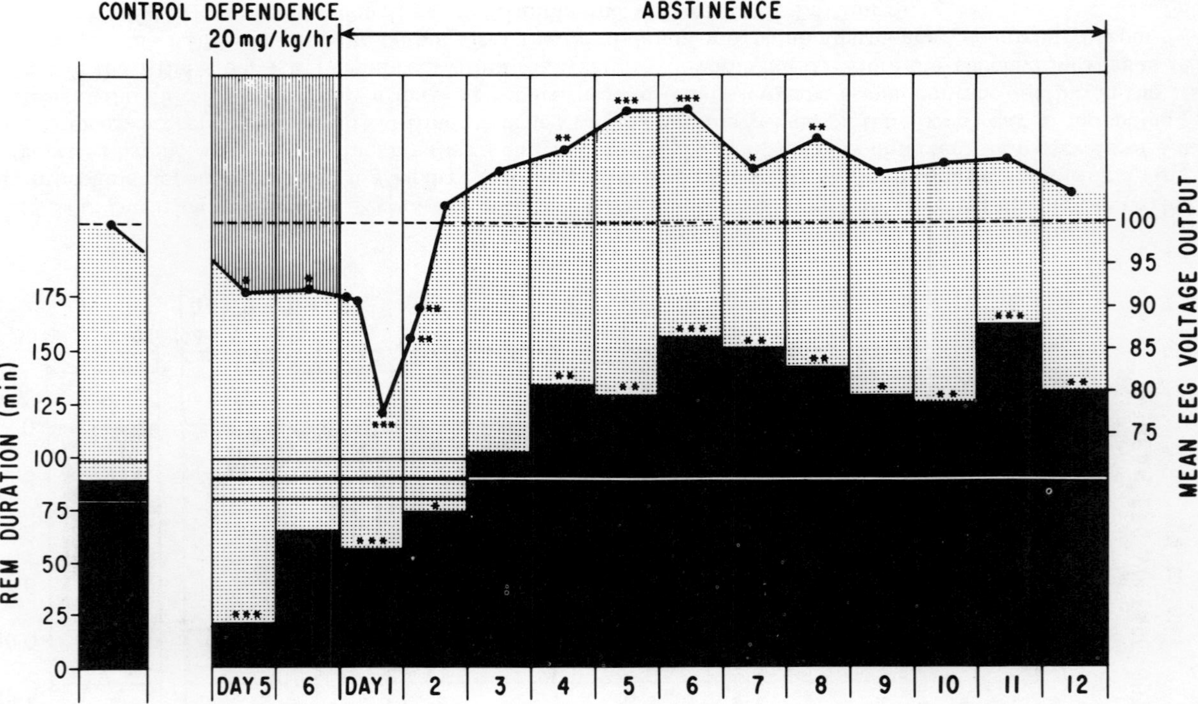

FIGURE 16. Changes in REM sleep time (lower solid black bars) and REM EEG voltage output (points on upper curve) in intervals of 1 day up to 12th day after withdrawal of morphine from dependent rats. Values for first 2 days of morphine abstinence represent periods of 0–4, 4–8, and 8–24 hr. The REM EEG voltage output remained significantly elevated on 8th day of abstinence, after which a trend toward higher levels continued. The postwithdrawal rebound in REM sleep time, which became manifest on 4th day, was still evident on 12th day of the experiment. (Each value represents the mean for 5 rats up to the 6th day and for 3 rats up to the 12th day; * signifies $P < 0.05$; **, $P < 0.01$; ***, $P < 0.001$.) (Reprinted from Khazan and Colasanti [84], p. 29, by courtesy of Williams and Wilkens Co., Baltimore.)

to man. The deprivation of REM sleep resulting from the administration of certain agents such as the tricyclic antidepressants imipramine and amitriptyline [87], and the monoamine oxidase inhibitor phenelzine [88], was followed by a rebound similar in extent to that after nonpharmacological REM deprivation.

Our results showed that the rebound increases in the REM sleep time of morphine-abstinent rats extended to 180% of the baseline value. Since the total loss of REM time during the addiction cycle and early withdrawal is 60% of the baseline value, we should expect a rebound of no more than 65-75% of this REM loss, which would amount to 140% of the baseline value. Since the actual gain in the REM sleep of morphine-abstinent rats was 80% above the baseline rather than the maximal 40% expected on the basis of Dement's work [86], this gain in REM sleep after withdrawal of morphine extended to twice the anticipated gain.

Another investigation was undertaken to explore the effects of imipramine, which suppresses REM sleep [89-91], on this phenomenon of delayed rebound excess of REM sleep in dependent rats withdrawn from morphine. After maintenance of dependent rats on the highest dose of morphine (20 mg/kg/hr) for 2 days, injections were discontinued. Chronic imipramine administration (10 mg/kg/6 hr) initiated upon the withdrawal of morphine was followed by REM sleep suppression throughout the 7 days of treatment. During this period the abstinence symptoms were highly intensified and prolonged. In a second group of animals, imipramine treatment initiated on the fourth day after morphine withdrawal likewise suppressed REM sleep but had minimal effects on the gross behavior of the abstinent rats [92] and on the protracted REM rebound following imipramine withdrawal (Fig. 17). It was assumed that the above modifications of morphine abstinence were due to the interaction of imipramine with the altered central adrenergic and cholinergic activities that follow the withdrawal of morphine.

The suppressant effect of opiates on sleep and REM sleep in experimental animals was also demonstrated in clinical studies [81,93]. Kay et al. [93] reported evidence of a delayed rebound excess of REM sleep subsequent to the initial suppression resulting from acute morphine administration. Moreover, after self-administration of heroin on a chronic basis, Lewis et al. [81] found that, although a gradual restoration of normal REM sleep time occurred during the period of administration, a long-term rebound in REM sleep remained evident for 2-3 months after the treatment. Our results obtained in the rat were in agreement with the clinical findings and supported the viewpoint of the existence of different mechanisms underlying the phenomenon of REM rebound resulting from addictive and nonaddictive agents [82,83].

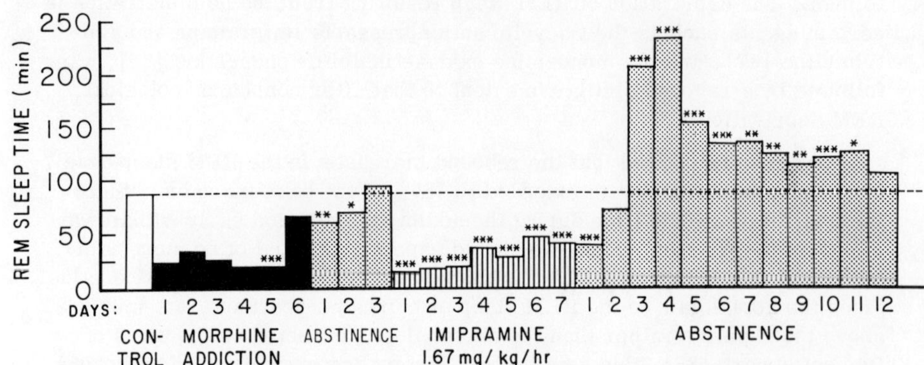

FIGURE 17. Changes in REM sleep time in morphine-abstinent rats treated with imipramine. Note the significant delay of REM rebound due to imipramine administration. Imipramine appears not to alter the course of protracted REM rebound phenomenon encountered with morphine abstinence (* signifies $P < 0.05$; **, $P < 0.01$; ***, $P < 0.001$). (Constructed from published data [92].)

D. Morphine Dependence: Pellet Implantation vs Intravenous Administration

In order to assess whether different methods used for the induction of dependence on morphine may yield different degrees of addiction and abstinence, the following experiments were undertaken. Rats prepared with chronic electrodes for recording the direct and the voltage-integrated EEG as well as the integrated EMG were made dependent on morphine by the technique of subcutaneous (sc) pellet implantation. This technique, originally described by Maggiolo and Huidobro [94] and subsequently modified by Way et al. [95], has been much used in recent studies on morphine dependence.

Two pellets, each containing 100 mg of morphine base, were implanted below the dorsal neck region of each rat and were then removed 72 hr later. The EEG and EMG recordings collected continuously revealed a marked suppression of the REM stage of sleep during the first 2 days after the implantation. By the third day, however, the duration of REM sleep had returned to the baseline values. Upon the removal of the morphine pellets, REM sleep time again became reduced within the first day but returned to the baseline levels by the second day of abstinence. A significant but short-lived rebound in REM sleep subsequently occurred on the third day, after which REM sleep duration returned to control values. These changes in

REM sleep time during abstinence were much less pronounced than those reported earlier for rats withdrawn from morphine administered iv [84]. The results of this study indicate that the changes resulting from addiction by these two different routes of morphine administration are qualitatively similar. However, a somewhat greater magnitude of change was observed in rats made dependent on morphine by the iv method [96].

E. Studies in Morphine Postaddicts

Altered responses to drugs in postaddict Macaca mulatta were reported to occur [97]. Effects of morphine addiction persisting for a long period after withdrawal in both experimental animals and man have been reported. These long-term effects of morphine encompass various physiological and behavioral changes. Cochin and Kornetsky [98] reported that loss of tolerance to morphine analgesia in the hot-plate procedure in previously addicted rats was not complete even up to 12 months after withdrawal of morphine. In a comprehensive study of morphine effects in the rat, Martin et al. [33] reported that the postaddict rat has greater spontaneous locomotor activity as well as slight elevations of body temperature and metabolic rate for as long as 4-6 months after morphine withdrawal. In man, physical signs of morphine abstinence persisted for at least 6 months [99]. Martin et al. [100] studied changes in the sensitivity of the respiratory center to CO_2 occurring upon withdrawal of morphine from human addicts. Whereas the state of hyposensitivity of this center persisted from the seventh through the thirteenth week after withdrawal, a marked increase in the sensitivity was initially manifested by 16-20 hr after withdrawal. In a biochemical study, Eisenman et al. [101] reported that human postaddicts excreted elevated levels of urinary epinephrine for at least 17 weeks following morphine withdrawal. More recently, a comparative study of several physiological parameters during tolerance and early and protracted abstinence in man was reported [102]. Pharmacological redundancy as an adaptive mechanism has been postulated and discussed [103].

Moreover, after a single dose of morphine, human postaddicts have shown some degree of behavioral stimulation, which is in contrast to the overall depressant effects seen in normal subjects. In other behavioral studies on postaddicts, a pattern of mental stimulation and euphoria following morphine administration was likewise reported [104,105]. A comparative study of the EEG and behavioral responses of naive and formerly addicted rats to acute morphine in our animal model was therefore initiated to examine such long-term morphine effects.

Predrug control recordings of the EEG and EMG of these rats were collected over a period of 2 hr. Then, a 10 mg/kg test dose of morphine or an equivalent volume of saline was administered ip, and polygraphic and behavioral correlates were collected over an additional period of 3-4 hr; this period often extended to the appearance of the first EEG, EMG, and behavioral sleep. As mentioned earlier, a morphine injection of 10 mg/kg into the naive rat was followed by a biphasic pattern of initial behavioral depression and subsequent stimulation. Morphine challenge to postaddict rats on the second day after the withdrawal of morphine induced a less pronounced effect wherein the duration of action was decreased by about 50%. The CNS depressant phase was only one-fourth that of the naive rats; the CNS stimulant phase, on the other hand, appeared to be relatively less affected. In contrast, morphine challenge to postaddict rats withdrawn for 7, 14, or 21 days induced an almost continuous state of behavioral arousal.

The postaddict rats given a morphine challenge 2, 4, or 6 months after morphine withdrawal were readily distinguishable from the naive rats simultaneously challenged. The EEG and behavioral correlates of these postaddicts did not show the typical biphasic pattern of depression and stimulation seen in the naives. Instead, episodes of EEG slow bursts and stuporous behavior alternated with periods of behavioral arousal. The rats challenged with morphine at the longer intervals after withdrawal showed progressively longer periods of initial behavioral stupor associated with EEG slow bursts, and their overall responses to morphine tended to approach the biphasic pattern seen in the naive rats [53], as shown in Fig. 18. In contrast to this group receiving only one morphine challenge, postaddict rats given repeated challenges during periods of up to 1 year after morphine withdrawal showed a more persistent arousal phase.

Follow-up studies were conducted with rats exposed to morphine (10 mg/kg) only twice weekly for 3 weeks [106]. Ten days after the last injection of morphine or saline a 10 mg/kg test dose of morphine was administered to both groups. Rats previously exposed exhibited an attenuation of the depressant phase, which was succeeded by the excitatory phase. Hence, the results of these experiments indicated a distinct difference in the EEG and behavioral responses to morphine challenge between rats having previous exposure to morphine and morphine-naive rats. This difference was clearly manifest in spite of a short period of exposure to morphine with a 10-day intervening period before the final morphine test dose.

A recent EEG study in the rat has supplied direct evidence of activation of the reward system and simultaneous depression of the punishment system following morphine administration [107]. This report also indicated that an "incubation period" of 2-7 days is required for the development of single-dose tolerance. In addition, the work of Kornetsky and Bain [108] demonstrated that tolerance became more pronounced at longer time intervals after the initial morphine injection.

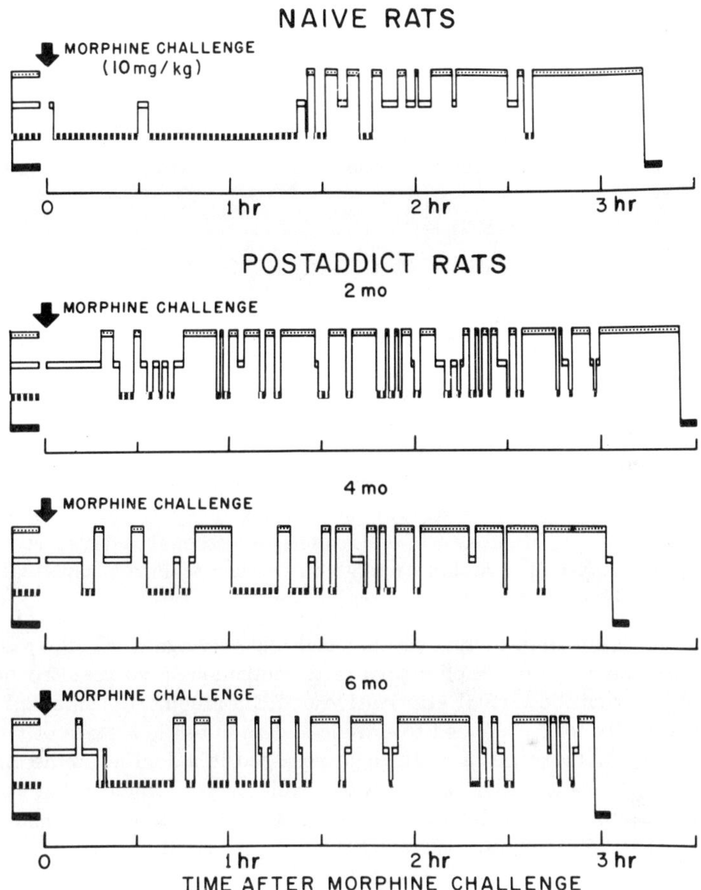

FIGURE 18. The responses of a naive and postaddict rat to a 10 mg/kg morphine test dose. Note the biphasic pattern of response of the naive rat in contrast to postaddicts. (See key in Fig. 9.)

Earlier, Cochin and Kornetsky [98] speculated the involvement of an antigen-antibody reaction that needed an incubation period for development and was strengthened by repeated exposure to single doses of morphine. A recent report has indicated that the mouse can be made to develop antibodies to morphine immunogen and that these antibodies can potentially modify the pharmacological effects of morphine [109]. Increased immunoglobulin M (IgM) concentrations, however, were recognized as a common immunological accompaniment to narcotic addiction [110]. Since the IgM changes decreased during methadone maintenance treatment [111], the clinical characteristics of patients with normal vs high serum IgM levels were further studied [112]. This study concluded that high serum IgM levels in methadone-treated addicts were associated with continuing drug abuse with laboratory evidence of continuing mild liver disease, or with both.

F. Studies with Other Addictive Agents

1. Methadone: EEG and Sleep-Awake Effects

In analogy to our morphine EEG studies, we have also evaluated the EEG correlates and the sleep-awake activity in rats during a cycle of methadone dependence and abstinence [113,114]. Tolerance and physical dependence to methadone were induced by automatic iv injections through chronic jugular cannulas, over a period comparatively longer than that for morphine, 8-10 days. The initial dose of methadone was 0.15 mg/kg given hourly for 24 hr. This dose was increased on successive days, reaching 2 mg/kg bihourly on the eighth or tenth day, when a state of physical dependence was achieved.

The initial dose of methadone induced high-voltage EEG slow waves during the awake state. Such exposure to methadone also resulted in decreased SWS and the virtual elimination of REM sleep. Repeated administration of methadone produced tolerance and resulted in a state of physical dependence. Withdrawal of methadone resulted in a decline in the EEG voltage output of the entire sleep-awake cycle, a phenomenon that correlated with the behavioral hyperirritability of the abstinent rat. The duration of SWS and REM sleep was enhanced from the fourth to the tenth hour during abstinence. Both sleep and REM sleep time then declined to minimal levels and remained below control baseline values up to the third day, after which a protracted REM rebound became evident and extended to the end of the twelfth and final day studied. The EEG and behavioral findings presented here provide evidence of the analogous states of dependence and abstinence induced by methadone and morphine following automatic iv administration and withdrawal [115] (see the reports of Henderson et al. [116], Kay and Martin [117], and Martin et al. [118] in this regard).

Such a model of addiction enabled us to assess the EEG effects and self-administration properties of the narcotics methadone and L-α-acetylmethadol (LAAM) when substituted for morphine in self-maintained dependent rats [118a]. While the pattern of sleep-awake distribution was analogous to that of morphine (Fig. 12), the duration of the interinjection intervals was distinctly different with these three narcotics. L-α-Acetylmethadol exhibited the longest interinjection intervals in the dependent rats that have free access to the lever, self-injecting the drug and titrating the dosage they need.

Furthermore, methadone administered by the iv route in the rat exhibited the shortest duration of effect, reflected by shorter interinjection intervals than morphine, similar to earlier findings in rhesus monkeys.* It is of interest to note that methadone exhibited a narrower margin of safety than morphine in self-maintained dependent rats.

2. Long-Term Effect of Ethanol Ingestion

In view of the long-term effects that persist after administration of morphine, an experiment was undertaken to determine whether alterations in CNS function persist after ethanol ingestion. Rats were fed 20% ethanol every 8 hr for 4-6 weeks. The total daily dosage was 1-9 mg/kg. After a 2-week period of gradual withdrawal, the animals were maintained with a naive group (unexposed to ethanol) for 6-8 months. The body weights of the naive and ethanol groups were comparable throughout the experiment. Both groups were then subjected to implantation of electrodes for chronic EEG and EMG recording. Administration of a 4 mg/kg test dose of ethanol by single oral injection resulted in a markedly greater suppression of REM activity in rats previously exposed to ethanol. A difference in both number and duration of episodes of REM sleep persisted during the 6 hr following ethanol challenge [119]. With the use of EEG, EMG, and sleep-awake activity studies in the chronic rat preparation, long-term modification in the CNS response to ethanol after ingestion of relatively modest doses of ethanol was demonstrated.

G. Studies with Nonaddictive CNS Active Agents: Marihuana Extract (Δ^8- and Δ^9-THC)

With the use of our chronic experimental animal, the administration of either marihuana extract, Δ^8-, or Δ^9-trans-tetrahydrocannabinol (Δ^8-THC or Δ^9-THC) was found to produce polyspike discharges in the EEG during the awake as well as the REM sleep state [120,121] (see Fig. 19). In the awake state, these high-voltage discharges in the EEG are superimposed on lower-voltage EEG tracings and were more plentiful upon repeated injections. Our findings, as well as the findings of others [122-124], with these psychotamimetic agents support and extend earlier observations in the rat, rabbit, and cat [125].

*C. Schuster, personal communication, 1973.

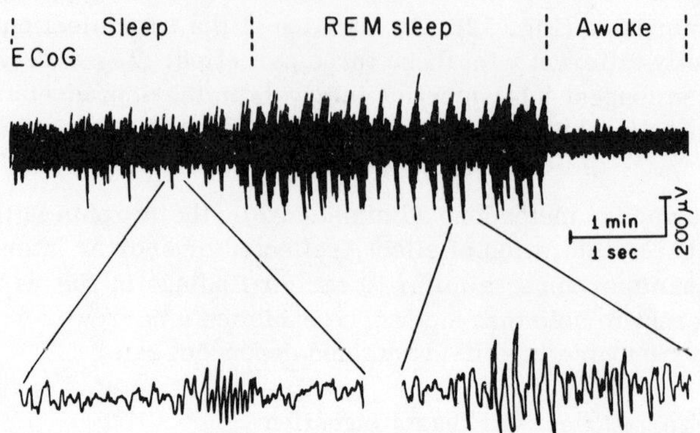

FIGURE 19. The development of rhythmic polyspike EEG discharges in the REM sleep state after Cannabis extract treatment. In this example, these bursts override the entire duration of the REM sleep episode. The higher-speed tracing compares the sleep spindle and the marihuana-induced burst. (Reprinted from Masur and Khazan [120], p. 1278, by courtesy of Pergamon Press, Elmsford, New York.)

IV. COMPARISON WITH OTHER PROCEDURES

The EEG technique we have been using enabled us to view the total process of addiction on morphine in the rat starting with the development of tolerance and physical dependence, to self-maintained addiction, up to the abstinence state. The EEG changes elucidated by these addiction studies in the rat are well defined and bear a close resemblance to those found in man. For example, the high-voltage EEG slow bursts induced by morphine in naive rats have also been reported to follow morphine administration in man. A protracted rebound in REM sleep time, reported in man to follow withdrawal of heroin, has been detected in our morphine-abstinent rats. Long-term effects of morphine explored in postaddict rats have been defined in EEG and behavioral terms and are reminiscent of the behavioral stimulation of human ex-addicts given morphine.

Many investigators have utilized the behavioral and self-administration technique in their studies of drug dependence in experimental animals [126-131]. However, only minor effort was made to incorporate the EEG-EMG correlates with the addiction and abstinence parameters [132]. On the other hand, clinical investigators have included the EEG correlates in their studies of narcotics and of narcotic antagonists in human subjects.

The efficacy and duration of action of a pure narcotic antagonist, such as naloxone, were ensured by determining the degree of blockade of the subjective "euphoria" and the EEG effects of heroin challenges in treated post-addict volunteers [133,134]. Analogous to these findings, naloxone blocked the EEG and behavioral effects of morphine in our experimental animal. These EEG studies offer valuable information of basic as well as applied importance, pertinent to the recent concept of the treatment of drug dependence, not with opioids [135,136], but rather with an opiate antagonist [137-141]. (See also studies of Wikler [142], Wikler and Pescor [143], and Goldberg and Schuster [144] on the involvement of conditioning in opiate addiction and relapse.)

Our method for the study of the EEG as a parameter representing brain activity during dependence and abstinence may be contrasted with other methods employing indirect parameters such as spontaneous motor activity, analgesia, pupil diameter, body weight, temperature and metabolic rate, jumping response, flexor reflexes, subjective ratings and reports, and respiratory sensitivity to CO_2 (for review, see Lewis et al. [145]). We feel, however, that the study of EEG correlates and sleep-awake pattern of activity offers a continuum of information that should help to further delineate the pharmacodynamics of opiates, opioids, and narcotic antagonists and postulate their possible clinical attributes.

V. SUMMARY AND CONCLUSIONS

The use of the rat model of opiate addiction described in this chapter permitted further insight into the pharmacodynamics of drug dependence. The longitudinal monitoring of the EEG-EMG and the sleep-awake activity of control, dependent, and abstinent rats made possible a thorough characterization of the process of the development of tolerance and physical dependence, the state of drug-seeking behavior, and the states of immediate and protracted abstinence. By means of the EEG-EMG parameters, long-term effects of morphine were determined. With this animal model, protracted REM sleep rebound, reported in man to follow abstinence from addictive agents, was reproduced in morphine- and methadone-dependent rats following withdrawal. The induction of EEG slow bursts by morphine, morphine-like narcotics, and morphine antagonist-analgesics was postulated to be an agonistic property of these agents. In contrast to narcotic antagonists with agonistic activity, such as nalorphine, the "pure" narcotic antagonist naloxone, while blocking morphine EEG effects, failed to induce these same effects. The probable involvement of brain amines in the EEG effects of morphine was also demonstrated.

In conclusion, repeated drug administration in conjunction with longitudinal recording of the EEG and EMG and analysis of sleep-awake activity should be applicable to the assessment of the basic properties and addictive liability of an analgesic agent. With these parameters, the relative potency, duration of effect, development of tolerance and physical dependence, intensity of drug-seeking behavior, severity of abstinence state, future relapse, and protracted abstinence can be simultaneously delineated. These parameters should provide a basis for the evaluation of the efficacy and duration of action of narcotic antagonists in the "deconditioning" process and suppression of drug-seeking behavior in postaddict rats relapsing to morphine self-administration. It also appears that the adaptation of this tool to the study of experimental addiction to drugs other than narcotics should prove beneficial. In addition, it is proposed that by the use of this experimental model, the study of acute and chronic EEG and behavioral correlates of nicotine, for example, should offer further insight into the pharmacodynamics of this agent.

ACKNOWLEDGMENTS

The author is extremely grateful to Dr. G. H. Acheson and Dr. J. E. Moreton for their critical evaluation in reviewing this chapter. Special thanks are due to Miss S. R. Tillett for her excellent assistance in the preparation of this manuscript.

REFERENCES

1. R. Caton, Brit. Med. J. 2:278 (1875).

2. H. Berger, Arch. Psychiat. Nervenkr. 87:527-570 (1929).

3. G. Moruzzi and H. W. Magoun, Electroencephalogr. Clin. Neurophysiol. 1:455-473 (1949).

4. P. B. Bradley and J. Elkes, Brain 80:77-117 (1957).

5. V. G. Longo, Electroencephalographic Atlas for Pharmacological Research. Rabbit Brain Research, Vol. 2. Amsterdam: Elsevier, 1962.

6. W. R. Adey, R. T. Kado, and J. M. Rhodes, Science 141:923-933 (1963).

7. M. A. B. Brazier, Clin. Pharmacol. Ther. 5:102-116 (1964).

8. N. Khazan, I. Kandalaft, and F. G. Sulman, Psychopharmacologia 10: 226-236 (1967).

9. A. Rechtschaffen and A. Kales, eds., A Manual of Standardized Terminology, Techniques and Scoring System for Sleep Stages of Human Subjects, National Institutes of Health Publ. no. 204. Washington, D.C.: Public Health Service, U. S. Govt. Printing Office, 1968.

10. W. R. Klemm, Animal Electroencephalography. New York: Academic Press, 1969.

11. N. Khazan, in An Introduction to Psychopharmacology (R. H. Rech and K. E. Moore, eds.). New York: Raven, 1971, pp. 175-211.

12. A. Wikler, Proc. Soc. Exp. Biol. Med. 29:261-265 (1952).

13. F. Rinaldi and H. E. Himwich, Arch. Neurol. Psychiat. 73:387-395 (1955).

14. W. Dement, Electroencephalogr. Clin. Neurophysiol. 10:291-296 (1958).

15. C. D. Clemente, Exp. Neurol. Suppl. 4:1-141 (1967).

16. M. Jouvet, in Psychopharmacology: A Review of Progress, 1957-1967 (D. H. Efron, ed.), Public Health Service Publ. no. 1836, Washington, D. C.: U. S. Govt. Printing Office, 1968, pp. 523-540.

17. E. Hartmann, ed., Sleep and Dreaming, Int. Psychiat. Clin., Vol. 7, Boston: Little, Brown, 1970, pp. 1-444.

18. E. Aserinsky and N. Kleitman, Science 118:273-274 (1953).

19. D. C. Kay, Psychosomatics 14:108-118 (1973).

20. N. Khazan and C. H. Sawyer, Proc. Soc. Exp. Biol. Med. 114:536-539 (1963).

21. N. Khazan, M. Kawakami, and C. H. Sawyer, Pharmacologist 5:266 (1963).

22. N. Khazan and C. H. Sawyer, Psychopharmacologia 5:457-466 (1964).

23. C. K. Himmelsbach, G. H. Gerlach, and E. J. Stanton, J. Pharmacol. Exp. Ther. 53:179-188 (1935).

24. S. Kaymakcalan and L. A. Woods, J. Pharmacol. Exp. Ther. 117:112-116 (1956).

25. L. M. Gunne, Arch. Int. Pharmacodyn. Ther. 129:416-428 (1960).

26. C. Hanna, Arch. Int. Pharmacodyn. Ther. 124:326-329 (1960).

27. A. Wikler, P. C. Green, H. D. Smith, and F. T. Pescor, Fed. Proc. Fed. Amer. Soc. Exp. Biol. 19:22 (1960).

28. J. R. Weeks, Science 138:143-144 (1962).

29. W. M. Davis and J. R. Nichols, Psychopharmacologia 3:139-143 (1962).

30. E. W. Maynert and G. I. Klingman, J. Pharmacol. Exp. Ther. 135: 285-295 (1962).

31. J. W. Sloan, J. W. Brooks, A. J. Eisenman, and W. R. Martin, Psychopharmacologia 3:291-301 (1962).

32. J. R. Weeks, Fed. Proc. Fed. Amer. Soc. Exp. Biol. 20:397 (1961).

33. W. R. Martin, A. Wikler, C. G. Eades, and F. T. Pescor, Psychopharmacologia 4:247-260 (1963).

34. J. R. Weeks, Science 138:143-144 (1962).

35. N. Khazan, in Drug Addiction: Experimental Pharmacology (J. M. Singh, L. H. Miller, and H. Lal, eds.), Vol. I. Mount Kisco, N.Y.: Futura, 1972, pp. 159-172.

36. J. R. Weeks, in Methods in Psychobiology (R. O. Myers, ed.), Vol. 2. New York: Academic Press, 1972, pp. 155-168.

37. D. Sutton and J. M. Miller, Science 140:988-989 (1963).

38. Z. Drohocki, Rev. Neurol. 80:619 (1948).

39. C. Munoz and L. Goldstein, J. Pharmacol. Exp. Ther. 132:354-359 (1961).

40. L. Goldstein, H. B. Murphree, and C. Pfeiffer, Ann. N. Y. Acad. Sci. 107:1045-1056 (1963).

41. L. Goldstein, H. B. Murphree, A. A. Sugarman, C. C. Pfeiffer, and E. H. Jenney, Clin. Pharmacol. Ther. 4:10-21 (1963).

42. W. R. Martin and C. G. Eades, Psychopharmacologia 1:303-335 (1960).

43. N. Khazan and B. Colasanti, J. Pharmacol. Exp. Ther. 177:491-499 (1971).

44. N. Khazan, J. R. Weeks, and L. A. Schroeder, J. Pharmacol. Exp. Ther. 155:521-531 (1967).

45. B. Colasanti and N. Khazan, Neuropharmacology 12:463-469 (1973).

46. H. L. Andrews, Psychosom. Med. 3:399-409 (1941).

47. R. L. Cahen and A. Wikler, Yale J. Biol. Med. 16:239-244 (1944).

48. A. Wikler and S. Altschul, J. Pharmacol. Exp. Ther. 98:437-446 (1950).

49. C. H. Sawyer, B. V. Critchlow, and C. A. Barraclough, Endocrinology 57:345-354 (1955).

50. L. Goldstein and J. Aldunate, J. Pharmacol. Exp. Ther. 130:204-211 (1960).

51. H. Isbell and H. F. Fraser, Pharmacol. Rev. 2:355-397 (1950).

52. A. Wikler, Pharmacol. Rev. 2:435-506 (195[illegible]).

53. N. Khazan and B. Colasanti, Psychopharmacologia 22:56-63 (1971).

54. B. Colasanti and N. Khazan, Fed. Proc. Fed. Amer. Soc. Exp. Biol. 31:304 (1972).

55. B. Colasanti and N. Khazan, Neuropharmacology 12:619-627 (1973).

56. B. Koe and A. Weissman, J. Pharmacol. Exp. Ther. 154:499-516 (1966).

57. E. Eidelberg and A. S. Schwartz, Nature (London) 225:1152-1153 (1970).

58. G. G. Yarbrough, D. M. Buxbaum, and E. Sanders-Bush, Life Sci. 10:977-983 (1971).

59. D. M. Buxbaum, G. G. Yarbrough, and M. E. Carter, J. Pharmacol. Exp. Ther. 185:317-327 (1973).

60. S. Spector, A. Sjoerdsma, and S. Udenfriend, J. Pharmacol. Exp. Ther. 147:86-95 (1965).

61. E. L. Way, H. H. Loh, and F. H. Shen, Science 162:1290-1292 (1968).

62. S. Algeri and E. Costa, Biochem. Pharmacol. 20:877-884 (1971).

63. D. L. Cheney and A. Goldstein, Science 171:1169-1170 (1971).

64. E. L. Way, Fed. Proc. Fed. Amer. Soc. Exp. Biol. 31:113-120 (1972).

65. W. D. M. Paton, Brit. J. Pharmacol. Chemother. 12:119-127 (1957).

66. E. A. Gyang and H. W. Kosterlitz, Brit. J. Pharmacol. Chemother. 27:514-527 (1966).

67. C. Pinsky and R. C. Fredrickson, Nature (New Biology) 231:94-96 (1971).

68. D. Beleslin and L. Polak, J. Physiol. (London) 177:411-419 (1965).

69. W. D. M. Paton, Can. J. Biochem. Physiol. 41:2637-2653 (1963).

70. M. Sharkawi and M. P. Shulman, J. Pharm. Pharmacol. 21:546-547 (1970).

71. E. F. Domino and A. Wilson, J. Pharmacol. Exp. Ther. 184:18-32 (1973).

72. E. F. Domino, M. Vasko, and A. Wilson, in Neurobiology (H. Lal and J. Singh, eds.). Mount Kisco, N. Y.: Futura, in press.

73. J. R. Weeks, L. A. Schroeder, and N. Khazan, Pharmacologist 6:183 (1964).

74. N. Khazan and J. R. Weeks, Pharmacologist 10:189 (1968).

75. J. R. Weeks and R. J. Collins, Psychopharmacologia 6:267-279 (1964).

76. R. J. Collins and J. R. Weeks, Arch. Exp. Pathol. Pharmakol. 249: 509-514 (1965).

77. W. R. Martin, Amer. J. Hosp. Pharm. 22:133-139 (1965).

78. N. Khazan, Fed. Proc. Fed. Amer. Soc. Exp. Biol. 29:780 (1970).

79. V. Synek, Int. Pharmacopsychiat. 2:99-109 (1969).

80. A. Wikler, J. Nerv. Ment. Dis. 120:157-175 (1954).

81. S. A. Lewis, I. Oswald, J. I. Evans, M. O. Akindele, and S. L. Thompsett, Electroencephalogr. Clin. Neurophysiol. 28:374-381 (1970).

82. A. Kales, E. J. Malmstrom, M. B. Scharf, and R. T. Rubin, in Sleep: Physiology and Pathology (A. Kales, ed.). Philadelphia: Lippincott, 1968, pp. 331-343.

83. I. Oswald, J. I. Evans, and S. A. Lewis, in Scientific Basis of Drug Dependence (H. Steinberg, ed.). London: Churchill, 1969, pp. 243-257.

84. N. Khazan and B. Colasanti, J. Pharmacol. Exp. Ther. 183:23-30 (1972).

85. N. Khazan and B. Colasanti, Psychophysiology 9:90 (1972).

86. W. Dement, Science 131:1705-1707 (1960).

87. E. Hartmann, Psychophysiology 5:207 (1968).

88. M. O. Akindele, J. I. Evans, and I. Oswald, Electroencephalogr. Clin. Neurophysiol. 29:47-56 (1970).

89. N. Khazan and P. Brown, Pharmacologist 11:255 (1969).

90. N. Khazan and P. Brown, Life Sci. 9:279-284 (1970).

91. A. Wasserman and N. Khazan, Pharmacologist 13:255 (1971).

92. M. Gold, B. Colasanti, and N. Khazan, Paper presented at the Fifth International Congress on Pharmacology, San Francisco, July 1972, p. 83.

93. D. C. Kay, R. B. Eisenstein and D. R. Jasinski, Psychopharmacologia 14:404-416 (1969).

94. C. Maggiolo and F. Huidobro, Acta Physiol. Lat. Amer. 11:70-78 (1961).

95. E. L. Way, H. H. Loh, and F. H. Shen, J. Pharmacol. Exp. Ther. 167:1-8 (1969).

96. N. Khazan, B. Colasanti, and A. Kirchman, Pharmacologist 13:314 (1971).

97. S. Irwin and M. H. Seevers, J. Pharmacol. Exp. Ther. 116:31-32 (1956).

98. J. Cochin and C. Kornetsky, J. Pharmacol. Exp. Ther. 145:1-10 (1964).

99. C. K. Himmelsbach, Arch. Intern. Med. 69:766-772 (1942).

100. W. R. Martin, D. R. Jasinski, J. D. Sapira, H. G. Franary, O. A. Kelly, A. K. Thompson, and C. R. Logan, J. Pharmacol. Exp. Ther. 162:182-189 (1968).

101. A. J. Eisenman, J. W. Sloan, W. R. Martin, and D. R. Jasinski, J. Psychiat. Res. 7:19-28 (1969).

102. W. R. Martin and D. R. Jasinski, J. Psychiat. Res. 7:9-17 (1969).

103. W. R. Martin, Fed. Proc. Fed. Amer. Soc. Exp. Biol. 29:13-18 (1970).

104. L. Lasagna, J. M. von Felsinger, and H. K. Beecher, J. Amer. Med. Ass. 157:1006-1020 (1955).

105. H. K. Beecher, Measurement of Subjective Responses: Quantitative Effects of Drugs, New York: Oxford Univ. Press, 1959.

106. P. Nash, B. Colasanti, and N. Khazan, Psychopharmacologia 29: 271-276 (1973).

107. J. M. Nelsen and C. Kornetsky, Paper presented at the Fifth International Congress on Pharmacology, San Francisco, July 1972, p. 166.

108. C. Kornetsky and G. Bain, Science 162:1011-1012 (1968).

109. B. Berkowitz and S. Spector, Science 178:1290-1292 (1972).

110. M. H. Grieco and C. Y. Chuang, J. Allergy Clin. Immunol. 51:152-160 (1973).

111. P. Cushman and M. H. Grieco, Amer. J. Med. 54:320-327 (1973).

112. P. Cushman, J. Allergy Clin. Immunol. 52:122-128 (1973).

113. T. Roehrs and N. Khazan, Pharmacologist 15:167 (1973).

114. N. Khazan and T. Roehrs, Pharmacologist 15:168 (1973).

115. N. Khazan and T. Roehrs, in Drug Addiction (H. Lal and J. Singh, eds.), Vol. 3. New York: Stratton Intercontinental Medical Book Corp., 1974, pp. 335-342.

116. A. Henderson, G. Nemes, N. B. Gordon, and L. Roos, Psychophysiology 7:346-347 (1970).

117. D. C. Kay and W. R. Martin, Psychophysiology 9:95 (1972).

118. W. R. Martin, D. R. Jasinski, C. A. Haertzen, D. C. Kay, B. E. Jones, P. A. Mansky, and R. W. Carpenter, Arch. Gen. Psychiat. 28:286-295 (1972).

118a. J. Moreton, T. Roehrs, and N. Khazan, Fed. Proc. Fed. Amer. Soc. Exp. Biol. 23:516 (1974).

119. S. Gitlow, S. Bentkover, S. Dziedzic, and N. Khazan, Fed. Proc. Fed. Amer. Soc. Exp. Biol. 32:729 (1973); Psychopharmacologia 33:135-140 (1973).

120. J. Masur and N. Khazan, Life Sci. 9:1275-1280 (1970).

121. B. Colasanti and N. Khazan, Pharmacologist 13:246 (1971).

122. E. S. Boyd, E. H. Boyd, J. S. Muchmore, and L. E. Brown, J. Pharmacol. Exp. Ther. 176:480-488 (1971).

123. J. E. Moreton and W. M. Davis, Neuropharmacology 12:897-907 (1973).

124. J. L. Martinez, Jr., S. W. Stadnicki, and U. H. Schaeppi, Life Sci. 11:643-651 (1972).

125. F. Lipparini, A. S. De Carolis, and V. G. Longo, Physiol. Behav. 4:527-532 (1969).

126. M. H. Seevers and G. A. Deneau, in Physiological Pharmacology (W. S. Root and F. G. Hofmann, eds.), Vol. 1. New York: Academic Press, 1963, pp. 565-640.

127. J. E. Villarreal, in Drug Dependence (R. T. Harris, W. M. McIsaac, and C. R. Schuster, eds.), Part II, Chap. 9. Austin, Texas: Univ. of Texas Press, 1970, pp. 83-116.

128. S. R. Goldberg, J. H. Woods, and C. R. Schuster, Science 166:1306-1307 (1969).

129. C. R. Schuster and T. Thompson, Annu. Rev. Pharmacol. 9:483-502 (1969).

130. R. D. Hindman, J. M. Miller, E. R. Meyer, and J. Cochin, Pharmacologist 13:262 (1971).

131. S. R. Goldberg, J. H. Woods, and C. R. Schuster, J. Pharmacol. Exp. Ther. 176:464-471 (1971).

132. H. Takagi, H. Aishita, and K. Yamatsu, Jap. J. Pharmacol. 19: 174-175 (1969).

133. M. Fink, A. Zaks, R. Sharoff, A. Mora, A. Bruner, S. Levit, and A. M. Freedman, Clin. Pharmacol. Ther. 9:568-577 (1968).

134. J. Volavka, A. Zaks, J. Roubicek, and M. Fink, Neuropharmacology 9:587-593 (1970).

135. V. P. Dole and M. E. Nyswander, J. Amer. Med. Ass. 193:646-650 (1965).

136. R. Levine, A. Zaks, M. Fink, and A. M. Freedman, J. Amer. Med. Ass. 226:316-318 (1973).

137. W. R. Martin, C. W. Gorodetzky, and T. K. McClane, Clin. Pharmacol. Ther. 7:455-465 (1966).

138. J. H. Jaffe and L. Brill, Int. J. Addict. 1:99-123 (1966).

139. J. H. Jaffe, Curr. Psychiat. Ther. 3:147-156 (1967).

140. D. R. Jasinski, W. R. Martin, and C. A. Haertzen, J. Pharmacol. Exp. Ther. 157:420-426 (1967).

141. W. R. Martin, D. R. Jasinski, and P. A. Mansky, Arch. Gen. Psychiat. 28:784-791 (1973).

142. A. Wikler, in Narcotics (D. M. Wilner and G. G. Kassebaum, eds.). New York: McGraw-Hill, 1965, pp. 85-100.

143. A. Wikler and F. T. Pescor, Psychopharmacologia 10:255-284 (1967).

144. S. R. Goldberg and C. R. Schuster, J. Exp. Anal. Behav. 14:33-46 (1970).

145. J. W. Lewis, K. W. Bentley, and A. Cowan, Ann. Rev. Pharmacol. 11:241-270 (1971).

Chapter 10

CONDITIONING TECHNIQUES IN THE STUDY OF REINFORCEMENT MECHANISMS AND THE SELF-ADMINISTRATION OF DEPENDENCE-PRODUCING DRUGS*

W. MARVIN DAVIS

Department of Pharmacology
School of Pharmacy
The University of Mississippi
University, Mississippi

STANLEY G. SMITH

Department of Pharmacology
Department of Psychology
The University of Mississippi
University, Mississippi

*Preparation of this manuscript was supported by USPHS Grant DA 00018-07 from the National Institute on Drug Abuse and by the Research Institute of Pharmaceutical Sciences, School of Pharmacy, The University of Mississippi, University, Mississippi.

I. INTRODUCTION

The use of conditioning methods for the analysis of behavioral control by dependence-producing drugs is an increasingly popular area of research [1]. As a consequence of this research activity, techniques have been developed for the direct study of the determinants and effects of drug-taking behavior [2]. The most fruitful of these have been the drug self-administration procedures which provide a paradigm of value for: (a) the experimental investigation of behavioral properties of dependence-producing drugs in lower organisms to obtain information which can be applied to human drug-taking behavior; (b) broad multidisciplinary efforts to elucidate the psychological, pharmacological, and neurochemical mechanisms underlying drug dependence; and (c) the classifying of new drugs and the prediction of their abuse potential in man. This chapter is a brief review of some of the self-administration methods with an emphasis on how to use conditioning techniques. It is intended not only to give the new researcher some background on the various techniques, but also to present practical aspects usually obtainable only from actual experience in a behavioral laboratory.

II. TECHNIQUES

Among the several different modes of administration utilized in the study of drug-taking behavior [2], three currently in use, the peroral, the intragastric, and the intravenous self-administration methods, are described briefly in this section.

A. Peroral Self-Administration

The peroral (po) approach (see Fig. 1 for an unautomated experimental setting) was one of the earliest and simplest laboratory techniques devised for the analysis of narcotic drug dependence [3-5]. The main problem with this procedure is that most narcotics such as morphine have a very bitter taste to man and are normally rejected by rats when offered in an aqueous solution. To circumvent this problem, procedures were developed for inducing the drinking of narcotic solutions through forced drinking trials following the preliminary development of a state of physical dependence.

One of the first procedures for obtaining morphine-drinking behavior was described by Nichols and co-workers [3]. Physical dependence was established via daily intraperitoneal injections of morphine. The injections were started at 20 mg/kg and increased progressively by equal increments to 160 mg/kg on the 29th day. Following the establishment of physical dependence, rats were given "escape training" which consisted of 24 hr without liquids (0), 24 hr access to 0.5 mg/ml morphine hydrochloride solution (M), and 24 hr access to tap water (W). The training proceeded in the above sequence for 9 days (i.e., 0, M, W, 0, M, W) during which the liquid container, a 100-ml graduated drinking tube (see Fig. 1), was randomly placed to the right or left side of the front of the cage. To test drug-taking behavior,

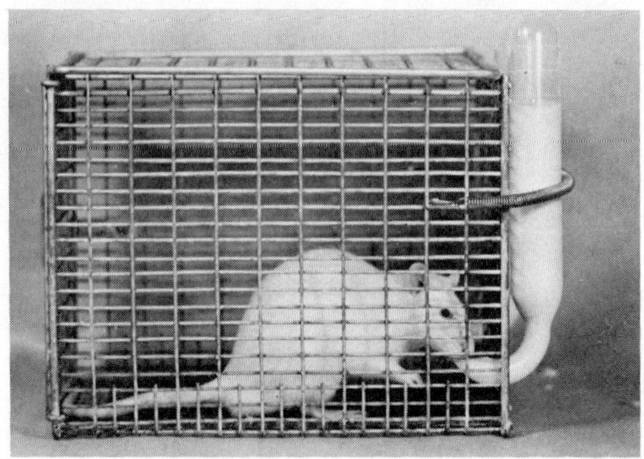

FIGURE 1. A typical arrangement for oral drug self-administration studies. In a choice situation two such graduated drinking tubes may be used to present both a drug solution and tap water. To facilitate photographic visualization, milk rather than an aqueous solution was placed in the tube.

five "choice tests" were given, each following a 9-day training sequence. For the choice days, two drinking tubes, one containing water and the other a morphine solution, were presented simultaneously (left and right positions on the front of the cage) for a 24-hr period and the amount of morphine solution selected was measured. In the same fashion, "relapse tests" were conducted after several weeks of abstinence from opiate and removal from the drinking environment. These revealed a lengthy retention of morphine drinking by some rats.

An oral procedure devised by Kumar et al. [6] did not require premedication to induce dependence. The animals were placed on a 7-hr access to water regime and quickly became accustomed to relieving their normal thirst during this period. Following this period, continuous access to a 0.5 mg/ml morphine solution in one group of subjects or to a quinine solution (0.5 mg/ml) in a second group was given for 7 hr daily for 1 month with no other liquid available. On the first and third days following the training, choice trials were given with both morphine and water available, as in Nichols' procedure. The results indicated that only the morphine access group developed a preference for morphine on the choice trials.

Experimenters who have used procedures similar to those described above record as their dependent variable the amount of drug solution imbibed, or in some cases the number of laps at the drinking spouts is determined by electronic drinkometers, which can be purchased commercially or easily constructed [7].

To validate the peroral self-administration procedure as a model for narcotic abuse behavior, it has been shown that rats greatly increase their ingestion of the drug solution following forced training, whereas they do not so respond to quinine solutions of bitterness equal to that of morphine [3, 8]. Therefore, the increase in morphine preference does not reflect merely a progressive desensitization of the taste mechanism to the aversive taste [9]. Also, experiments have shown that when rats were deprived of morphine after developing a morphine preference, they lost weight markedly [9]. The abrupt weight loss is one reliable sign of withdrawal in rats [10].

Probably the strongest validation of the po method was provided by Kumar et al. [11]. After establishing drug preference, various doses of morphine were given subcutaneously to different groups of rats 30 min before choice trials. There was a reduction in morphine ingestion that was directly proportional to the dosage of the preinjected drug, whereas the total fluid intake during the drinking period was unaffected. Therefore, the same stimulus (morphine) which elicited morphine-drinking behavior was shown upon prior injection to selectively inhibit this behavior, further attesting to the behavioral control properties of the drug.

An interesting procedure and one that extends previous methods in oral self-administration has been reported by Filewich.* The method employed a home-cage drink cycle and home-cage preference test based on the technique of Kumar et al. [6]. The procedure also employed a lever-press response for securing oral morphine or quinine in a self-administration chamber (see Fig. 2 for an illustration of a similar self-administration chamber and liquid delivery pump).

More specifically, water-satiated rats were given an opportunity to lever press for aqueous solutions of morphine (0.5 mg/ml) and quinine (0.5 mg/ml). All rats were maintained on a morphine or quinine drinking cycle in their home cage. Rats that received quinine solution in their home cage showed a continued preference for water when given preference tests of water vs quinine in the home cage. These same subjects maintained a low, stable rate of lever pressing for both morphine and quinine. In contrast, subjects that received morphine solution as the drug in the home cage developed a preference for it over water in the preference tests. These rats also displayed a relatively high and stable rate of lever pressing for morphine. Substitution of quinine resulted in extinction of lever-pressing behavior. Reacquisition and reextinction were also demonstrated for these animals. Thus, considerable evidence has been amassed to validate po self-administration as a laboratory method for the analysis of narcotic dependence.

B. Intragastric Self-Administration

The intragastric (ig) method is a relatively new self-administration technique that offers an interesting alternative to the po methods. It bypasses the oral sensory mechanisms and yet delivers the drug to essentially the same drug disposition chain: stomach, intestine, venous circulation of the viscera, and systematic blood stream. Being able to bypass the oral sensory system enables the study of drugs that have an aversive taste without using forced training procedures that previously were necessary to obtain good oral self-administration of drugs. The further requirement of establishing physical dependence or imposing liquid deprivation has prevented the study of completely self-initiated acquisition of narcotic-taking behavior by nondependent rats. With the ig technique it is now possible to develop a more complete paradigm taking into account conditioning principles governing the initial acquisition of drug-taking behavior. Research on ig self-administration of narcotic drugs has been carried out by Gotestam [12] and in our laboratory [13,14]. Gotestam's technique involves opening

*Personal communication, 1974.

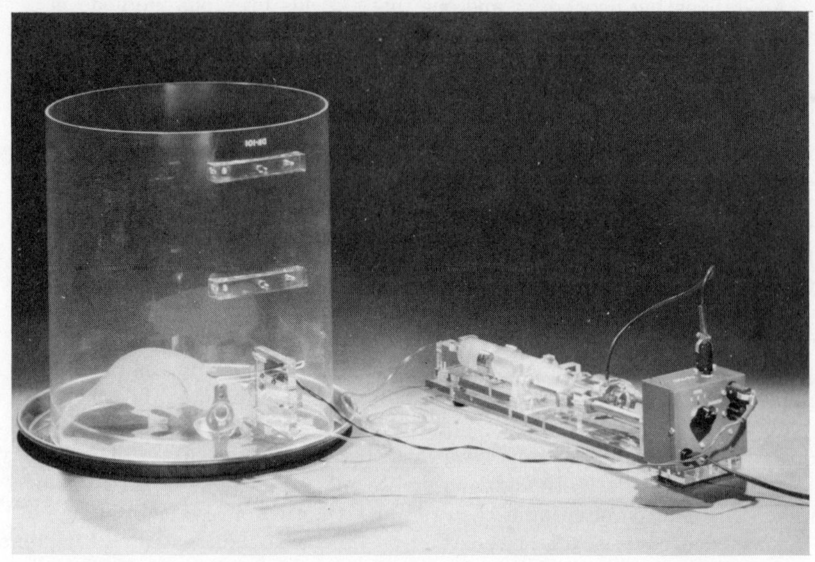

FIGURE 2. Simulated oral self-administration setting for morphine. A lever press activates the liquid pump (right side), which delivers the solution through clear vinyl tubing to a metal cup shown in the lower center of the experimental chamber. This setting is similar to that used by Filewich. (Photograph courtesy of Davis Scientific Instruments, 11116 Cumpston St., North Hollywood, California 91601.)

the abdomen to expose the stomach, making an incision in the stomach, and placing into the stomach a 12-mm diameter plastic button with a polyethylene tubing attached. After the stomach wound is closed, the tubing is brought out of the abdomen through the muscle incision; the abdomen is then closed and the tubing is carried under the skin to the dorsal neck region where it is anchored to neck muscles and brought out through a skin incision. The anchoring and exiting procedure is similar to Weeks' method [15] of neck anchoring and exiting for intravenous cannulas. The rats are allowed 1 week to recover from surgery; if they are introduced into the research setting earlier, they die from gastric hemorrhages. This preparation is said to have a life span of 2 months after catheterization [12].

We have developed a new surgical method that involves placing a considerably smaller ig catheter, the type II catheter described in Chapter 1, into the esophagus via the neck, not the mouth. The surgery required for this procedure is similar to that for a jugular catheter (procedure 2,

Chapter 1) except that the incision is made on the midline of the throat and the cannula is inserted into the esophagus rather than into the jugular vein. The procedure is simple, it allows the rats to eat and drink normally, and it can be used for long-term research. With this technique no damage to the stomach can occur and so no ulceration is possible. Therefore, a period of only 24-48 hr is required for recovery from surgery before beginning experimentation. Using this method we have demonstrated self-administration behavior for morphine in our laboratory [13,14].

C. Intravenous Self-Administration

Since the initial development of the intravenous self-administration technique [16], it has become the most widely used research method for the analysis of drug-taking behavior. Already much has been accomplished with this model that provides insight into the behavioral principles governing the acquisition and maintenance of, and the reacquisition or relapse to, drug-taking behavior. Several general reviews are available [1,2,9,17]. From this research, methods for eliminating drug-taking behavior have also come [18,19].

Researchers planning to use the intravenous self-administration technique should be aware that it requires much greater technical expertise than the oral procedures; that is, methodological knowledge of cannula construction, surgical skills, and more complex apparatus are necessary. Descriptions of cannula construction, surgery, and apparatus used for the rat are given by Weeks [15] and Smith and Davis (Chapter 1). A typical experimental setting is shown in Fig. 3.

III. NARCOTICS SELF-ADMINISTERED

As the model compound for opiate research, morphine has been the focus of most self-administration studies on the opium alkaloids; a representative selection of such studies can be found in Refs. 5, 6, 16, 20-23. Only a few reports are at hand concerning other opiates, namely heroin [24], codeine [25-27], and dihydromorphinone [27].

A greater number of the synthetic analgesics have been tested and found to be self-administered by laboratory animals. However, here also the extent of published research is limited, compounds reported being methadone [28,29], etonitazene [30,31], meperidine [32], propiram fumarate [33], pentazocine [33,34], propoxyphene [33,35,36], and profadol [37].

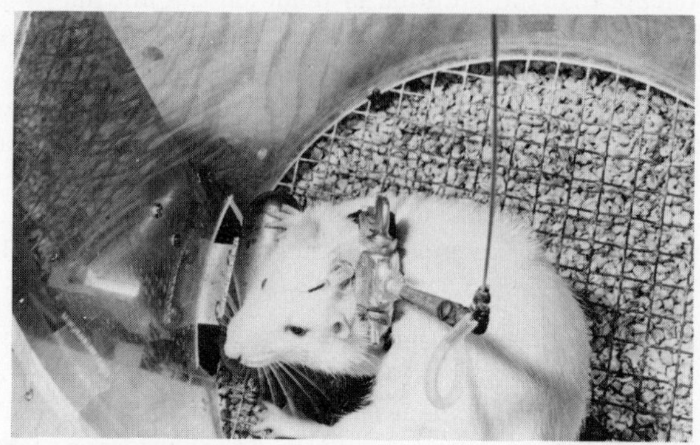

FIGURE 3. A typical arrangement for intravenous drug self-administration studies. Depression of the lever at the left causes the injection of a small quantity of drug solution. A pump located outside the sound-attenuating enclosure is attached to an injection system that leads to the animal via the needle tubing attached to the saddle worn by the rat. Attached to the injection system at the saddle is an implanted jugular cannula, visible at the midline between the ears of the rat.

IV. INITIAL RESPONSE TRAINING

In the past it was necessary for an experimenter to learn the "art of hand shaping" to obtain lever-pressing behavior for an intravenous or intragastric infusion of a drug. Hand shaping involved the paired presentation of a stimulus (e.g., buzzer, tone, or change in illumination) with an infusion of the drug. Usually 25-50 such pairings are presented. They are given randomly, usually dispersed over a 2- or 3-hr session. The pairings are given to enable an animal to learn to discriminate that the presentation of a buzzer (or another stimulus) is followed by a drug infusion. The experimenter then awaits the approach of a subject to the vicinity of the lever, upon which the buzzer and drug infusion are presented. This is repeated 15-20 times. The rats quickly learn to approach the lever. The experimenter next presents the buzzer and drug infusion only if the rat touches the lever and finally only for an actual depression of the lever. Rats can be thus hand shaped to lever press in one to three sessions. Because this procedure required the continuous presence of the experimenter to monitor behavior and to deliver buzzer and drug infusions (reinforcement), it was time-consuming, boring, and difficult for some to learn. A number of simple techniques have been used in our laboratory for obtaining lever-pressing behavior without hand shaping. Which procedure to adopt is a matter of personal preference and available equipment.

A. Method I: Autoshaping

An automated procedure for obtaining lever pressing for food [38] is also effective for drugs. The procedure is started with a fixed 40-sec intertrial interval (ITI) in which no manipulations are made, a dead period. At the termination of the ITI, a Plexiglas response manipulandum with a light inside of it is illuminated for 30 sec. Immediately following the 30-sec period, the light in the manipulandum is turned off and the drug is infused. However, if the subject responds on the lever during the lighted interval, the light is immediately turned off and the drug is infused. Some experience in our laboratory suggests that longer ITIs and longer illumination of the manipulandum may be of value. Such longer intervals would be more beneficial if the unit dosage of solution were medium or high, producing a rather extended duration of the reinforcing action of a drug. We have also found variable ITIs to be effective. The procedure for programming variable ITIs is identical to that for the variable interval reinforcement schedule discussed later in this chapter.

B. Method II: Response Elicitation

This method involves placing the animal on food deprivation (removing all food) for 24 hr before the experimental session. Prior to the session 3 or 4 Noyes food pellets (3.2-mm x 2.5-mm tablets weighing 45 mg which are employed as food reinforcements for small laboratory animals) are stuck to the response manipulandum with cellophane tape. In the process of securing the food pellets the subject activates the response manipulandum and causes the drug to be administered. A similar procedure that does not require deprivation is to place a highly preferred substance (e.g., a small amount of bacon grease) on the lever.

C. Method III: Small Experimental Chamber

In our laboratory we use self-administration chambers that are Plexiglas cylinders 24 cm in height and 25 cm in diameter. No hand shaping is required because the chambers are of optimal size for inducing an accidental lever-pressing rate high enough that self-administration is easily acquired by rats with drugs such as morphine or d-amphetamine. A very similar chamber can be purchased from Davis Scientific Instruments, 11116 Cumpston Street, North Hollywood, California 91601.

D. Method IV: Temporarily Reducing the Experimental Space

This method involves constructing a Plexiglas cubicle to use with existing equipment larger than that described above (method III) so as to force the subject into close proximity to the lever (see Cahoon and Crosby [39] for details on assembly of such a cubicle). By reducing the experimental space, the probability is increased for random contact with and depression of the lever. Once self-administration behavior has been acquired, the partition may be removed.

V. INTERMITTENT SCHEDULES OF DRUG REINFORCEMENT

Whenever delivery of a drug is contingent upon some, but not all, occurrences of lever-pressing behavior, an intermittent schedule of drug reinforcement is operating. That is, during intermittent reinforcement only selected responses are reinforced, i.e., followed by drug. The criteria for selecting such occurrences on intermittent schedules of drug reinforcement are either the number of responses (ratio schedule) or the period of time between availability of the drug (interval schedule). Each schedule of drug reinforcement has particular characteristics that exert a regular and orderly influence on the pattern of behavior emitted during self-administration. It is because of these characteristics and their predictability that schedules of reinforcement have become prominent in drug self-administration research.

Detailed information is not currently available in the pharmacology literature on how to program an intermittent schedule of reinforcement, or how to adjust the schedule requirement from continuous reinforcement (drug presentation following each response) to intermittent reinforcement. The methods constitute an "uncommunicated art" for those who have personally worked in an operant conditioning laboratory. Without such knowledge a researcher may be unable to obtain the schedule performance, and his subjects may stop responding. With some simple instruction this need not happen.

A. Ratio Schedules

Ratio schedules are operative when the animal must emit a certain number of responses before a reinforcer (drug) is presented. The term "ratio" refers to the total number of responses the organism must emit between successive reinforcements. There are two types of ratio schedules fixed ratios and variable ratios. The term fixed ratio (FR) indicates that a fixed number of responses must be emitted before each reinforcement. For example, FR 1 means that one response must be emitted before the next presentation of the reinforcer (also known as continuous reinforcement), FR 2 means that two responses must be emitted, and FR 50 means that 50 responses must be emitted before presentation of the reinforcer. Each time the subject is reinforced, the schedule requirement is renewed so that the subject must again emit the number of responses required by the ratio.

Difficulties may arise when a researcher new to this area reads that a FR 50 or FR 100 was used in a particular experiment. What is not stated, but always assumed to be understood by the reader, is that a progressively increasing ratio ("adjusting schedule") was used to achieve the FR 50 or FR 100. That is, the subject is first trained on FR 1 for part of a training session (25 or more reinforcements) to establish the self-administration behavior. Then the ratio requirement is established by slowly increasing the ratio, e.g., FR 2, FR 3, FR 5, FR 15, FR 25, FR 50, FR 70, etc., until the terminal requirement is achieved. The animal is usually given 10-20 reinforcements at each ratio requirement before moving on to the next. Without the adjusting schedule, a ratio requirement of 50 or 100 would be too high and the subject would just stop responding, i.e., extinguish. The performance characteristic for a fixed ratio is emission of the responses for the ratio requirement at an accelerated rate (one response following the other in rapid succession) and then a pause for a short period during and after the drug presentation (reinforcement). The final performance characteristics of the FR depend on: (a) how high the ratio requirement is, i.e., FR 50 vs FR 100; (b) the unit dosage of the drug maintaining each ratio, i.e., 60 μg/kg/injection vs 120 μg/kg/injection; and (c) the setting conditions, e.g., degree of physical dependence or interval since the last injection.

Another important point is that stable responding does not appear in a single session following achievement of the final FR requirement (i.e., FR 50 or FR 100). It may take 7-12 sessions or more before stable behavior is observed. The term stable refers to the behavioral characteristics of the FR described above that do not change over the period studied. A good experimental index for assessing when stability has been achieved is that of Schoenfeld et al. [40]. Self-administration of narcotic drugs on a fixed ratio has been demonstrated in a number of cases [16,22,32,41, 42].

A second type of ratio schedule is the variable ratio (VR). With the variable ratio a drug infusion (reinforcement) occurs after a given number of responses, the number varying randomly between successive reinforcements. The VR schedule is established around some mean number of responses. For example, VR 10 refers to the fact that, on the average, 10 responses will be required for reinforcement during the experimental session. To program a VR 10 schedule, the experimenter could reinforce responses (present the drug following a response) on a schedule similar to the following:

Unit Values for a VR 10 Schedule
(Total Responses Required
Following Each Reinforcement)

	1
	4
	8
	12
	16
	20
Total	61
Mean = 10 (VR 10)	

The unit values are then randomized to form a series comprised of at least three different complete sequences of the unit values. The random series is necessary to prevent the animals from learning the ratio requirements of a fixed series. An example of a random series is: 1, 4, 8, 12, 16, 20; 20, 16, 12, 8, 4, 1; 8, 12, 4, 16, 1, 20. This series would be repeated throughout the experiment.

Initially, the variable ratio (like the FR) must be presented on an adjusting schedule, e.g., VR 3, 5, 10, 15, 20, ..., N similar to the FR. If the VR requirement is advanced too rapidly the behavior of an animal will become erratic, and the response may be extinguished. Should this occur, one must return to FR 1 or to a lower VR requirement and progress upward again more slowly. Another means for adjusting a ratio behavior before placement on a VR schedule is to train the animal to a FR value higher than the highest ratio requirement of the terminal series of the VR, and then to transfer the subject to the VR. For example, if the terminal VR value is to be VR 20, the lowest value in the schedule might be 1 and the highest value 40. Therefore, the subject would be trained to FR 50 before switching to VR 20.

The characteristic performance observed with VR schedules is a very high rate of responding with no pauses between reinforcements. To date the only study using a VR schedule for drug self-administration of which we are aware is one with morphine carried out in our laboratory in which good VR schedule control was observed.*

*S. G. Smith and W. M. Davis, unpublished data, 1972.

B. Interval Schedules

An interval schedule is one in which a given interval of time elapses before a response will be reinforced. The temporal interval can be measured from any event, but reinforcement is the usual reference point. With drug self-administration the reference point should be the end of the drug infusion interval. There are two types of interval schedules, fixed interval (FI) and variable interval (VI). The FI schedule requires that a fixed time period must elapse, followed by a response, before reinforcement (drug) is provided. Thus, an FI 1 min refers to the fact that following the previous reinforcement 1 min must elapse, and a response must be emitted before presentation of the reinforcer.

The FI performance differs from the previous schedules in that a "scallop pattern" of responding emerges. That is, a pause occurs following reinforcement, and as the time interval progresses the response rate increases progressively so that the highest rate is emitted just prior to reinforcement. To obtain FI performance, an adjusting FI schedule of some sort may be required for long FIs (i.e., above FI 5 min), but not for short FIs (i.e., below FI 5 min). For long FIs, adjustment in 2-min increments can be used up to 10 min. Rarely is an FI over 10 min used in research.

Research on fixed-interval self-administration has been carried out by Dougherty and Pickens.* A number of different FI values were used in their study, and the amount of scallop (pause after drug presentation) was directly related to the value of the FI (i.e., the longer the FI, the more pronounced the scallop). To assess FI or VI stability one may use the index of Schoenfeld et al. [40].

The second type of interval schedule, the VI schedule, is one in which the time intervals between reinforcement vary randomly. This schedule is designed to produce a constant, moderate rate of lever pressing. To program a VI the several intervals, like unit ratios of a VR, are arranged around a mean, in this case the mean interval. For example, VI 60 sec refers to a VI schedule which has a mean interval of 60 sec and for which the lowest interval might be 0 and the highest interval might be 120 sec. Thus, the necessary array of intervals could be chosen as follows:

---

*J. Dougherty and R. Pickens, personal communication, 1973.

Unit Intervals in Series, i.e., Response Reinforced after Interval of	
	0 sec
	20 sec
	40 sec
	60 sec
	80 sec
	100 sec
	120 sec
Total	420 sec
Mean = 60 sec (VI 60)	

Like the VR, the VI should be programmed as a randomized series composed of at least three different sequences of the individual units. An example is: 0, 20, 40, 60, 80, 100, 120; 20, 60, 120, 100, 0, 40, 80; 120, 100, 80, 60, 40, 20, 0. This is done to ensure that the subject does not learn to discriminate the schedule sequence. To obtain the desired VI performance, an adjusting schedule should be used. For example, begin with VI 8.5 sec, move up to VI 30 sec and then to VI 60 sec or until the terminal VI requirement is reached. Some researchers would place the subject on an adjusting FR to reach FR 50 and then change to the terminal VI requirement.

Research with the VI schedule during self-administration of opioids has been limited [26,43]. Because the use of intermittent schedules of reinforcement in self-administration research is becoming more prevalent, any researcher interested in this area of experimentation should become familiar with the schedules of reinforcement.

VI. PROBLEMS OF ASSESSING DRUG INTERACTION

A. Baseline Techniques

A number of studies in recent years have measured the effect that treating an organism with another drug might have on opioid self-administration behavior. Such efforts are intended to determine whether the test drug can exert an interactive effect. Such research has been conducted with the narcotic antagonists naloxone and nalorphine [33,44], with an inhibitor of brain serotonin synthesis, p-chlorophenylalanine [45], with a general inhibitor of brain catecholamine synthesis, α-methyltyrosine [45], and with a specific brain dopamine receptor blocking agent, haloperidol

[45,46]. This research indicated that the narcotic antagonists, the amine biosynthesis inhibitors, and the dopamine receptor blocking agent all suppressed opiate self-administration.

These results may or may not permit the inference that the drug interactions observed involve the brain reinforcement mechanism, for the basic experimental design permits several possible alternative reasons for such suppression of self-administration behavior. First, the test agent may temporarily antagonize certain side effects or toxicity of the self-administered opiate which usually act to limit the amount of drug self-injection. This antagonism could thus cause an initially elevated rate; then as the effects of the test drug recede, there should follow a period of progressive response reduction because of the "extra" opiate. It has been clearly demonstrated that injecting additional opiate to a subject prior to or during a test session produces a proportional decrease in responding on an ongoing self-administration baseline [28].

Second, drugs tested for ability to suppress opioid self-administration might have activity-inhibiting actions that could decrease drug intake as a result of motor dysfunction. For example, those drugs that cause sedation or muscular relaxation could so inhibit motor behavior as to make it impossible for an animal to perform the lever-press behavior required for intravenous self-infusion. Obviously, because a drug produces heavy sedation or a neuromuscular deficit it should not be regarded as a specific blocking agent or antagonist to an opioid.

A third alternative explanation for a suppression of the ongoing baseline of self-administration responses could be the development of a nonspecific conditioned aversion to the opioid because of its interaction with the test agent; i.e., the test agent when interacting with the opioid could cause sickness or pain. For example, evidence pointing to the aversiveness of a large intravenous dose of morphine in the presence of α-methyltyrosine has been presented [47]. Thus, if the test agent should change the infusion of the self-administered opioid from a positive reinforcer to a painful or noxious event, the organism obviously would learn to inhibit responding. Therefore, to control for such alternative explanations as these, the experimenter who would assess a drug interaction by means of an ongoing baseline should consider the need for some additional verification of the results.

B. Control Procedures

1. Reacquisition Test

This procedure may be used to control for alteration of self-administration by means other than alteration of positive reinforcing properties, e.g., through antagonism of side effects or toxicity. The reacquisition procedure includes four steps: measuring operant level (baseline) responding for saline, allowing acquisition of the opiate self-administration response, extinguishing the response, and giving reacquisition trials. In this design the test agent is given prior to the reacquisition session. If a block of the primary reinforcing properties of the opioid occurs, no self-administration (i.e., responding significantly greater than baseline) will occur. Using a design that shows the effect of the test agent on an ongoing baseline with schedule-controlled responding for drug presentation, response suppression could reflect either extinction or satiation. However, if the drug-taking response is extinguished before the drug interaction test, the behavior will not be reestablished in the presence of an effective blocker of reinforcement. The required response will simply not be emitted at a rate significantly greater than baseline level. If self-administration behavior is observed, the test agent obviously does not block reinforcement. (For a detailed description of the reacquisition procedure see Davis and Smith [48].)

2. Conditioned Reinforcement Test

A second type of control procedure is for possible motor dysfunction as a result of the test agent. For this we have devised a conditioned reinforcement technique that permits development of the conditioned reinforcer independently of the subject's motor behavior. This technique enables presentation of the putative blocking agent and the reinforcing drug together at a particular time and testing of the results of their interaction at a later date in the absence of both drugs.

This procedure involves first taking an operant level (baseline of lever-pressing saline), then pretreating the organisms with the test agent (or a vehicle control) before a session of pairings of a buzzer with the presentation of the opiate. That is, the lever is removed from the chamber, a buzzer is sounded, and the subject is immediately infused intravenously with the drug independently of its behavior. The pairing procedure may be effective with as few as 50 repetitions; however, for some purposes 100 or more pairings may be desirable. Then 1, 4, or even 30 days later (depending on the duration of action of the test drug) the rat is again placed in the chamber and allowed to lever press, but only the buzzer stimulus is presented contingent to responses. For the vehicle group, the buzzer should have acquired conditioned reinforcing properties because of its association with the drug. The vehicle group should display a large increase in responding over the operant level. However, if the action of the opiate as a reinforcer was blocked during the pairing by pretreatment with the test agent, lever presses will not significantly exceed the operant level. To demonstrate the effectiveness of these procedures, it has been shown that extreme doses of haloperidol, up to 20 mg/kg [23], or of chlorpromazine* which induce almost complete motor suppression during pairings do not interfere

*S. G. Smith and W. M. Davis, unpublished data, 1972.

with acquisition of morphine-based conditioned reinforcement, as reflected in response levels tested 4 days after the pairings performed under the influence of these drugs.

Recently, we have instituted a program of research on the neurochemical basis of opiate reinforcement using the reacquisition test and the conditioned reinforcement test. This work first considered the possible involvement of brain catecholamines through use of α-methyltyrosine (AMT), a general depleter of brain catecholamines (i.e., both dopamine and norepinephrine). The results of this research indicated that acquisition of both primary (direct drug assessment) and conditioned (indirect assessment) reinforcement were blocked by pretreatment with AMT [19,48-50]. Subsequent research has concentrated on the role of the catecholamine norepinephrine through use of the dopamine-β-hydroxylase (DBH) inhibitors diethyl dithiocarbamate and 1-phenyl-3-(2-thiazolyl)-2-thiourea or U-14,624 [51,52]. This investigation indicated that DBH inhibitors blocked response acquisition based on either primary or conditioned morphine reinforcement, suggesting that the neurochemical reinforcement mechanism for opiates depends at least in part on norepinephrine as a transmitter for certain critical synapses. This inference would be unwarranted had not the reacquisition and conditioned reinforcement procedures been used for the analysis of the test effects, for in some cases definite motor deficits were produced by the DBH inhibitors.

3. Acquired Conditioned Suppression Test

Even though the reacquisition and conditioned reinforcement techniques control for the factors most likely to confuse the interpretation of results from drug interaction research, the acquired conditioned suppression technique is yet another good control procedure. It can control for conditioned aversion arising from pretreatment with the test agent and its subsequent interaction with the self-administered drug.

A good example of how this type of aversion can be induced in a drug interaction setting is the reaction when alcohol is ingested following pretreatment with disulfiram. In man, the resulting reaction is characterized by nausea, vomiting, flushing, hypotension, anxiety, and palpitations [53]. Thus, while alcohol alone may be a positive reinforcer, it becomes an extremely aversive stimulus in the presence of disulfiram. If a test drug induces a noxious state every time the organism self-administers the maintenance drug, responding will quickly stop (extinguish) because the reinforcer has changed from a positive event to a negative event. In many cases, this would change the interpretation that one should place on the results.

The acquired conditioned suppression procedure requires that the subject first be given standard VI 1 min (discussed in schedule of intermittent drug reinforcement) training for milk or food reinforcement until stable performance is observed. Next, the putative conditioned stimulus (buzzer) is presented to the animal on a random schedule to induce adaptation to possible response-disrupting characteristics of a novel stimulus. In a session on the day after completion of adaptation, the subject is injected with the proposed opioid blocking agent, placed in a different experimental environment containing an intravenous infusion system and the buzzer, and given 50-100 buzzer-opiate pairings. Twenty-four hours later, the subject is replaced on VI training. One, four, or even 30 days later, depending on the characteristic of the blocking drug, buzzer presentations are randomly superimposed on the VI baseline. If response suppression, compared to a vehicle control, is observed during the buzzer, the blocking agent has interacted with the opioid to produce aversive effects. However, if suppression is not observed, no aversion was produced to become associated with the buzzer when the blocking agent interacted with the opioid. The acquired conditioned suppression procedure actually controls for two unwanted problems: (a) motor inhibition, because the test is carried out when the test drugs are no longer present, and (b) a drug interaction which could convert a positive reinforcing stimulus into a negative reinforcing stimulus. Lyons has provided a complete review of conditioned suppression procedures and methods for computing a suppression ratio [54].

VII. CONCLUDING REMARKS

Although other test systems can provide valuable data concerning the pharmacology of dependence-producing drugs, only the self-administration paradigm permits replication of human behavior constituting drug abuse and study of the variables which control it. As the technologies and experimental designs associated with drug self-administration have advanced, there is an increased opportunity for elucidating important aspects of the opiate dependence problem by means of this animal model. It is to be anticipated that methods for eliminating self-administration behavior in the laboratory will prove to be applicable as new and improved therapeutic measures in narcotic dependence.

ACKNOWLEDGMENTS

The authors wish to express appreciation to Ms. Edith Pritchard, Toreen Werner, Wilma, Beeler, and Charlotte Delcambre for their assistance during preparation of this manuscript. The authors also wish to thank Mr. William C. Martin of the Science Education Resources Center at the University of Mississippi for photographic materials presented in this chapter.

REFERENCES

1. C. R. Schuster and J. E. Villarreal, The experimental analysis of opioid dependence. In Psychopharmacology: A Review of Progress 1957-1967 (D. H. Efron, J. D. Cole, J. Levine, and J. R. Wittenborn, eds.), Washington, D. C.: U. S. Government Printing Office, Public Health Service Publication no. 1836.
2. C. R. Schuster and T. Thompson, Self-administration of and behavioral dependence on drugs. Annu. Rev. Pharmacol. 9:483-502 (1969).
3. J. R. Nichols, C. P. Headlee, and H. W. Coppock, Drug addiction. I. Addiction by escape training. J. Amer. Pharm. Ass. Sci. Ed. 44: 788-791 (1956).
4. J. R. Nichols and W. M. Davis, Drug addiction. II. Variation of addiction. J. Amer. Pharm. Ass. Sci. Ed. 48:259-262 (1959).
5. W. M. Davis and J. R. Nichols, Physical dependence and sustained opiate directed behavior in the rat. Psychopharmacologia 3:139-145 (1962).
6. R. Kumar, H. Steinberg, and I. P. Stolerman, Inducing a preference for morphine in rats without premedication. Nature (London) 218: 564-565 (1968).
7. J. H. Hill and E. Stellar, An electronic drinkometer. Science 114: 43-44 (1951).
8. I. P. Stolerman and R. Kumar, Regulation of drug and water intake in rats dependent on morphine. Psychopharmacologia 26:19-28 (1972).
9. R. Kumar and I. P. Stolerman, Morphine dependent behavior in rats: Some clinical implications. Psychol. Med. 3:225-237 (1973).
10. W. R. Martin, A. Wikler, C. G. Eades, and F. T. Pescor, Tolerance to and physical dependence on morphine in rats. Psychopharmacologia 4:247-260 (1963).
11. R. Kumar, H. Steinberg, and I. P. Stolerman, How rats can become dependent on morphine in the course of relieving another need. In Scientific Basis of Drug Dependence (H. Steinberg, ed.). New York: Grune & Stratton, 1969.
12. K. G. Gotestam, Intragastric self-administration of medazepam in rats. Psychopharmacologia 28:87-94 (1973).
13. S. G. Smith, T. E. Werner, and W. M. Davis, Technique for intragesic delivery of solutions: Application for self-administration of morphine and alcohol by rats. Physiol. Psychol. 3:220-224 (1975).

14. S. G. Smith, T. E. Werner, and W. M. Davis, Morphine and ethanol: Intragastric and intravenous self-administration. Proceedings of the Society for Neuroscience, St. Louis, October 1974.

15. J. R. Weeks, Long-term intravenous infusion. In Methods in Psychobiology (R. D. Myers, ed.). New York: Academic Press, 1972.

16. J. R. Weeks, Experimental morphine addiction: Method for automatic intravenous injections in unrestrained rats. Science 138:143-144 (1962).

17. S. G. Smith and W. M. Davis, Self-administration research in the behavioral analysis of opiate dependence. In Neurobiology of Drug Dependence, Vol. 3: Behavioral Analysis (H. Lal and J. Singh, eds.). Mt. Kisco, N.Y.: Futura, in press.

18. S. G. Smith and W. M. Davis, Interrelationships of exteroceptive and interoceptive stimuli associated with morphine self-administration: Significance to elimination of drug-seeking behavior. In Drug Addiction, Vol. 3: Neurobiology and Influences on Behavior (J. M. Singh and H. Lal, eds.). New York: Stratton Intercontinental Medical Book Corp., 1974.

19. W. M. Davis and S. G. Smith, Alpha-methyltyrosine to prevent self-administration of morphine and amphetamine. Curr. Ther. Res. 14: 814-819 (1972).

20. T. Thompson and C. R. Schuster, Morphine self-administration, food-reinforced, and avoidance behavior in rhesus monkeys. Psychopharmacologia 5:87-94 (1964).

21. J. L. Claghorn, J. M. Ordy, and A. Nagy, Spontaneous opiate addiction in rhesus monkeys. Science 149:440-441 (1965).

22. N. Khazan, J. R. Weeks, and L. A. Schroeder, Electroencephalographic, electromyographic and behavioral correlates during a cycle of self-maintained morphine addiction in the rat. J. Pharmacol. Exp. Ther. 155:521-531 (1967).

23. S. G. Smith and W. M. Davis, Haloperidol effects on morphine self-administration: Testing for pharmacological modification of the primary reinforcement mechanism. Psychol. Rec. 23:215-221 (1973).

24. B. C. Blakesley, L. C. Dinneer, R. D. Elliott, and D. L. Francis, Intravenous self-administration of heroin in the rat: Experimental technique and computer analysis. Brit. J. Pharmacol. 45:181-182 (1972).

25. G. Deneau, T. Yanagita, and M. H. Seevers, Self-administration of psychoactive substances by the monkey. Psychopharmacologia 16: 30-48 (1969).

26. J. H. Woods and C. R. Schuster, Opiates as reinforcing stimuli. In Stimulus Properties of Drugs (T. Thompson and R. Pickens, eds.). New York: Appleton-Century, 1971.

27. R. J. Collins and J. R. Weeks, Relative potency of codeine, methadone, and dihydromorphinone to morphine in self-maintained addict rats. Naunyn-Schmiedebergs Arch. Exp. Pathol. Pharmakol. 249:509-514 (1965).

28. T. Thompson and R. Pickens, Drug self-administration and conditioning. In Scientific Basis of Drug Dependence (H. Steinberg, ed.). New York: Grune & Stratton, 1969.

29. C. R. Schuster and R. L. Balster, Self-administration of agonists. In Agonist and Antagonist Actions of Narcotic Analgesic Drugs (H. W. Kosterlitz, H. O. J. Collier, and J. E. Villarreal, eds.). Baltimore: University Park Press, 1973.

30. A. Wikler, W. R. Martin, F. T. Pescor, and C. G. Eades, Factors regulating oral consumption of etonitazene solution by morphine-addicted rats. Psychopharmacologia 5:55-76 (1963).

31. A. Wikler, Conditioning factors in opiate addiction and relapse. In Narcotics (D. M. Wilner and G. G. Kassebaum, eds.). New York: McGraw-Hill, 1965.

32. R. J. Collins and J. R. Weeks, Lack of effect of dexoxadrol in self-maintained morphine dependence in rats. Psychopharmacologia 42: 563-570 (1967).

33. F. Hoffmeister and U. U. Schlichting, Reinforcing properties of some opiates and opioids in rhesus monkeys with histories of cocaine and codeine self-administration. Psychopharmacologia 23:55-74 (1972).

34. J. H. Woods and C. R. Schuster, Self-administration of pentazocine by the rhesus monkey. Paper reported to the Committee on Problems of Drug Dependence, Palo Alto, California, February 1969.

35. R. L. Balster, C. R. Schuster, and M. C. Wilson, The substitution of opiate analgesics in monkeys maintained on cocaine self-administration. Paper reported to the Committee on Problems on Drug Dependence, Toronto, February 1971.

36. W. H. Talley and I. Rosenblum, Self-administration of dextropropoxyphene by rhesus monkeys to the point of toxicity. Psychopharmacologia 27:179-182 (1972).

37. J. E. Villarreal, Contributions of laboratory work to the analysis and control of drug dependence. In Drug Abuse: Data and Debate (P. H. Blachly, ed.). Springfield, Ill.: Thomas, 1970.

38. S. G. Smith, L. A. Borgen, W. M. Davis, and H. B. Pace, Automatic magazine and bar-press training in the rat. J. Exp. Anal. Behav. 15: 197-198 (1971).

39. D. D. Cahoon and R. M. Crosby, A technique for the automatic shaping of escape and avoidance behavior in the operant conditioning chamber. Psychol. Rec. 19:431-432 (1969).

40. W. N. Schoenfeld, W. W. Cumming, and E. Hearst, On the classification of reinforcement schedules. Proc. Nat. Acad. Sci. U.S. 42: 563-570 (1957).

41. R. Pickens and C. R. Plunkett, Morphine reinforcement in rats: Confounding activity effects. Paper presented at American Psychological Association, Miami, September 1970.

42. B. E. Jones and J. A. Prada, Relapse to morphine use in dogs. Psychopharmacologia 30:1-12 (1973).

43. C. R. Schuster and J. H. Woods, The conditioned reinforcing effects of stimuli associated with morphine reinforcement. Int. J. Addict. 3: 223-230 (1968).

44. S. R. Goldberg, F. Hoffmeister, U. U. Schlichting, and W. Wuttke, Aversive properties of nalorphine and naloxone in morphine-dependent rhesus monkeys. J. Pharmacol. Exp. Ther. 179:269-276 (1971).

45. J. Pozuelo and F. W. Kerr, Suppression of craving and other signs of dependence in morphine-addicted monkeys by administration of alpha-methyl-para-tyrosine. Mayo Clin. Proc. 47:621-628 (1972).

46. H. Hanson and C. Cimini-Venema, Effects of administration of haloperidol on morphine self-administration in the rat. Clin. Toxicol. 7:273 (1974).

47. W. R. Coussens, W. F. Crowder, and W. M. Davis, Morphine induced saccharin aversion in α-methyltyrosine pretreated rats. Psychopharmacologia 29:151-157 (1973).

48. W. M. Davis and S. G. Smith, Blocking of morphine based behavioral reinforcement by alpha-methyltyrosine. Life Sci. 12:185-191 (1973).

49. W. M. Davis, M. Babbini, W. R. Coussens, S. G. Smith, and W. F. Crowder, Antagonism of behavioral effects of morphine by alpha-methyltyrosine. Pharmacologist 13:280 (1971).

50. W. M. Davis, S. G. Smith, and W. F. Crowder, Morphine based conditioned reinforcement. Paper presented at the Fifth International Congress on Pharmacology, San Francisco, July 1972; p. 52 in abstracts of papers.

51. W. M. Davis and S. G. Smith, Noradrenergic basis for reinforcement associated with morphine action in non-dependent rats. In Drug Addiction, Vol. 3: Neurobiology and Influences on Behavior (J. M. Singh and H. Lal, eds.). New York: Stratton Intercontinental Medical Book Corp., 1974.

52. W. M. Davis, S. G. Smith, and J. H. Kalsa, Noradrenergic role in the self-administration of morphine or amphetamine. Pharmacol. Biochem. Behav., in press.

53. J. M. Ritchie, The aliphatic alcohols. In The Pharmacological Basis of Therapeutics (L. S. Goodman and A. Gilman, eds.). New York: Macmillan, 1970.

54. D. O. Lyons, Conditioned suppression: Operant variables and aversive control. Psychol. Rec. 18:317-338 (1968).

Part IV

TOLERANCE, DEPENDENCE, AND WITHDRAWAL

Chapter 11

APPLICATION OF THE PELLET IMPLANTATION TECHNIQUE FOR THE ASSESSMENT OF TOLERANCE AND PHYSICAL DEPENDENCE IN THE RODENT*

EDDIE WEI

School of Public Health
University of California
Berkeley, California

E. LEONG WAY

Department of Pharmacology
School of Medicine
University of California
San Francisco, California

*Much of the work described in this review was supported by research grants DA00037 and DA00091 from the National Institute of Drug Abuse.

I. INTRODUCTION

Many investigators have used the rodent for assessing tolerance to and physical dependence on morphine because the procedures are simple and inexpensive. The rodent model appears to have validity since the classic effects of morphine such as analgesia (antinociception), tolerance, and physical dependence can easily be demonstrated. In the past, quantitative studies on tolerance and physical dependence development have been limited because frequent, repeated injections of high doses of morphine over several weeks were required to render the animals sufficiently tolerant and dependent [1]. In recent years, the morphine pellet implantation procedure has been widely used to produce within 3 days a high degree of tolerance and physical dependence in the mouse, rat, and guinea pig.

II. PRINCIPLE

The morphine-tolerant-dependent state is generally considered to be a consequence of a counteradaptive action to repeated administrations of the drug. A simple schematic representation of the phenomenon of narcotic tolerance and dependence is illustrated in Fig. 1: (a) A normal physiological function is maintained at some set point. (b) A single dose of morphine disrupts the physiological function (white arrow). (c) Homeostatic mechanisms develop (black arrow) that counteract the effects of morphine. The set point is back to normal, but after repeated morphine administration the consequence of the counteradaptive response is an altered state in which the organism is tolerant to and dependent on morphine. The degree of tolerance and dependence is determined by the magnitude and temporal pattern of the morphine dose. (d) The abrupt withdrawal of morphine or the administration of antagonists removes the acute morphine effects so that homeostatic mechanisms overshoot (black arrow). This exaggerated rebound accounts for the abstinence syndrome.

Within this framework, the investigator can assess tolerance and physical dependence quantitatively. The measurement of tolerance is the difference in the dose-response curve produced by a narcotic (white arrow) in condition (c) vs (b). Physical dependence, on the other hand, is measured by the magnitude of the overshoot of the black arrow in (d) vs (c).

III. INDUCTION OF TOLERANCE AND PHYSICAL DEPENDENCE

A large number of methods have been devised for inducing narcotic tolerance and dependence in the rodent. These different techniques may be distinguished by the route, frequency, and method of drug delivery to the

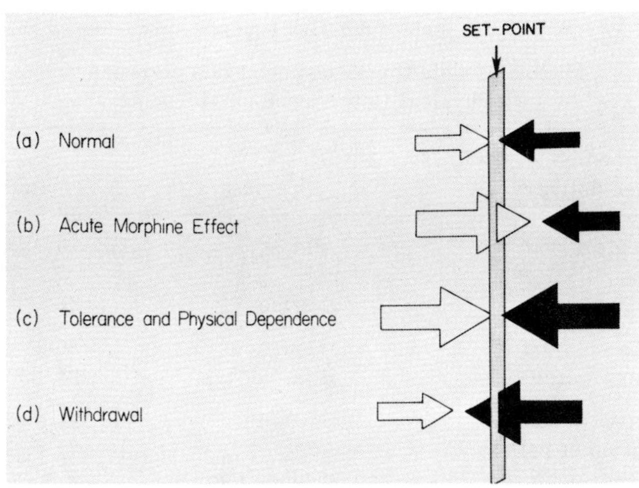

FIGURE 1. Biological mechanisms of morphine effects.

animal. The objectives of these experimental maneuvers are to minimize acute toxicity while effecting a sufficiently high narcotic intake so that a high degree of tolerance and dependence will rapidly develop. A summary of some of the more extensive and thorough investigations of rodent models is given in Table I. With perhaps the exception of Collier's [2] method, none of these procedures rivals the pellet method in convenience and rapidity of induction of a high degree of tolerance and physical dependence. The simplicity of the technique is such that in mice, two persons can implant as many as 200 mice within 1 hr.

The implantation technique was originated by Maggiolo and Huidobro [3], who made a pellet by compressing 75 mg of morphine base under high pressure. Such a pellet, however, is cumbersome to make and its absorption is not rapid enough to produce physical dependence of a magnitude that can be measured by abrupt withdrawal, although striking abstinence signs could be precipitated by injecting nalorphine [3]. With the cooperation of two colleagues [4], a morphine pellet was formulated that enabled us to develop procedures for the quantitative assessment of tolerance and physical dependence [5-8]. The implantation procedure has gained considerable popularity because of its suitability for rapidly inducing a high degree of tolerance and physical dependence. Moreover, the procedure is adaptable for assessing tolerance and physical dependence in the same animal [5].

TABLE I

Murine Models for Assessment of Tolerance to or Physical Dependence on Morphine

Method of morphine delivery	Species	Reference
Daily parenteral injections	Rat	15, 19, 22, 26-28
	Mouse	23, 29
Oral intake via food or drinking water	Mouse	30
	Rat	31-33
Subcutaneous implantation of pellets	Mouse	3, 5, 24
	Rat	7, 8, 11, 16, 34
	Guinea pig	9
Tissue depots of drug	Rat	2, 35
Intraventricular injection	Rat	36

A. Morphine Pellet Formulation

The Gibson pellets consist of morphine base (Mallinckrodt, St. Louis, Mo.), 75 mg; fumed silicone dioxide (Cab-O-Sil, Cabot Corp., Boston, Mass.), 0.75 mg; microcrystalline cellulose (Avicel, SMC Corp., Los Angeles, Calif.), 75 mg; and calcium stearate (impalpable powder, Grade A, Mallinckrodt, St. Louis, Mo.), 1.5 mg. The pellets are formulated according to the following directions: Screen the morphine base, microcrystalline cellulose, fumed silicone dioxide, and calcium stearate through 60-mesh screen. Slug, using 1.91-cm FFBE punch and die, obtaining thin, firm wafers. Screen with no. 16 mesh using a Stokes oscillating granulator. Mix well in a twin shell blender. Compress via Colton tablet press model 330 to obtain a tablet 3 mm thick with a hardness of 15 Strong-Cobb units. In placebo pellets, 75 mg of microcrystalline cellulose is substituted for the morphine base [4]. Ready-made pellets may be obtained from the Pharmaceutical Technology Laboratory, University of California, San Francisco, Calif. 94143.

B. Pellet Implantation Procedure

To implant the pellets, it is preferable to use light ether anesthesia for rats and guinea pigs. Mice may be implanted without anesthesia if manually restrained. If ether should complicate the interpretation of the experimental results, rats and guinea pigs will also tolerate the operation without anesthesia if lightly restrained. The pellet is implanted subcutaneously in the back or in the lower abdominal wall. After the skin is shaved (optional), a small incision is made with a pair of scissors. The blades of the scissors are then inserted into the incision and the subcutaneous tissue gently parted. The pellet is inserted approximately 2-4 cm into the pocket made by the scissors. If the pellet is inserted at a sufficient depth in the tissue, it is not necessary to close the incision with thread or wound clips. However, to ensure that the pellet remains in the subcutaneous tissue, one may wish to surgically close the incision.

In experiments where the dissolution rate of the pellet was measured, it has generally been observed that 25-50% of the morphine in the pellet is absorbed in the first two days, after which the rate of absorption of morphine tends to plateau [5,9,10]. Plasma levels of morphine also correlate with the time course for the dissolution of the pellet [9].

C. Behavior After Implantation

After implantation of the morphine pellets, animals exhibit the characteristic signs of acute morphine effects. In mice this consists of the typical Straub tail and increased motor activity within 30 min after implantation. By 24 hr, the acute effects have largely subsided and the general behavior of the morphine-implanted mice resembles that of placebo-implanted controls. The mortality in morphine-treated mice is generally less than 15% in animals weighing at least 20 g, but the ability to tolerate an implant may vary considerably with different strains. When smaller or less resistant mice are used, animals should be primed a day earlier with 2 or 3 injections of morphine. This pretreatment should make susceptible animals more tolerant to the implanted pellet. Maximum tolerance and dependence require 3-4 days to develop; in our laboratory, we routinely allow 3 days.

In rats, the typical acute narcotic effects are also observed shortly after implantation of the morphine pellet. Some of the signs are a cataleptic state, exophthalmos, Straub tail, and shallow respiratory movements. The rat usually remains immobile with its belly resting on the bottom of the cage. Occasionally, however, especially during the onset of catalepsy, the rat will manifest a startle response and sporadically scurry about inside the cage. The belly of the rat may become matted with dried urine because of its immobile posture. The animal gradually recovers from the acute effects of morphine so that by the third day after implantation, the morphinized rat grooms itself and appears normal when compared to placebo-implanted controls; tolerance to and dependence on morphine are maximal between 3 and 5 days after implantation [6,8,11].

When animals are maintained at 16-27°C, we have practically no mortality after implantation of a single pellet. A 2-10% mortality may be observed if rats are placed in cages containing sawdust. The immobile posture of animals placed with their nose in sawdust apparently results in the death of some animals from suffocation. For this reason, rats should preferably be placed in cages with wire bottoms after implantation. The mortality rate may change drastically, however, under different environmental conditions. For example, during a heat wave, when the ventilation system was inadequate and our laboratory temperatures rose to 35-38°C, approximately 25-30% of morphine-implanted rats died. The elevated body temperature in rats tolerant to morphine [12] may have accounted for the increased susceptibility to heat.

In the guinea pig, after implantation of 4 morphine pellets, the animals become tranquilized for 24 hr and have a decreased reaction time when tested by the hot-plate method. Reaction times return to normal 14 hr after implantation. A biphasic change in body temperature and some body weight loss were also observed during the first two days after implantations [10]. No other adverse effects were observed when guinea pigs, weighing approximately 350-400 g, were implanted with up to 4 morphine pellets [10].

The optimum time for obtaining a tolerant and dependent state after implanting a morphine pellet is 3 days. In the mouse, tolerance and dependence were noted to be maximum 3-4 days after implanting the pellet, after which there was a decrease in these parameters because the pellet becomes encapsulated with fibrous tissue [5]. Similarly, in the rat, tolerance and precipitated withdrawal signs become maximal 3-5 days after a single pellet implant [8,11]. Likewise, in the guinea pig, dependence was maximal 3 days after the simultaneous implantation of 4 morphine pellets; but, surprisingly, tolerance to the antinociceptive effect of morphine could not be determined although tolerance to the hypothermic effects of morphine could be measured [10]. Further details on the kinetic relationship of morphine dose to abstinence behavior can be found in the exhaustive study by Blasig et al. [9].

D. Assessment of Tolerance

The measurement of tolerance as an entity poses problems that are difficult to surmount. In theory and practice, tolerance to morphine can be assessed for any morphine effect. However, for each of the many effects of morphine, there may be a different rate at which tolerance develops and lasts, and the degree of tolerance that develops can also vary. Moreover, the biochemical basis for each morphine action may also differ, and it is not known whether the mechanisms of tolerance development for each morphine action have a common underlying basis. It is important, therefore, for the investigator assessing tolerance to bear in mind constantly these aspects that are often ignored.

Tolerance to morphine after its repeated administration can be evaluated by graded assay procedures where a decrease in sensitivity of an animal to a given dose of morphine can be measured, or by quantal assays that determine the increase in the amount of morphine required to produce a given effect.

Examples of narcotic effects that have been assessed in mice are analgesia (antinociception), hypothermia, respiratory depression, and the stimulant effects of narcotics on locomotor activity. Practicalities, however, limit the number of narcotic effects that can be measured. In our laboratory, we routinely use the classic D'Amour and Smith [13] tail-flick method to determine the increase in the median "analgetic" dose (AD_{50}) of morphine that invariably occurs after morphine pellet implantation. A 2.5-sec delay in the tail reaction time to thermal stimulus is used as a quantal response to varying doses of morphine. The test is performed 6-8 hr after pellet removal to allow for elimination of residual active morphine. By this time the tail-flick reaction returns to predrug baseline level. The morphine AD_{50} is then calculated according to Litchfield and Wilcoxon [14].

Development of tolerance after morphine pellet implantation is discernible within 24 hr and becomes maximal on the third or fourth day. The results obtained by Way et al. [5] are shown in Table II. The morphine AD_{50} nearly doubled after 24 hr and increased about 5-fold after 72 hr of implantation; more recently the increase in morphine AD_{50} we generally note is about 10-fold, and we have obtained as high as a 20-fold increase. This wide variation in the increase in morphine AD_{50} necessitates paired studies using a control group implanted with placebo pellets. After the fourth day, there is a loss in tolerance because encapsulation of the pellet restricts the absorption of morphine. Thus, the morphine AD_{50} very nearly returns to the control level by the sixth day. To prevent the loss in tolerance, a second pellet can be implanted. Blasig et al. [9] have successfully implanted in a single rat 39 pellets over a period of 15 days.

TABLE II

Effect of Morphine Pellet Implantation on Tolerance and Physical Dependence Development[a,b]

Length of implantation (hr)	Morphine AD_{50} mg/kg sc	Morphine AD_{50} 95% confidence limits	Naloxone ED_{50} mg/kg sc	Naloxone ED_{50} 95% confidence limits
0	10.7	9.8-11.6	12.0	
3			3.20	2.99-3.42
6			1.60	1.10-2.32
12	13	11.7-14.4	0.42	0.36-0.48
24	22	20.5-23.5	0.26	0.20-0.34
48	39	35.1-43.3	0.058	0.049-0.067
72	53	49.5-56.7	0.045	0.040-0.049

[a] From Way et al. [5].

[b] Results show effect as measured respectively by the median effective dose (AD_{50}) of morphine required to inhibit the tail-flick response to thermal stimulus and the median effective dose (ED_{50}) of naloxone required to precipitate withdrawal jumping.

E. Assessment of Physical Dependence

The withdrawal syndrome is represented by a constellation of behavioral signs. Not all the abstinence signs will appear in one animal and some of the signs may be exhibited by a nondependent animal. In any assessment procedure, therefore, some degree of arbitrariness needs to be imposed not only in selecting the signs that are to be included, but also in weighing or ranking the relative importance of each sign.

Objective or subjective criteria that have been used for measuring abstinence signs are summarized in Table III. Judging from the reported data, objective criteria appear more amenable to quantification.

For each withdrawal sign, several dimensions may be measured. The parameters include the frequency of occurrence, the intensity of each event, and finally, the probability that such a sign would occur in a population of animals. For example, withdrawal jumping is a prominent abstinence sign in the mouse; to quantify this response, the average number of jumps per mouse, the height of each jump, and the incidence of jumping may all be used as criteria of abstinence behavior.

TABLE III

Withdrawal Signs in the Rodent

Objective criteria	Subjective criteria
Body weight loss	Degree of emotionality in response to prodding
Frequency of jumping	Intensity of salivation
Incidence of jumping	Piloerection
Frequency of wet shakes	Nonpurposive motor activity
Reaction threshold to foot shock	
Vocalization	
Fighting behavior	
Struggling response to restraint	

A basic problem in estimating the intensity of the abstinence syndrome is how to equate one withdrawal sign with another. For example, one may ask: If an animal salivates and has diarrhea during withdrawal, is it more or less severely affected than another animal that only manifests a few escape attempts? To resolve some of these difficulties, point scoring systems and ranking systems have been proposed for quantifying withdrawal intensity [8,15,16]. Alternatively, some investigators [6] have chosen to study only one or two signs, such as the incidence of jumping or body weight loss, because these signs can be measured more precisely. At present, it appears that the choice of a particular set of withdrawal signs for quantifying abstinence should be dictated by the nature of the experimental question.

In selecting any particular sign of withdrawal for assessing dependence intensity, consideration must always be given to the possibility that any experimental manipulation of the dependent state might selectively affect only the withdrawal sign and not the total syndrome. This criticism can be met by using several withdrawal signs for quantal assay of dependence with naloxone. If the total dependent state is altered by some experimental maneuver, parallel changes in the naloxone ED_{50} should be effected in most of the behavioral parameters that are assessed. However, the rate of development of some withdrawal signs is not always parallel and certain intense abstinence signs may suppress the appearance of other withdrawal signs [9].

Most investigators have found the abrupt withdrawal syndrome difficult to quantify because the protracted course of abstinence requires extended periods of continuous observation. For example, when saline is substituted for the normally scheduled morphine injections, withdrawal signs such as aggressive behavior [17,18], irritability, deranged thermoregulation, sneezing, yawning, wet shakes, and loss of body weight develop gradually over a period of 1-4 days after the last morphine dose [19]. For the assessment of drugs with opiate-like activity, suppression of abrupt withdrawal signs may be a sensitive bioassay [5,15,20].

A convenient procedure for assessing the degree of dependence after abrupt withdrawal is to follow the changes in body weight [21,22]. Dependent animals lose considerable body weight over a 24-hr period after abrupt withdrawal, and this can be recorded conveniently at 6-hr intervals for 1-2 days. Figure 2 shows the loss in body weight that occurs after the removal of 2 placebo pellets, 1 morphine pellet, and 2 morphine pellets implanted for 72 hr [6]. It is clear from the data that the loss in body weight provides a reliable index of dependence intensity.

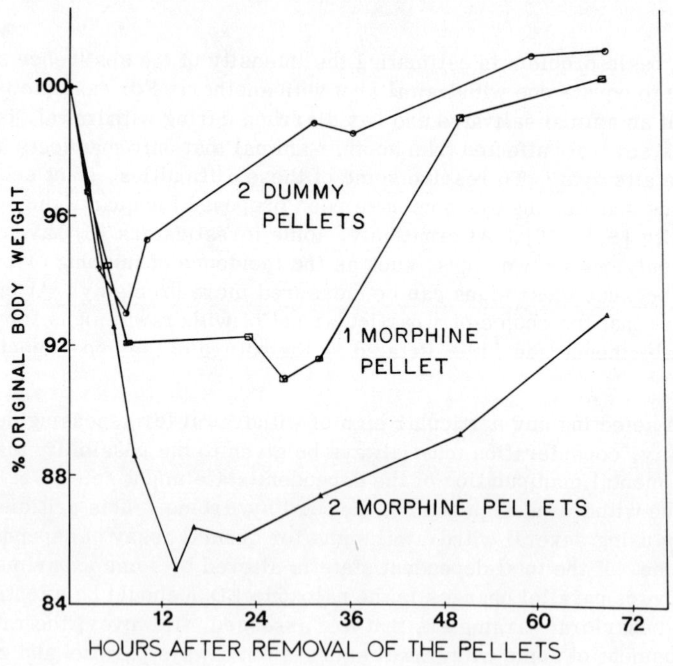

FIGURE 2. Percent loss in mean body weight of morphine-dependent mice after abrupt withdrawal. Dependence was produced by pellet implantation for 3 days, and abstinence was induced by pellet removal. (From Ho et al. [6].)

The delayed onset and protracted course of abrupt morphine withdrawal have led to the increasing use of antagonist-precipitated withdrawal for the assessment of physical dependence. The withdrawal syndrome precipitated by opiate antagonists, in contrast to abrupt withdrawal, is a rapid, explosive event that appears to condense, in a short time period, the abstinence signs of abrupt withdrawal. The precipitated withdrawal syndrome in the mouse, rat, and guinea pig has been fully described by many investigators (see Table I for references).

Precipitated abstinence in the mouse is characterized by defecation, urination, sniffing, increased motor activity with exploratory behavior, stereotyped jumping, tremors, and sometimes convulsions [3]. The stereotyped jumping is a highly characteristic behavior and can be used as an index for estimating the degree of physical dependence on morphine [5]. The degree of dependence can be assessed without removal of the pellet by estimating the amount of naloxone required to precipitate jumping from a circular platform such as a stool. Using jumping as a quantal response to varying doses of naloxone, the ED_{50} can easily be determined. An inverse relationship exists between the two parameters, the higher the degree of dependence, the lower the naloxone ED_{50}. In Table II, it can be seen that the naloxone ED_{50} after morphine pellet implantation decreased with increasing time up to 3 days. A 70-fold decrease in the naloxone ED_{50} was noted to occur between the time of the first estimation at 3 hr and the final estimation at 72 hr. Alternatively, dependence intensity can be quantified by a graded response. The total jump attempts after a fixed dose of naloxone can be counted [20,23,24]. In this procedure it is necessary to use several animals and note the average jumps per group, since some animals may not jump at the dose of naloxone that is selected.

The more prominent withdrawal signs in the rat rendered dependent by pellet implantation are the following:

1. Blanching of ears: loss of coloration during withdrawal.
2. Teeth chattering: an audible, loud, and distinct noise apparently due to fasciculations of the mandibular muscles; this sound is identical to the gnawing sound produced by an animal eating food pellets.
3. Escape attempts or jumping: the animal attempts to escape from its cage or container, or leaps into the air like a frog.
4. Wet shakes: vigorous rotational body movements similar to those produced by an animal when wetted with water.
5. Abnormal posturing: slouching posture of the thorax or abdomen, or crossing of front paws.

6. Swallowing movements: a licking movement of the tongue, usually accompanied by salivation and rhinorrhea.

7. Ptosis: in contrast to a normal animal, which may close its eyes during the experiment, ptosis in the abstinent animal is not reversed by a light noise produced by tapping the container with a pencil.

8. Diarrhea: the presence of a formless stool, usually adhering to the base of the tail.

9. Vocalization: may be elicited by lightly prodding the animal with a stick.

Other abstinence signs that occur less frequently are exophthalmos, chromodacryorrhea, penile erection, and seminal emissions [7].

A point scoring system may be used to quantify the degree of dependence but, as with the mouse, dependence can be quantified on an all-or-none basis by estimating the naloxone ED_{50} for a given withdrawal sign. The more reliable indices are diarrhea, abnormal posturing, ear blanching, swallowing movements, ptosis, teeth chattering, escape attempts, and wet shakes.

In order to obtain a common index for relating one abstinence sign to another, we have recently determined the naloxone thresholds for precipitating different withdrawal signs in the rat [7]. The results of our experiments indicate that the relationship between opiate antagonists and morphine dependence is highly complex. We found that in rats implanted with 1 morphine pellet, low doses of naloxone (0.02-0.1 mg/kg) elicited ear blanching, abnormal posturing, and diarrhea. At intermediate doses of naloxone (0.1-0.5 mg/kg), abstinence signs that also appeared were teeth chattering, swallowing movements, some escape behavior, and wet shakes. At high doses of naloxone (0.5-10 mg/kg) wet shakes or repeated attempts to escape were precipitated in almost all animals. Other signs of precipitated abstinence, such as the incidence of seminal emissions and chromodacryorrhea as well as the average number of wet shakes and escape attempts per responding animal, exhibited a poor dose-response relationship with increasing naloxone dosage in the tested range of 0.04-10 mg/kg. Loss of body weight correlated well to the log dose of naloxone. From these results, it appears that body weight loss, escape behavior, and wet shakes are the more precise indices of withdrawal intensity. However, with very severe dependence, the incidence of wet shakes may actually decrease [9].

F. Assessment of Factors Altering Tolerance Development

The biological processes concerned with the development of tolerance appear to be distinct from those associated with acute morphine action. Such a statement may seem obvious since an acute response to morphine can be elicited within minutes, whereas tolerance to morphine usually does not become apparent until after repeated, frequent administration of high doses for many days. However, in assessing experimental conditions that may alter the development of tolerance to morphine, it is not always easy to differentiate between an action that may represent a prolonged acute response and one concerned immediately with tolerance development.

To illustrate this point, suppose, for example, that the injection of a pharmacological agent A prior to morphine pellet implantation greatly reduces the increase in morphine AD_{50} that invariably occurs after 3 days of implantation. Does this mean that A has blocked the development of tolerance to morphine? Conceivably, A could have elicited a lowering of the morphine AD_{50} by at least three possible modes: (a) inhibition of a process concerned with tolerance development to morphine, (b) a long-lasting antagonism of morphine analgesia, or (c) facilitation of morphine access to its brain receptor sites (e.g., breakdown of blood-brain barrier to morphine or decreased metabolism or excretion of morphine). Before concluding, therefore, that A might be acting to block tolerance development, the latter two mechanisms should be excluded. To exclude the possibility that A does not alter the effects of morphine acutely, pretreatment with compound A would also have to be assessed in groups of animals receiving a placebo pellet implant. To exclude the possibility that A does not alter the disposition of morphine, the brain distribution of morphine under the imposed experimental conditions would have to be compared in the control and experimental groups.

G. Assessment of Factors Altering Dependence Development

The problems to be encountered in assessing dependence development on morphine are similar in many ways to those in evaluating tolerance development. To establish that an experimental treatment blocks dependence development, it is also necessary to establish that the manipulation does not alter the acute action and the brain disposition of morphine. Hence, experiments with placebo pellet animals and brain uptake studies are also required to control these complicating factors.

Using the above experimental approaches to exclude factors that are not involved in the development of tolerance to and dependence on morphine, it has been demonstrated that it is possible to alter the development of tolerance and dependence without necessarily modifying acute responses to morphine and, conversely, acute effects of morphine can be greatly modified without affecting processes associated with tolerance and dependence development [25].

IV. SUMMARY

A simple and rapid pellet implantation technique for inducing morphine tolerance and dependence in the rodent has been described. Various parameters used for assessing tolerance and dependence have also been briefly discussed. The development of quantitative animal models has greatly facilitated research on the neurochemical and neuroanatomical substrates of morphine dependence, and hopefully rapid advances may soon be made in understanding the biological mechanisms of narcotic addiction.

REFERENCES

1. H. Halbach and N. B. Eddy, Tests for addiction (chronic intoxication) of morphine type. Bull. W. H. O. 28:139-173 (1963).

2. H. O. J. Collier, D. L. Francis, and C. Schneider, Modification of morphine withdrawal by drugs interacting with humoral mechanisms: Some contradictions and their interpretation. Nature (London) 237: 220-223 (1972).

3. C. Maggiolo and F. Huidobro, Administration of pellets of morphine to mice: abstinence syndrome. Acta Physiol. Latinoamer. 11:70-78 (1961).

4. R. D. Gibson and J. E. Tingstad, Formulation of a morphine implantation pellet suitable for tolerance-physical dependence studies in mice. J. Pharm. Sci. 59:426-427 (1970).

5. E. L. Way, H. H. Loh, and F. H. Shen, Simultaneous quantitative assessment of morphine tolerance and physical dependence. J. Pharmacol. Exp. Ther. 167:1-8 (1969).

6. I. K. Ho, S. E. Lu, S. Stolman, H. H. Loh, and E. L. Way, Influence of p-chlorophenylalanine on morphine tolerance and physical dependence and regional brain serotonin turnover studies in morphine-tolerant-dependent mice. J. Pharmacol. Exp. Ther. 182:155-165 (1972).

7. E. Wei, H. H. Loh, and E. L. Way, Quantitative aspects of precipitated abstinence in morphine-dependent rats. J. Pharmacol. Exp. Ther. 184:398-403 (1973).

8. E. Wei, Assessment of precipitated abstinence in morphine-dependent rats. Psychopharmacologia 28:35-44 (1973).

9. J. Blasig, A. Herz, K. Reinhold, and S. Zieglgansberger, Development of physical dependence on morphine in respect to time and dosage and quantification of the precipitated withdrawal syndrome in rats. Psychopharmacologia 33:19-38 (1973).

10. A. Goldstein and R. Schultz, Morphine tolerant longitudinal muscle strip from guinea pig ileum. Brit. J. Pharmacol. 48:655-666 (1973).

11. T. J. Cicero and E. R. Meyer, Morphine pellet implantation in rats: quantitative assessment of tolerance and dependence. J. Pharmacol. Exp. Ther. 184:404-408 (1973).

12. L. M. Gunne, The temperature response in rats during acute and chronic morphine administration. A study of morphine tolerance. Arch. Int. Pharmacodyn. 129:416-428 (1960).

13. R. E. D'Amour and D. L. Smith, A method for determining loss of pain sensation. J. Pharmacol. Exp. Ther. 72:74-79 (1941).

14. J. T. Litchfield and F. Wilcoxon, A simplified method of evaluating dose-effect experiments. J. Pharmacol. Exp. Ther. 96:99-113 (1949).

15. W. R. Buckett, A new test for morphine-like physical dependence (addiction liability) in rats. Psychopharmacologia 6:410-416 (1964).

16. L. Grumbach, M. Shelotsky, and J. E. Boston, Characteristics of physical dependence to morphine in the rat. In Proceedings of the 32nd NAS-NRC Committee on Problems on Drug Dependence pp. 6844-6859 (1970).

17. H. Lal, J. O'Brien, and S. K. Puri, Morphine-withdrawal aggression: Sensitization by amphetamines. Psychopharmacologia 22:217-223 (1971).

18. D. H. Thor and B. G. Teel, Fighting of rats during post-mortem withdrawal; effect of pre-withdrawal dosage. Amer. J. Psychol. 81:439-442 (1968).

19. W. R. Martin, A. Wikler, C. G. Eades, and F. T. Pescor, Tolerance to and physical dependence on morphine in rats. Psychopharmacologia 4:247-260 (1963).

20. J. K. Saelens, F. R. Granat, and W. K. Sawyer, The mouse jumping test: A simple screening method to estimate the physical dependence capacity of analgesics. Arch. Int. Pharmacodyn. Ther. 190:213-218 (1971).

21. E. Hosoya, Some withdrawal symptoms of rats to morphine. Pharmacologist 1:77 (1959).

22. T. Akera and T. M. Brody, The addiction cycle to narcotics in the rat and its relation to catecholamines. Biochem. Pharmacol. 17:675-688 (1968).

23. I. Marshall and D. G. Grahame-Paige, Evidence against a role in brain 5-hydroxytryptamine in the development of physical dependence upon morphine in mice. J. Pharmacol. Exp. Ther. 179:634-641 (1971).

24. Y. Maruyama and A. E. Takemori, The role of dopamine and norepinephrine in the naloxone-induced abstinence of morphine-dependent mice. J. Pharmacol. Exp. Ther. 185:602-608 (1973).

25. E. Leong Way, Brain neurohormones in morphine tolerance and dependence. Proc. Int. Congr. Pharmacology 5th 1:77-94 (1973).

26. C. K. Himmelsbach, G. H. Gerlach, and E. J. Stanton, A method for testing addiction tolerance and abstinence in the rat. J. Pharmacol. Exp. Ther. 53:179-188 (1935).

27. S. Kaymakcalan and L. A. Woods, Nalorphine-induced "abstinence syndrome" in morphine tolerant albino rats. J. Pharmacol. Exp. Ther. 177:112-116 (1956).

28. W. R. Coussens, W. F. Crowder, and S. G. Smith, Acute physical dependence upon morphine in rats. Behav. Biol. 8:533-543 (1973).

29. H. Loh, F. Shen, and E. L. Way, Inhibition of morphine tolerance and physical dependence and brain serotonin synthesis by cycloheximide. Biochem. Pharmacol. 18:2711-2721 (1969).

30. L. Shuster, R. V. Hannam, and W. E. Boyle, Jr., A simple method for producing tolerance to dihydromorphinone in mice. J. Pharmacol. Exp. Ther. 140:149-154 (1963).

31. A. Wikler, W. R. Martin, F. T. Pescor, and C. G. Eades, Factors regulating oral consumption of an opioid (etonitazene) by morphine-addicted rats. Psychopharmacologia 5:55-76 (1963).

32. I. P. Stolerman and R. Kumar, Preferences for morphine in rats: Validation of an experimental model of dependence. Psychopharmacologia 177:137-150 (1970).

33. M. E. Risner and K. A. Khavari, Morphine dependence in rats produced after 5 days of ingestion. Psychopharmacologia 28:51-62 (1973).

34. H. A. Tilson, R. H. Rech, and S. Stolman, Hyperalgesia during withdrawal as a means of measuring the degree of dependence in morphine dependent rats. Psychopharmacologia 28:287-300 (1973).

35. P. G. Goode, An implanted reservoir of morphine solution for rapid induction of physical dependence in rats. Brit. J. Pharmacol. 41: 558-566 (1971).

36. H. Watanabe, The development of tolerance to and of physical dependence on morphine following intraventricular injection in the rat. Jap. J. Pharmacol. 21:383-391 (1971).

Chapter 12

SCREENING OF DEPENDENCE LIABILITY OF DRUGS USING RATS

EIKICHI HOSOYA

Department of Pharmacology
Keio University, School of Medicine
Shinjuku-ku, Tokyo, Japan

I. INTRODUCTION

In developing new drugs that act on the central nervous system, it is necessary to determine before the drugs are used in clinical investigations whether their repeated administration results in dependence production.

A method using monkeys for the prediction of physical and psychological dependence on morphine was introduced by Seevers [1] in 1936. It was accepted in 1963 by WHO [2] and in 1966 by the NRS-NAS committee [3] on the problems of drug dependence in the United States as the standard method for this purpose (revised in 1972 [4]).

However, elaborate and expensive facilities are needed for this method and accordingly not every laboratory can afford to keep satisfactory facilities and personnel. Moreover, a fairly large amount of the test drug is necessary to carry out the procedure satisfactorily, in spite of the fact that the number of drugs to be tested is very large and the number of synthesized drugs is usually very small. Accordingly, other simpler methods using small animals are essentially needed and several methods have been proposed.

In 1955, the Japanese Ministry of Welfare asked the author to establish a simple but reliable method for the screening of physical dependence liability of drugs using small animals such as rats or mice. In March 1958 at the 31st meeting of the Japanese Pharmacological Society, the author first offered the idea [5], based on his experimental data, that the sharp decrease in body weight of morphinized rats caused by the withdrawal of morphine could be regarded as a useful tool for the screening of physical dependence on morphine-type drugs, although the phenomenon itself had been observed by Fichtenberg [6] in 1951.

Since then, this idea has been studied and applied to the investigation of many kinds of CNS drugs such as analgesics, hypnotics, tranquilizers, etc., by the author and his colleagues [7-15]. It is now generally agreed that this method can be applied satisfactorily to the screening of morphine-type analgesics and to some extent to hypnotics and tranquilizers.

At the same time, the author has been looking keenly for papers published in and out of Japan concerning the screening of dependence liability using small animals. Among many interesting papers, the author feels that those of Martin [16], Buckett [17], and Lorenzetti and Sancilio [18] are particularly outstanding.

It was further found that weight loss due to the precipitation of abstinence by the administration of antagonists such as nalorphine and naloxone could be regarded as a good indicator for the screening of dependence as well as withdrawal.

The significance of the changing pattern of both body temperature and spontaneous locomotor activity of rats [19-21,23,25-27] was also studied carefully on many kinds of dependence-producing drugs, and it was concluded that these two indicators were valuable as supplementary criteria for the screening of dependence liability.

As for the jumping and wet dog phenomena of rats or mice after the administration of naloxone, the author is of the opinion [29] that they cannot be regarded as true abstinent phenomena.

Improvement of the procedures for the screening of dependency has been achieved in our laboratory continuously in the past 15 years. It was found that the substitution [30,32] of the test drug for morphine in morphine-tolerant rats could supply additional useful information for this purpose and this substitution became one of the indispensable procedures in our method.

Until a few years ago, the body weight of animals was measured before the time of each drug administration and 6, 8, 12, or 24 hr after the last administration, and the loss (decreased ratio) of weight due to withdrawal, precipitation, or substitution was calculated.

However, Nozaki [30,33,34] carefully observed the changing pattern of the body weight of rats for 72 consecutive hours in normal and morphinized rats. She found that the body weight of normal rats decreases from morning to evening continuously and increases from evening to morning without stopping or with a small valley at midnight; that is, decrease during the day and increase at night are the general pattern of body weight changes in normal rats; it is not affected by illumination of the room (Fig. 1). However, this pattern is significantly altered by the repeated administration of dependence-producing drugs (Figs. 2 and 3), by their withdrawal, by the injection of antagonists, and/or by the substitution thereafter (Fig. 4). Nozaki concluded that the comparison of the changing pattern of body weight could supply more useful information for the screening of dependence production than the mere comparison of body weight before and after withdrawal.

In order to compare the changing pattern of body weight, it became necessary to measure the body weight of rats not only in the daytime but also through the night. This is because the tendency of body weight to decrease in the morning due to drug withdrawal cannot be fully differentiated from the normal diurnal decrease in the daytime and vice versa, and the tendency toward increasing body weight due to the repeated administration of the test drug cannot be fully clarified at night since the body weight of normal rats increases at night. This is one of the reasons why the automatic determination of body weight was necessary.

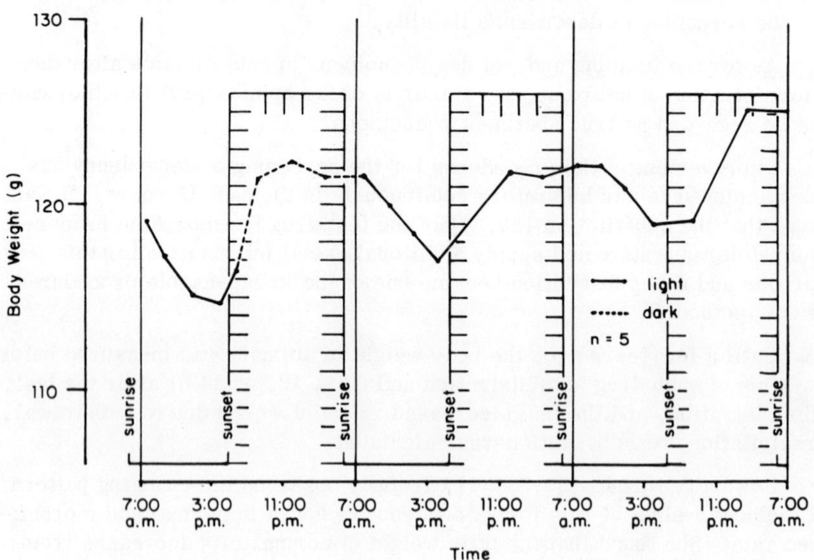

FIGURE 1. Changes of the body weight of normal rats for three consecutive days in a Koitotron (a finely conditioned cabinet). Changing patterns of body weight are similar whether the room is light or dark.

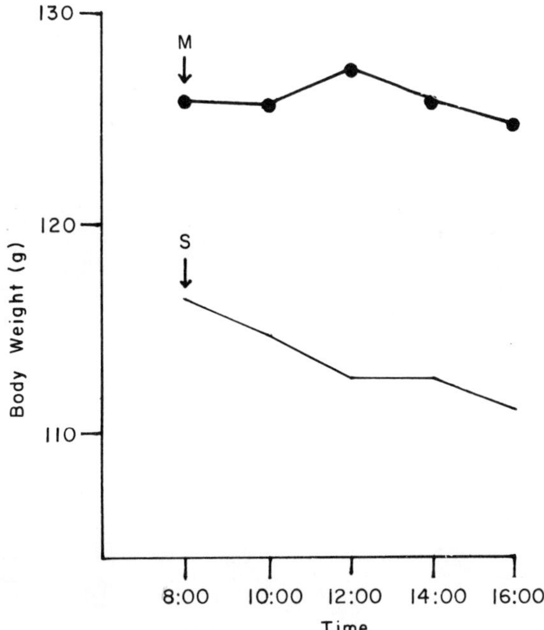

FIGURE 2. Changes of the body weight of rats after the first administration of morphine HCl (20 mg/kg sc) in daytime. Thin line shows the case of physiological saline solution; thick line shows the case of morphine injection.

After many trials and errors, in which several pharmacologists, physiologists, electronic specialists, and technicians participated, a nearly satisfactory (not yet 100%) instrument was devised for the automatic determination and printing of the body weight of each of six rats every 30 min without the movement of animals affecting the results.

This instrument made it possible to clarify the changing pattern of body weight of rats all day for 2-3 days continuously without touching the animal for the measurement of weights and to save manpower in obtaining the correct weight at midnight while the intake of food and water does not disturb the weighing.

Another problem to be solved was how to make rats tolerant to and dependent on the drug. As far as morphine is concerned several procedures have been proposed, such as repeated injection, implantation of a pellet [35], implantation of a capsule [36], and continuous injection. Through our 15

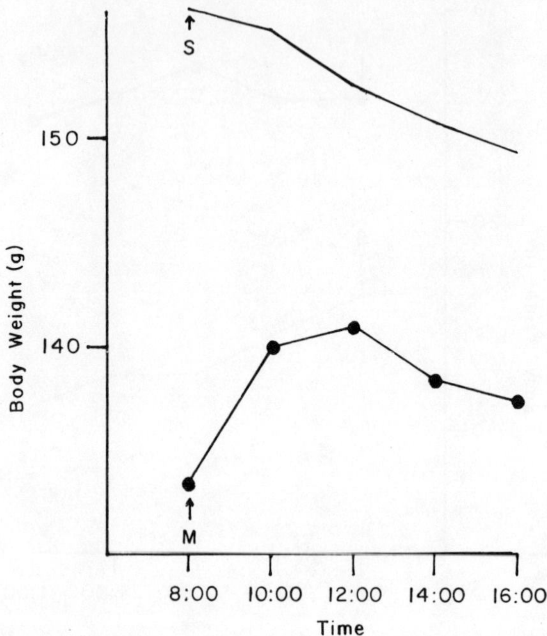

FIGURE 3. Changes of the body weight of Donryu rats after the repeated administration of morphine HCl (20 mg/kg) twice daily for 7 days. Thin line is the case of saline solution (0.5 ml/100 g); thick line is the case of morphine injection. (Room temperature, 20° ±0.1°C.)

years of experience, the author believes that the repeated hypodermic (or intraperitoneal) injection of drugs, at two or three definite times in the day, 7 days a week, for 7 weeks, is the easiest method for bringing the animals into a state of dependence.

As for pellet implantation, although it is simple, the author cannot dispel the following suspicions:

1. The absorption of the morphine contained in the pellet is largest at the beginning of implantation and it decreases day by day due to several factors. If one wants to make the animal dependent on morphine with certainty, one has to add the pellets gradually and to measure the concentration in the blood daily.

2. The withdrawal procedure is difficult since complete removal of the pellet and, accordingly, the rapid cessation of absorption is

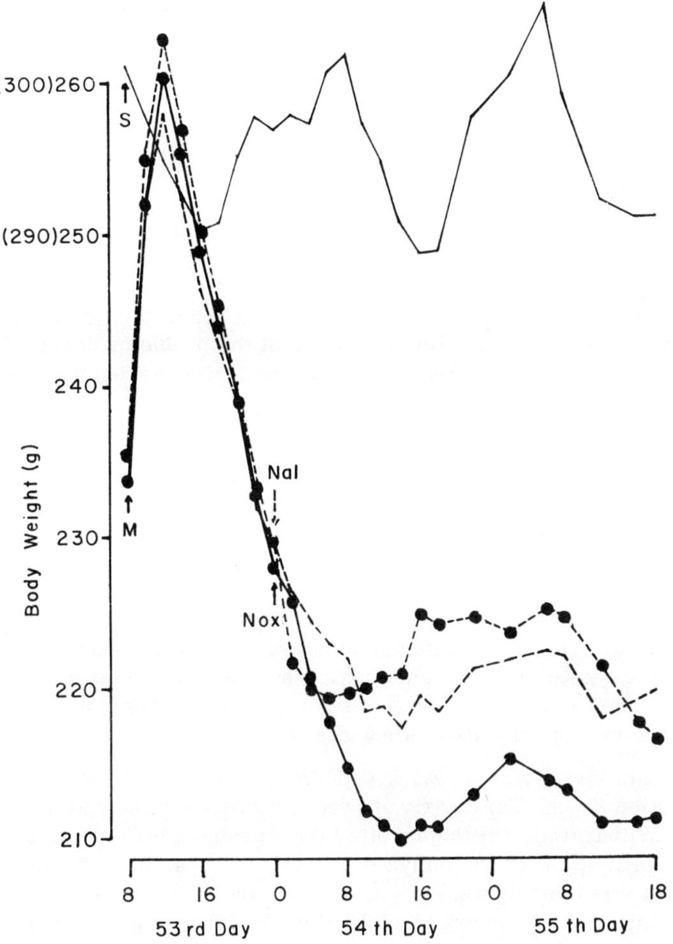

FIGURE 4. Changes in body weight of Donryu rats (n = 5) every 2 hr after repeated administration of morphine HCl (100 mg/kg, 2 times daily) for 53 days and its modification by injection of naloxone HCl (10 mg/kg) or nalorphine HCl (10 mg/kg) or by withdrawal on 54th day. Key: ___, body weight of control rats injected with NaCl solution twice daily for 53 days; ●—●, body weight of morphinized rats injected with morphine at 8:00 a.m. on the 53rd day and naloxone (10 mg/kg) at 0:00 on the 54th day; ●---●, body weight of morphinized rats injected with morphine at 8:00 a.m. on the 53rd day and nalorphine (10 mg/kg sc) at 0:00 a.m. on the 54th day; ----, body weight of morphinized rats injected with morphine at 8:00 a.m. on the 53rd day and receiving no injection (withdrawal) thereafter. (Room temperature, 20° ±1°C.) Note significant increases of body weight by injection of morphine to morphinized rats in daytime, when normal rats lose their weight, and sharp decrease of body weight by withdrawal or administration of antagonists at night.

impossible. This necessitates adopting the procedure of precipitation by antagonists which sometimes might lead to false conclusions, as will be discussed later.

3. The pellet might be broken for some reason in the animal's body. However, if the pellet is very compact, absorption will be slow.

The implantation of a morphine-containing reservoir proposed by Goode [36] seems ideal and may eliminate some of the problems described above. If obtaining and implanting the reservoir are easily carried out, the method might be worthwhile.

At present we are studying the continuous injection procedure [37] without interfering with the animals' movements whether or not it fulfills our expectation of shortening the time necessary for the production of dependence. Although our studies are still in progress, the following facts have been found:

1. Continuous intraperitoneal injection of 50 mg/kg morphine HCl per 12 hr caused a significant decrease in the body weight of rats after the cessation of the injection. The grade of the decrease in body weight is similar to that of the repeated administration of morphine 50 mg/kg twice daily for 6 weeks.
2. Similarly, withdrawal of pethidine after 12 hr of continuous injection (50 mg/kg) clearly showed a decrease in body weight of rats. Withdrawal of pethidine after its repeated administration twice daily for 7 weeks did not cause any decrease in body weight, and it was the only weak point in our method. Therefore, the continuous injection procedure in addition to the substitution procedure may be a useful tool for the screening of dependence liability of pethidine-type drugs.

Recently, Nozaki presented an interesting hypothesis [37,38] that the grade of physical dependence on morphine might be measured in rats by the following product: (percent body weight decrease by withdrawal) x (length of time until body weight returns to prewithdrawal level). The author thinks that many more experimental results are needed before Nozaki's hypothesis can be accepted, but such experiments seem to be worth doing.

The author has explained the chronological development of his 15-year study on the screening of dependence liability using small animals. Unfortunately, almost all of our experimental results and opinions were presented to the general or regional meetings of the Japanese Pharmacological Society in Japanese and very few of them were published in English. Thus, the author will give a detailed explanation of the method used in his laboratory and a summary of the results. Of course, the study is only half-completed, and there may be some claims and opposite opinions in the future, but the author now believes that physical dependence liability of morphine-type drugs can be simply and reliably screened by the careful observation of changes in the body weight of rats and that this method may be applied to some extent to other types of dependence-producing drugs.

II. EXPERIMENTAL ANIMALS

Male rats of Donryu strain (Nippon Rat Co., Saitama, Japan), initially weighing about 120 g and raised for a week in our laboratory, are used throughout the experiments. Young rats less than 100 g should not be used and old rats over 300 g are not adequate for the experiments. Donryu is a strain bred in Japan and originating from the Wistar rat that shows very stable and steady increase of body weight with little individual deviation. Growth curves are shown in Fig. 5.

III. MAINTENANCE OF RATS

Five rats are usually housed in one cage, but for automatic balancing and determinations of temperature and activity one rat is kept in one cage.

Rat chow, NMF (made by Oriental Co., Tokyo), and water are allowed to be taken freely. A wooden cabinet (2.1 m x 2.1 m x 1.13 m) called a Koitotron accepts 18 cages and has a space for the measurement of body weight and injection. A Koitotron placed in the laboratory room has its own control system for temperature (20° ± 0.5°C) and humidity (65 ± 10%) and shuts out the outside noise and all light except that which enters through a small peep window.

Electronic devices such as the amplifier and the recorder for the automatic determinations of body weight, body temperature, and spontaneous locomotor activity are placed outside the Koitotron and are connected by wires through the wooden wall (Fig. 6).

In this way, rats receive few stresses and are not touched. Researchers are asked only to inspect the rats through the window of the Koitotron whether or not the automatic instruments are in their correct positions, except during drug injection.

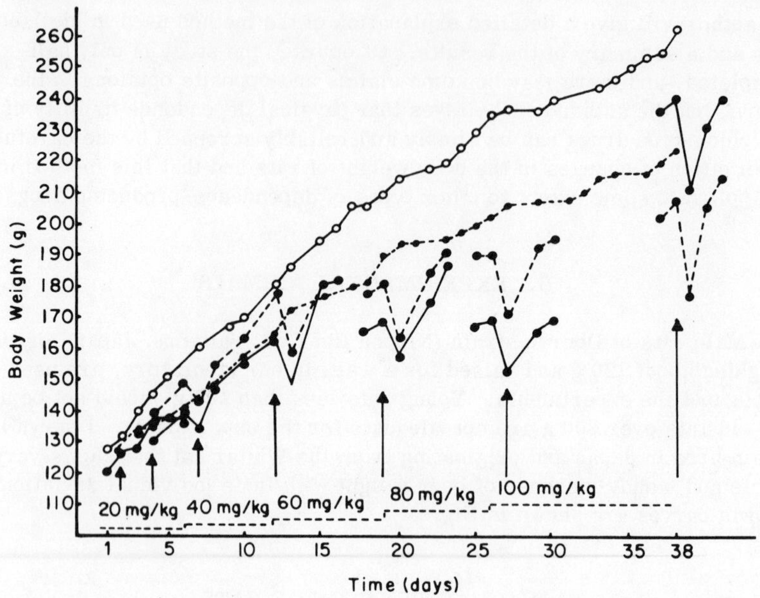

FIGURE 5. Key: o___o, normal growth curve; •...•, chronic morphine with dosages indicated at arrows; •---•, chronic morphine with injections of NaCl; •___•, chronic morphine with injections of nalorphine. Arrows indicate injection of morphine at indicated dose, NaCl, or nalorphine, 10 mg/kg. The latter two injections were designed to precipitate withdrawal. A different rat was used for each determination of effect of NaCl or nalorphine in causing change in weight loss due to withdrawal. Note that the extent of decrease in body weight upon withdrawal increased with the duration of morphinization; the longer the morphine is administered the greater the degree of body weight loss due to withdrawal or to antagonist injection.

IV. MEASUREMENT OF BODY WEIGHT

A. Standard Method

The usual measurement of the body weight of rats is done by putting the animal on the balance by hand individually, in the morning at 8:00-9:00 a.m. and in the evening at 4:00-5:00 p.m. (or 8:00-9:00 p.m. if possible), both just before drug administration. In cases of withdrawal, precipitation, or substitution the body weight is measured every 2-4 hr, sometimes throughout the night until the next morning.

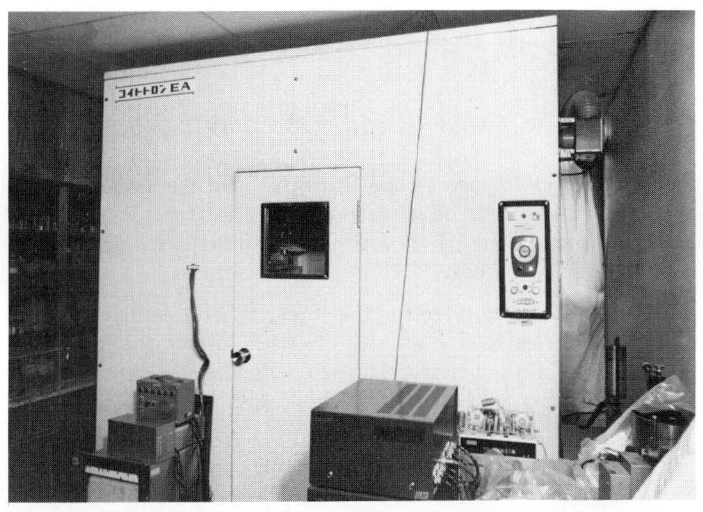

FIGURE 6. The Koitotron, a finely conditioned cabinet for temperature, humidity, lighting, ventilation, and noise, placed in laboratory room.

B. Simplified Method

If it is too difficult to measure the body weight every 2-4 hr for 12-24 hr after withdrawal, precipitation, or substitution, one may measure the body weight of rats at 12 and 24 hr after the above procedure and compare the values with those obtained at the same time of the previous day. Details concerning this point will be discussed later.

C. Automatic Measurement

The principle of this measurement is to change the weight pressure into electricity by a transducer; the current is amplified and printed by number every 30 min. The most difficult point to be overcome was how to eliminate the disturbing effects due to the rats' movements being accurate to the 0.5 g level. The more sensitive the instrument, the more difficult it is to determine the correct body weight because of the vibration of movement. This problem was solved by attaching a special electronic controller which communicates the electricity only when the rats are in a still condition; i.e., unless the rats stop moving no electrical current is transmitted. Accordingly, the body weight may not be recorded at every 30 min punctually but with some delay, which is not a major factor for our purpose. This device proved to be very useful in conserving manpower through the night and getting six to twelve data every time (Figs. 7-9).

V. ADMINISTRATION OF DRUGS

Morphine hydrochloride, as the standard, and the drug to be tested are injected subcutaneously or sometimes intraperitoneally by hand, taking care not to leak more than 0.5-1.0 ml at one time, twice daily after weighing, 7 days a week repeatedly.

For the purpose of disinfecting the injection site, it is advisable to avoid wiping with an excessive amount of ethanol since the licking of alcohol was found to increase the body weight to a significant extent. We recommend the use of cotton with the alcohol well squeezed out.

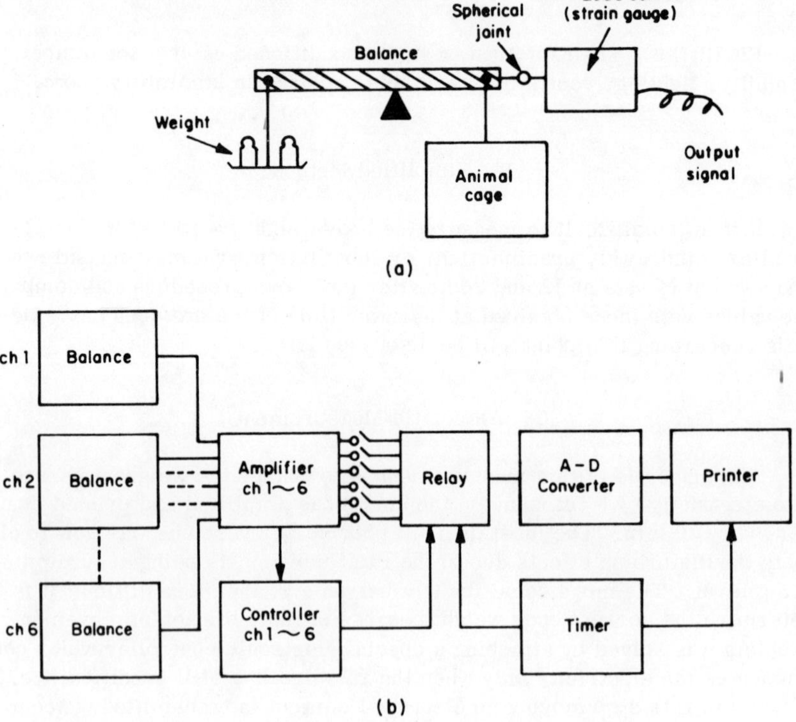

FIGURE 7. (a) Automatic balance. (b) Schematic connection.

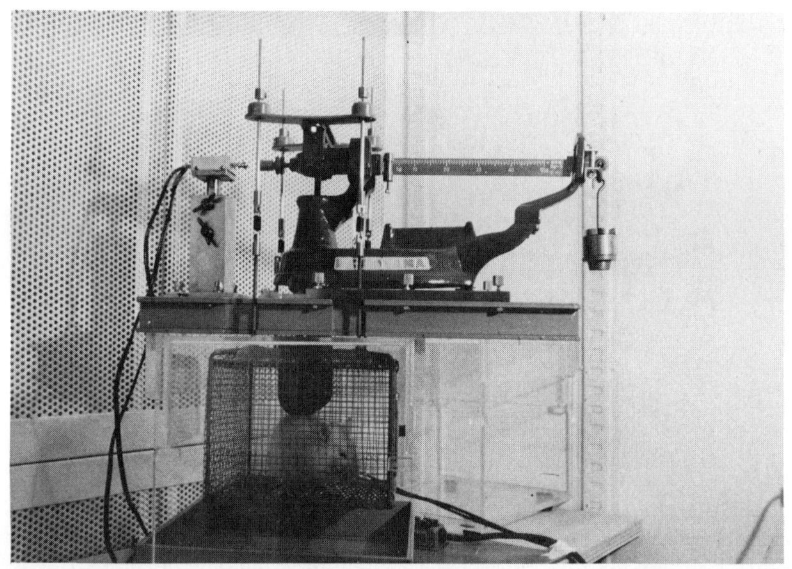

FIGURE 8. Automatic balance. At the start, the balance is kept in a balanced situation with the weight of the cage (~ 900 g) including the rat. When the body weight of the rat is increased or decreased, the difference in the weight pushes or pulls the strain gauge, which transforms the power into electrical current proportionally. The current is then amplified and printed by number. Weights of food, water, feces, and urine are independent from that of the cage.

Drugs to be tested are dissolved in distilled water. If they are insoluble in water, the following steps are taken: (a) Some of the drugs are suspended in the water by means of ultrasonic waves and injected subcutaneously or intraperitoneally. (b) Some of them may be dissolved in some solvent. For this kind of drug, the solvent itself must be tested as another control parallel to NaCl solution to determine its influence on the animals. (c) Some of them are suspended in 2% arrowroot solution and infused into the stomach via a stomach tube.

The amount of drug to be administered varies, needless to say, according to the ED_{50}, LD_{50}, and also the route of administration. In our experience, it is practical and convenient to administer the therapeutic dose of the test drug for the human adult as the dose per kilogram of rat body weight. For instance, if the therapeutic dose of an analgesic for the human adult is 100 mg, the dose of the drug for rat is 100 mg/kg. Of

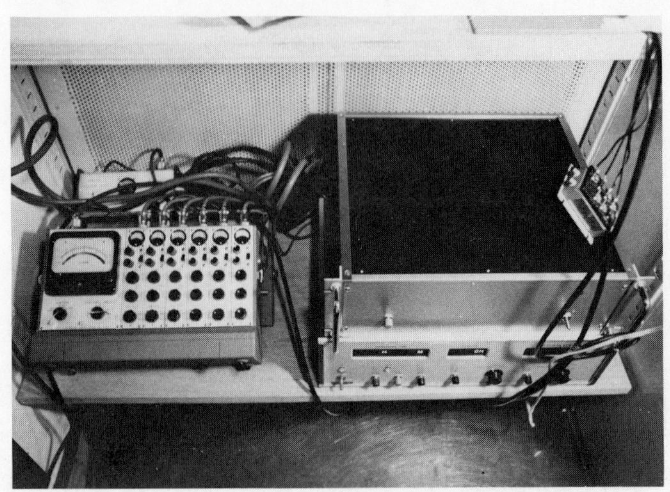

FIGURE 9. Automatic balance. The amplifier and the electronic controller that pass the electrical current only when the rat is in a still condition. Lacking this control instrument, the balance becomes like a motility meter, and cannot measure the correct weight. The interval of weighing is preset about 30 min, depending on the activity of the animal.

course, such calculation may not always be applied to every kind of drug, but we usually adopt this calculation for new compounds about which we know little. Making this dose the standard, 5-10 times or 1/5-1/10 the amount of the standard dose is administered for tests.

At the same time, two different ways of dosing are always tried for the screening of dependence: (a) administration of the fixed amount of the test drug and (b) administration of the increasing dose of the test drug. As for (b), the ratios of the increasing dose are 20, 50, or 100% every week, with modifications according to the toxic reactions that appear.

Usually we make rats tolerant to and dependent on morphine as follows:

1. Morphine HCl, 50 mg/kg, is injected sc twice daily, 7 days a week for 6-7 weeks repeatedly.
2. Morphine injection is begun twice daily at the rate of 20 mg/kg and the dose is increased every week to 40, 60, 80, and finally 100 mg/kg of body weight; this amount (100 mg/kg) is maintained over 10 days until the next procedure.

3. Control group is injected with 0.5-1.0 ml of physiological saline solution and solvent if necessary, the same as drug solution.

The continuous injection method is discussed in Sec. XI.

VI. ANTAGONISTS

As the best antagonist to morphine-type drugs, naloxone is recommended for use. Nalorphine or levellorphan can also be used in areas where naloxone is not available. However, the reactions by naloxone are not always of the same grade as those by the latter group.

The amount of naloxone is usually 1/50 of the test drug and that of nalorphine may be 1/10; that of levallorphan would be a little more. (The author has no experience with levallorphan.)

One must be aware that the more severe the dependence on morphine, the more severe the reaction (antagonism) caused by the same amount of antagonist.

Figure 5 clearly shows this situation. As can be seen in the figure, the decrease in rat body weight caused by nalorphine (10 mg/kg) or withdrawal becomes larger as the number of injection days increases, such as 6th, 12th, 20th, 26th, and 38th day of repeated administration of morphine.

VII. MEASUREMENT OF BODY TEMPERATURE

A thermistor is put ~ 30 mm into the rectum of a freely moving rat (one rat in one cage) and the temperatures of six rats are determined and recorded electronically every 30 min throughout 24 hr without touching the animal. The instrument was made by Takara Electronic Co., Yokohama, Japan (Fig. 10). All of the apparatus except the thermistor is located outside the Koitotron, in which temperature, humidity, illumination, and noise are kept stable. Telemetry of body temperature is not difficult, but the oscillator is too big to place under the peritoneum of rats. The rectal temperature of normal rats goes down after the first injection of morphine (20 mg/kg) (Fig. 11). However, with the repeated administration of morphine, body temperature goes up after injection and then goes down. The more the number of morphine injections is increased, the more the body temperature goes up and the sooner it goes up. After withdrawal or the injection of antagonist the body temperature of morphinized rats goes down (Fig. 12). It is interesting to note that the body temperature of morphinized rabbits goes up after withdrawal or antagonist injection. This is a significant difference between rats and rabbits in terms of body temperature

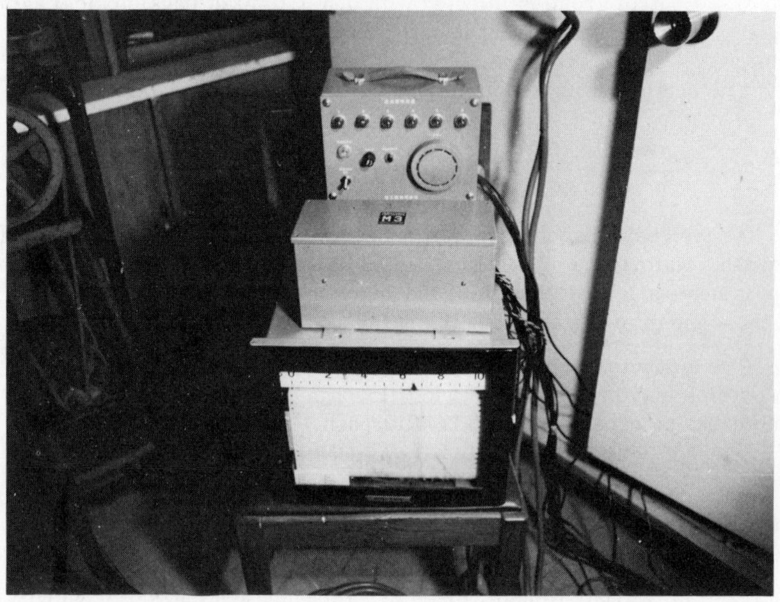

FIGURE 10. Device for automatic determination and recording of body temperature.

changes in the case of abstinence, although the body weight of both species apparently falls.

VIII. MEASUREMENT OF SPONTANEOUS LOCOMOTOR ACTIVITY

Spontaneous locomotor activity is measured and recorded by an Animal Motility Meter 40FC (Motron Products, Stockholm).

The activity of normal rats decreases with the first injection of morphine (20 mg/kg) (Fig. 13). With repeated administration, the amount of activity apparently increases after morphine injection and decreases significantly after withdrawal (Fig. 14) or after the injection of antagonist. The changing pattern of spontaneous locomotor activity of rats very much resembles that of body temperature as far as morphine is concerned. Both of them can sometimes be used as indicators of abstinence. However, they cannot be considered good indicators for pethidine and other similar drugs. Therefore, we utilize the changes of body temperature and spontaneous activity as supplementary factors.

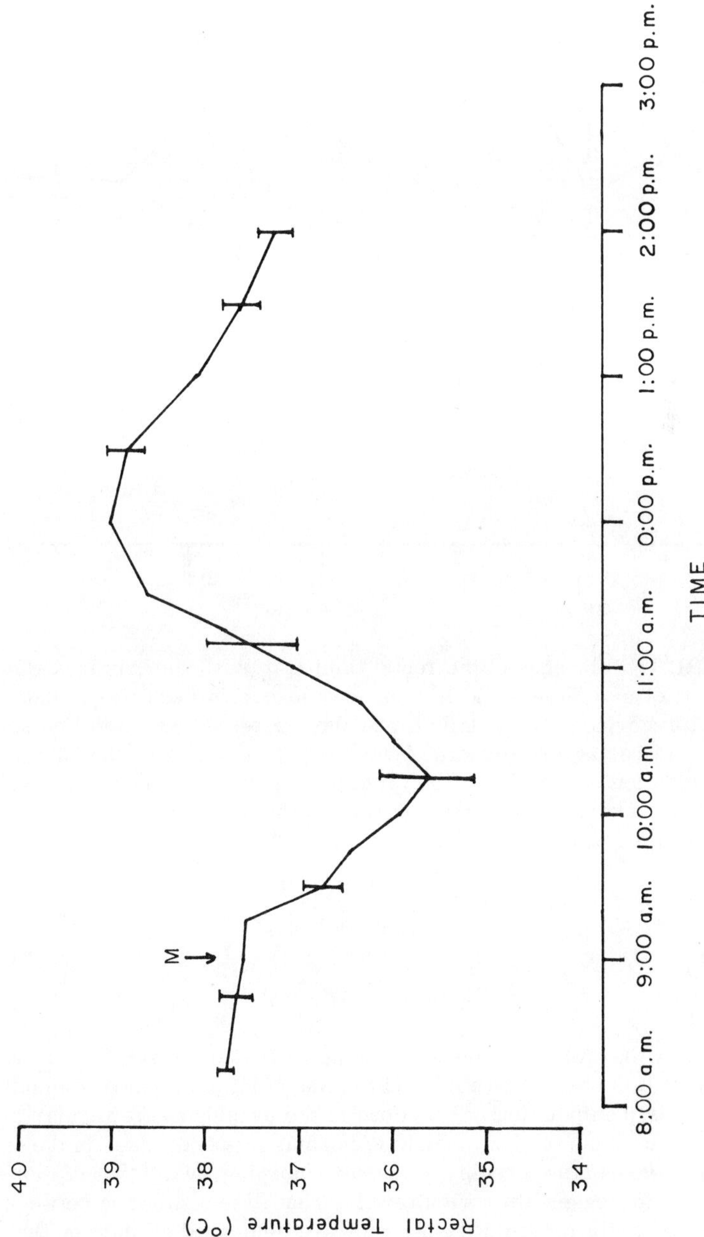

FIGURE 11. Changes of the rectal temperature of rat by the first administration of morphine HCl (20 mg/kg sc) in daytime. (Room temperature, 20° ±1°C; body weight 123 ±2.8 g; n = 6.)

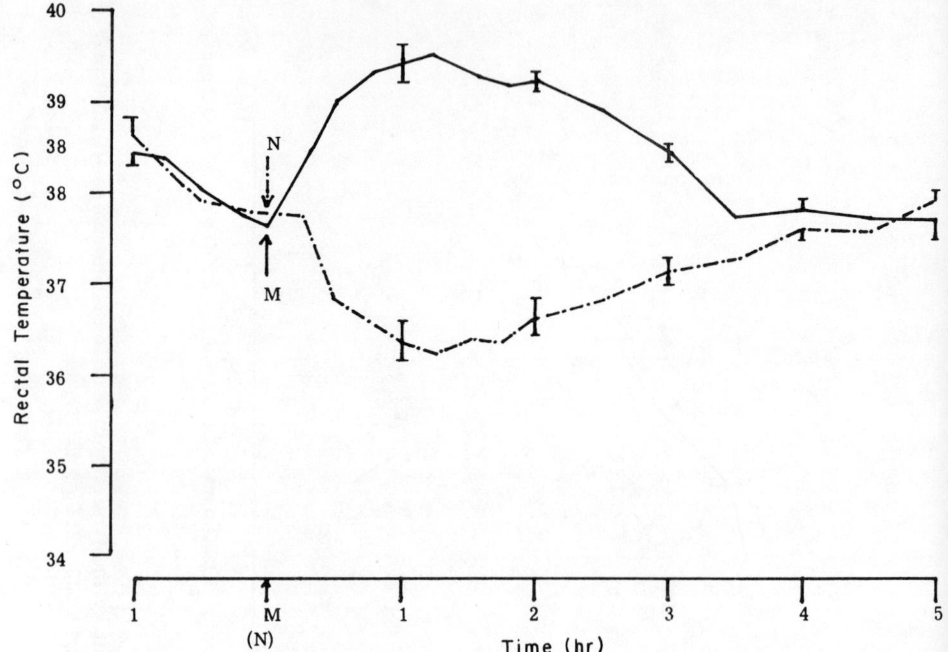

FIGURE 12. Changes of the rectal temperature of morphinized rats by the injection of morphine (solid line) or of naloxone (broken line). Rats are injected with morphine twice daily for 50 days repeatedly. Solid line shows the changes of rectal temperature of the morphinized rats on the 50th day after the injection of morphine (100 mg/kg). Broken line shows the changes of the rectal temperature of the same rats on the 51st day after the injection of naloxone (5 mg/kg). (Room temperature, 20° ±1°C; n = 6.)

IX. ABSTINENCE

A. Natural Withdrawal

Natural withdrawal is achieved by stopping the administration of the drug or by the injection of physiological saline solution in place of the drug solution. This manipulation is best done in the evening at the regular injection time, because the body weight of normal rats decreases in the daytime and increases from evening to the next morning, while that of morphinized rats decreases after withdrawal. Thus, the difference between them is more easily recognized when they are compared at night or the next morning, 10-16 hr after withdrawal.

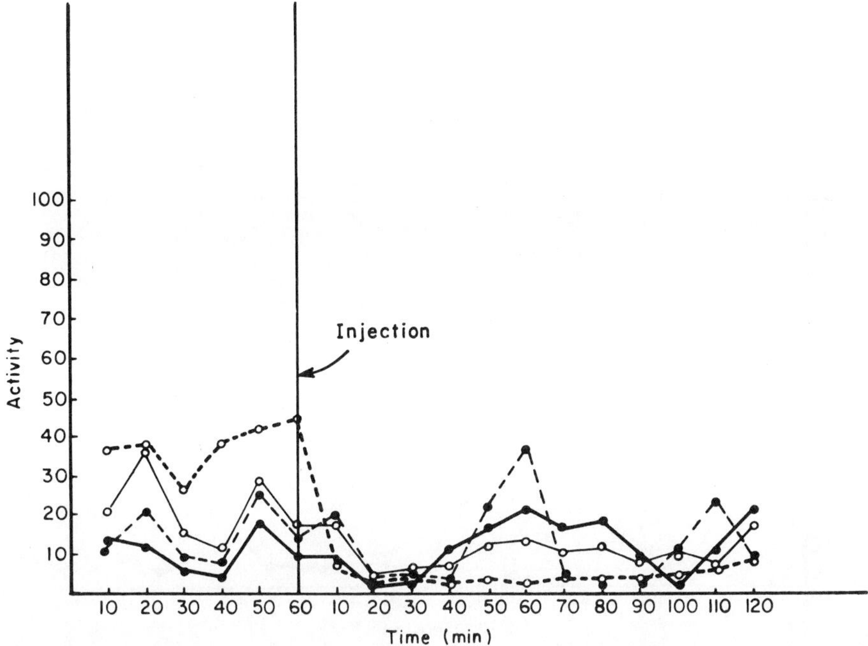

FIGURE 13. Changes of the spontaneous locomotor activity of normal rats by the injection of physiological saline solution or of morphine solution (20 mg/kg). Activity of rats decreases by the injection of morphine (•, NaCl; o, morphine).

For this purpose an automatic balance is very useful. If it is impossible to measure the body weight so often at night, one can abbreviate the measuring to four times as follows:

A. Body weight of morphinized rat in the morning at 8:00-9:00 a.m.

B. Body weight of morphinized rat just before withdrawal at 4:00-5:00 p.m. or 8:00-9:00 p.m.

C. Body weight of withdrawn rats the next morning at 8:00-9:00 a.m.

D. Body weight of rats 24 hr after withdrawal (4:00-5:00 p.m. or 8:00-9:00 p.m.).

When $A \leqq C$ and $B < C$ and $B \leqq D$, we may presume that the rats are not dependent on the drug. If, on the contrary, $A > C$ and $B > C$ and $B > D$, we may presume that the rats are dependent on the drug. Of course, the

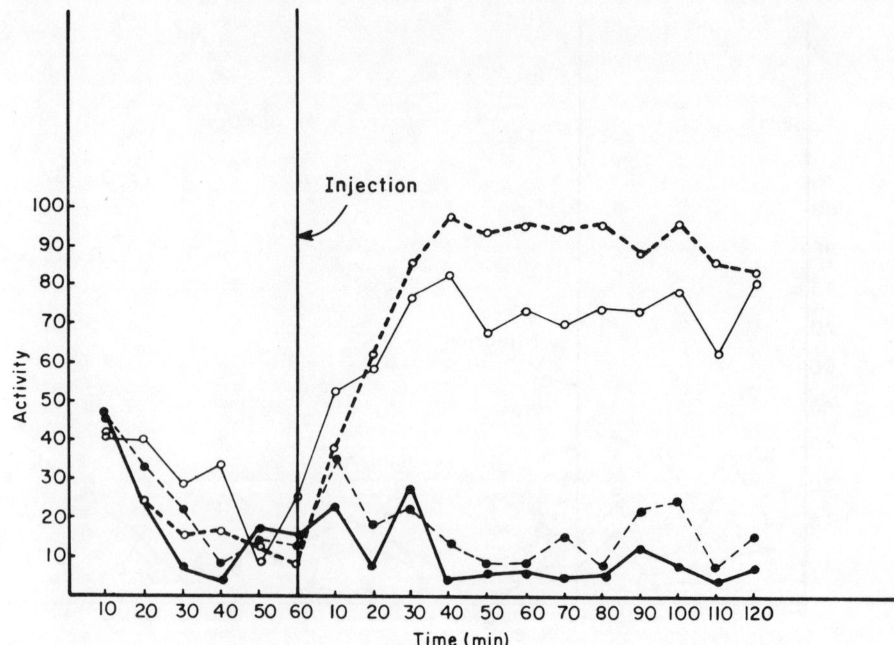

FIGURE 14. Changes of the spontaneous locomotor activity of morphinized (20-100 mg/kg twice daily for 35 days) rats by the injection of saline solution (withdrawal) or of morphine (•, NaCl; o, morphine).

results would not always be as above. There may be several combinations of the results, and accordingly no judgment could be done in these cases. In such cases the following experiments become necessary.

B. Precipitation by Antagonists

In this procedure, naloxone is usually injected subcutaneously in place of the test drug (1/50 amount of the test drug) at the regular injection time. Where the use of naloxone is impossible, nalorphine or levallorphan may be used as previously stated. The judgment is done the same as in the case of natural withdrawal.

C. Interpretation of Jumping and Wet Dog Phenomena Caused by the Administration of Antagonist to Morphine-Implanted Rats

Some researchers [39,40] insist that jumping and wet dog phenomena caused by the administration of naloxone to morphine-implanted rats or mice can be regarded as good signs of abstinence. However, the author does not fully agree with this interpretation for the following reasons:

As far as we could determine, the number of jumping and wet dog phenomena depends on the duration between the last administration of morphine and the injection of naloxone. When naloxone is injected at the same time as, or very soon after, the last morphine administration, jumping and wet dog phenomena are recognized most often. However, if naloxone is injected 4-8 hr after the last morphine administration, very few jumping or wet dog phenomena can be observed. As is well known, withdrawal symptoms of morphinized rats occur most significantly 6-8 hr after the last morphine administration. Therefore, if naloxone does accelerate or precipitate the withdrawal symptoms, and if jumping and wet dog phenomena are the withdrawal symptoms, the effect of naloxone, namely jumping and wet dog phenomena, should occur most frequently 6-8 hr after the last administration of morphine. But this is not the case. The fact is that the sooner naloxone is injected after morphine, the greater the number of jumping and wet dog phenomena observed.

By this line of thought and with the consideration of Weissman's paper [41], the author suggests that jumping and wet dog phenomena are the integrated results of acute antagonism to large amounts of morphine by antagonist and that they cannot be regarded as indicators of true dependence, even if their changes seem to be parallel to the grade of dependence.

X. SUBSTITUTION

Rats are made dependent on morphine by the repeated administration of morphine twice a day for 6-7 weeks, increasing the dose gradually from 20 mg/kg to a final dose of 100 mg/kg and maintaining the 100 mg/kg level for over 10 days.

On one evening of the seventh week at 5:00 p.m., various amounts of the test drug are administered in place of morphine, and the changing pattern of body weight is carefully observed, if possible, every 2-4 hr.

If this is difficult to do, the following weighing schedule should be used:

A. Body weight of morphinized rats just before morphine injection at 8:00-9:00 a.m.

B. Body weight of morphinized rats just before substitution at 4:00-5:00 p.m. or 8:00-9:00 p.m.

C. Body weight of rats 12-16 hr after substitution at 8:00-9:00 a.m. the next morning

If the tendency of the test drug to produce dependence in the rat is similar to that of morphine, C > B and C ≧ A, and if the test drug is not dependence producing, B > C.

XI. CONTINUOUS INJECTION

A small polyethylene tube (1.0 mm i.d.) with a 1/2 needle at the top is inserted under the skin of the rat's back and is fixed with a cloth band. The swivel attached to the ceiling of the cage can rotate in every direction without resistance and allows the rats to move freely. Part of the tube, accessible to the rat's mouth, is protected from biting by winding wire (Fig. 15).

Morphine solution in various concentrations is infused continuously for 12 hr by an electronic injector at the rate of 0.1 ml/hr, by which the absorption of morphine is readily accomplished.

Upon cessation of the continuous injection the body weight of rats decreases at a rate similar to that after withdrawal in morphinized rats (50 mg/kg twice daily for 7 weeks repeatedly). The decreases are observed both in the daytime and at night. However, normal rats continuously injected with physiological saline solution also show a fairly sharp decrease in body weight after the cessation of the continuous injection at night. This phenomenon suggests that continuous injection gives much stress to rats. Therefore, one must be careful in interpreting the results and must not draw conclusions until after careful comparison with the results of the control group.

Although we cannot omit the repeated injection for 7 weeks, it seems likely that in this way we can save many days, necessary for the production of dependence by repeated administration, and compress them into 12 hr to get similar effects on body weight. Moreover, we could prove the decrease in body weight of rats by the cessation of continuous injection (12 hr) of pethidine (50 mg/kg), which was impossible to confirm by repeated administration twice daily for 7 weeks. Accordingly, we may adopt continuous injection as a supplementary method. Further studies are necessary for the final decision as to whether continuous injection can satisfactorily replace repeated administration for 7 weeks.

XII. SIGNIFICANCE OF THE INCREASE IN BODY WEIGHT BY REPEATED ADMINISTRATION OF MORPHINE

The body weight of morphine-tolerant rats increases even in the forenoon by the administration of morphine, whereas it always decreases at this time of day in normal rats. This increase in body weight as well as in

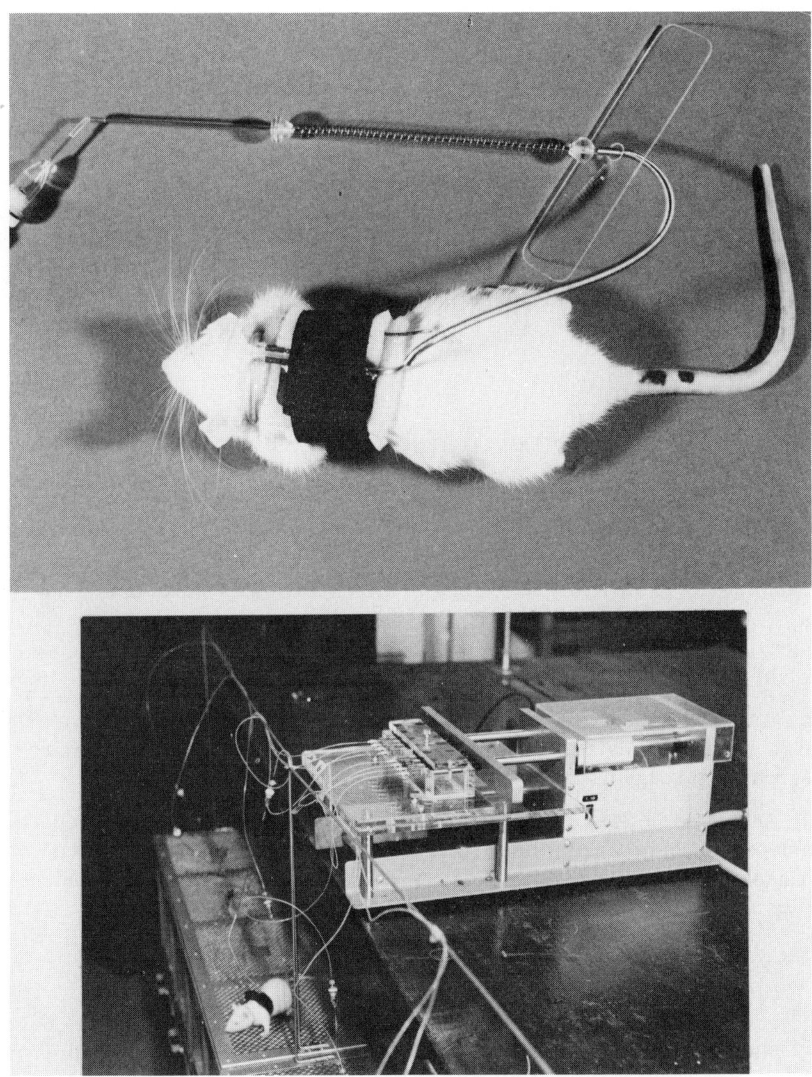

FIGURE 15. Apparatus for continuous injection.

locomotor activity appears much more clearly and earlier as the administration is repeated further.

What does this phenomenon mean? At present we have no answer, but the author assumes that tolerance develops to the depressive action of morphine, whereas no tolerance develops to its stimulating effect, and overall action results in the increases of body weight and activity.

Recently, the author learned that oral administration of propranolol (60 mg per person) was effective for the treatment of heroin (morphine) addiction in man. Several experiments were done by the author and his colleagues [42] in which it was found that propranolol inhibited the increases in body weight and spontaneous locomotor activity due to morphine injection to morphine-tolerant rats but that propranolol did not affect the decrease in body weight caused by withdrawal. Therefore, the effectiveness of propranolol, if any, is assumed by the author to be due to the depressant effects against the stimulating actions of morphine and not to any alleviation of withdrawal symptoms.

XIII. EXPERIMENTAL RESULTS FOR SOME CNS DRUGS

Table I shows the results of our experiments on the dependence-producing liability of some CNS drugs, details of which are omitted for reasons of space. The classification of A, B, C, and D and their subdivisions is done exclusively according to the experimental results and not by the similarity of their actions nor of their chemical structures. Morphine glucuronide, after its repeated administration, caused no change in body weight by withdrawal or by antagonist.

As can be seen, the table is not complete in some respects. We expect these gaps in the data to be filled in the future by the efforts of many researchers throughout the world.

As stated in Sec. I, the author has been compiling worldwide reports on dependence-producing liability using small animals and particularly on changes in the body weight of rats. Almost all of them favor the contention of the author, who is very grateful for such information.

XIV. DETAILED DESCRIPTION OF THE PROCESS

As stated previously, our method is not yet complete. Minor improvements are always carried out in the next experiments, but endless development is the fate of science, and therefore the author believes it may be helpful to describe our present process and to invite reexamination by researchers in the same field.

Since some details have been described in each section, main procedures will be written in the order of our experimentation.

TABLE I

Changes in Rat Body Weight Produced by Repeated Drug Administration, Withdrawal, and Substitution for Morphine[a]

Agent	Repetition for 40-50 days	Withdrawal after repetition	Naloxone after repetition	Substitution
A_1				
Morphine HCl	↑	↓	↓	↑
Codeine phosphate	↑	↓	↓	↑
d-Propoxyphene napsylate	↑	↓	↓	↑
A_2				
Azabicyclane	↑	↓	↓	↑
Pethidine HCl	↑	↑	↓	↑
Methadone HCl	↑	↑	↓	↑
Thienylaminobutene	↑	↑	↓	↑
B				
Nalorphine HCl	↑	↑	↓	↓
Pentazocine (base)	↑	↑	↓	↓
C				
Barbital sodium	↑	-	-	(↑)
Meprobamate	↑	-	-	(↑)
D_1				
Sulpyrine	(↑)	-	-	↓
Aminopyrine	↑	-	-	↓
D_2				
Chlorpromazine	-	-	-	↓
Acetaminophen	-	-	-	↓
Sodium salicylate	-	-	-	↓
d-Methorphan	-	-	-	↓
Dipropyl acetate	-	-	-	↓
Niflumic acid	-	-	-	↓
Simetride	-	-	-	↓
Cocaine HCl	-	-	-	↓
Δ^9-THC	-	-	-	↓

[a] ↑, increase; ↓, decrease; -, same as the control; (↑), a slight change.

1. Feed rats (male, ~ 120 g) for several days in a well-conditioned room.
2. Divide rats into necessary groups at random. Each group should consist of at least five rats.
3. Several groups are necessary as controls, such as the group receiving saline solution, the group receiving only the solvent in which the test drug will be dissolved, the group receiving morphine or other dependence-producing drug which has pharmacological action similar to that of the test drug, if any, etc.
4. Measure the body weight of rats at least twice a day, at almost the same time in the morning and in the evening at the gram level. If automatic balances are available, set to record the weight every half-hour for 36 hr.
5. Administer drugs after each measurement of body weight by hand, twice a day, 7 days a week for 6-7 weeks repeatedly, except in the case of continuous injection.
6. Modify the amounts of the test drug according to the LD_{50}, ED_{50}, and route of administration. When the decrease in body weight becomes apparent after some repeated administrations, the amount should be reduced. As already described, two kinds of doses, fixed and increasing, must be tried.
7. Observe the changes in the behavior of the rat before and after drug administration as well as the changes in body weight and, if possible, those in body temperature and spontaneous activity. Observations must be done particularly carefully at the time of the first administration and once a week during the repeated administration.
8. Withdraw the drug or inject the antagonist after 6-7 weeks of repeated administration at the regular injection time in the evening for at least five rats each. The changing pattern of body weight every 2-4 hr should be determined for 24 hr at least. If it is difficult to measure the body weight so often and at night, the schedule may be simplified as follows: Measure the body weight of rats at (a) 8:00-9:00 a.m. of the 50th day of repeated administration, (b) 4:00-5:00 p.m. or 8:00-9:00 p.m. of the same day as above (withdrawal or precipitation should be done just after the weight measurement), (c) 8:00-9:00 a.m. of the 51st day; (d) 4:00-5:00 p.m. or 8:00-9:00 p.m. of the 51st day. Compare the changes of body weight in 2 days. An automatic balance is very useful for this purpose.

9. Changes in body temperature and spontaneous locomotor activity should be measured.
10. Substitute various amounts of the test drug for morphine in the rats, to which morphine is administered twice a day for 6-7 weeks. The changes in body weight should be determined in a manner similar to that described in 8.
11. Compare the results obtained on the test drug caused by repeated administration, withdrawal, precipitation, and substitution with Table I, which may supply reliable proof for the prediction of dependence-producing liability.
12. As far as pethidine-like drugs are concerned, however, withdrawal after continuous injection would be necessary in addition to the above procedures in order to clarify their dependence liability. (Continuous injection may replace long-term repeated administration of the drug in the future but our present knowledge and experience are too limited to declare its certainty.)

Table II shows the instance of a new analgesic (X-100) studied for its dependence liability by our method. As can be understood by the comparison of the results with those of some analgesics in the table, X-100 may have some dependence liability similar to that of pentazocine, and a monkey test showed results quite similar to ours. Accordingly, a final decision was committed to clinical investigation.

XV. EVALUATION OF THE METHOD

As far as we have examined on new drugs, no results or claims contrary to our conclusions have yet been reported. Of course, there were cases in which we could not decide by our method alone whether the test drug should be listed on the narcotic list. As stated in Sec. I, our method aims to screen the dependence-producing liability of many specimens simply. The monkey test is absolutely necessary for further decision on the application of a drug to man. However, there were cases in which monkey tests were not superior to our rat tests. The author believes, therefore, that the two methods using monkeys and rats have their own "raison d'etre."

The following statement is made in the WHO Technical Report No. 287 [2] about tests using rodents: "A convenient procedure for assessment of the degree of dependence through abrupt withdrawal is to follow the body weight. Dependent animals lose considerable weight over 24 hours period." The author was pleased to read it and thought at the same time that the changing pattern of body weight of rats, not only after withdrawal but also

TABLE II

Changes in Rat Body Weight Produced by Repeated Drug Administration, Withdrawal, and Substitution for Morphine[a]

Agent	Repetition for 40-50 days	Withdrawal after repetition	Naloxone after repetition	Substitution
Morphine HCl	↑	↓	↓	↑
Codeine phosphate	↑	↓	↓	↑
d-Propoxyphene napsylate	↑	↓	↓	↑
Azabicyclane	↑	↓	↓	↑
Pethidine HCl	↑	↑	↓	↑
Methadone HCl	↑	↑	↓	↑
Thienylaminobutene	↑	↑	↓	↑
Nalorphine HCl	↑	↑	↓	↓
Pentazocine (base)	↑	↑	↓	↓
X-100	↑	↑	↓	↓

[a]↑, increase; ↓, decrease; (↑), slight increase.

in cases of repeated administration, precipitation, and substitution, supplies much more information for the prediction of dependence production of drugs.

REFERENCES

1. M. H. Seevers, Opiate addiction in the monkey, J. Pharmacol. Exp. Ther. 56:147-165 (1936).

2. Evaluation of dependence producing drugs. WHO Technical Report Series No. 287, 1964.

3. Testing for dependence-liability in animals and man, Addendum 1 of minutes, Committee on the Problems of Drug Dependence. 28th Meeting NAS-NRC, February 1966.

4. Testing for dependence-liability in animals and man (revised 1972). Bull. Narcotics 25:25-39 (1973).

5. E. Hosoya and S. Otobe, Withdrawal symptoms of morphinized rats. Folia Pharmacol. Jap., p. 120 (1958).

6. D. G. Fichtenberg, Study of experimental habituation to morphine. Bull. Narcotics 3:19-42 (1951).

7. E. Hosoya and S. Otobe, Effects of repeated administration of morphine upon the bodyweights of rats. Folia Pharmacol. Jap. 54:118 (1958).

8. E. Hosoya and S. Otobe, Studies on the addiction-liability of rats to some analgesics. Folia Pharmacol. Jap. 54:000 (1958).

9. E. Hosoya, Some withdrawal symptoms of rats to morphine. Pharmacologist 1:77 (1959).

10. E. Hosoya and A. Oguri, Effects of repeated administration of some tranquilizers and hypnotics upon the bodyweights of rats. Folia Pharmacol. Jap. 56:159 (1960).

11. E. Hosoya and A. Oguri, Effects of some tranquilizers upon the spontaneous locomotor activities of rats under peculiar conditions. Folia Pharmacol. Jap. 57:77 (1960).

12. E. Hosoya and A. Oguri, Screening of dependence liability of tranquilizers. Folia Pharmacol. Jap. 57:78 (1960).

13. E. Hosoya, Studies on the addiction liability of morphine on rats (4th report). Folia Pharmacol. Jap. 57:3 (1962).

14. E. Hosoya, Does the administration of nalorphine shorten the duration of the tolerance to morphine already formed in a rat's body? Folia Pharmacol. Jap. 58:10 (1962).

15. E. Hosoya, Effects of the repeated administration of morphine and the withdrawal thereafter upon rats. Folia Pharmacol. Jap. 58:149 (1962).

16. W. R. Martin, Tolerance to and physical dependence on morphine in rats. Psychopharmacologia 4:247-260 (1963).

17. W. R. Buckett, A new test for morphine-like physical dependence (addiction liability in rats). Psychopharmacologia 6:410-416 (1964).

18. O. J. Lorenzetti and L. F. Sancilio, Morphine dependent rats as a model for evaluating potential addiction liability of analgesic compounds. Arch. Int. Pharmacodyn. Ther. 183:391-402 (1970).

19. E. Hosoya and A. Oguri, Changes of the spontaneous activities of rats by the administration of morphine (in English). Keio J. 12:83-97 (1963).

20. E. Hosoya and H. Akita, Catecholamine level in brain and the spontaneous activities of morphinized rats (in English). Keio. J. Med. 12: 127-130 (1963).

21. I. Anan and E. Hosoya, Effects of the repeated administration of morphine, its withdrawal and nalorphine-injection upon the body temperature of rats (in Japanese). Keio Igaku 46:471-480 (1969).

22. E. Hosoya, Relationship between the biogenic amines in rat brain and the phenomena of tolerance to and dependence on morphine (in Japanese). Report to the Ministry of Education for its research grant, 1963.

23. E. Hosoya, Screening of physical dependence liability of drugs using small animals: Drug-abuse. Report of U.S.-Japan Cooperative Researches on Drug Abuse (in English). Tokyo: Japan Society for the Promotion of Sciences, 1968, pp. 217-230.

24. T. Akera and T. M. Brody, The addiction cycle to narcotics in the rat and its relation to catecholamines. Biochem. Pharmacol. 17:675 (1968).

25. I. Anan and E. Hosoya, Effects of the repeated administration of cocaine and its withdrawal upon the body temperature of rats (in Japanese). Keio Igaku 47:555 (1970).

26. T. Oka and E. Hosoya, Effect of paraphenyl alanine and cholinergic antagonists on body temperature changes induced by the administration of morphine to non-tolerant and morphine tolerant rats. J. Pharmacol. Exp. Ther. 180:136 (1972).

27. T. Oka and E. Hosoya, The effect of cholinergic antagonists on increases of spontaneous locomotor activity and body weight induced by the administration of morphine to tolerant rats (in English). Psychopharmacologia 23:231 (1972).

28. M. Nozaki and E. Hosoya, Hourly changes of the body temperature of rats by the repeated administration of some analgesics. Paper presented at the 45th regional meeting of the Japanese Pharmacological Society, November, 1971.

29. M. Nozaki and E. Hosoya, Studies on wet dog phenomena (in Japanese). Paper presented at the 45th regional meeting of the Japanese Pharmacological Society, October 1971.

30. M. Nozaki and E. Hosoya, Hourly changes of the body weight of rats by the administration of antipyretic analgesics and the effect of substitution with such analgesics for morphine on the bodyweight of morphinized rats. Paper presented at the 44th regional meeting of the Japanese Pharmacological Society, June 1971.

31. E. Hosoya and M. Nozaki, Physical dependence liability of marihuana compared with cocaine. Report of U.S.-Japan Cooperative Research on Marihuana (in English). Tokyo: Japan Society for the Promotion of Sciences, 1971.

32. M. Nozaki and E. Hosoya, Hourly changes of the body weight of rats by the repeated administration of some tranquilizers, their withdrawal and the substitution with them for morphine in morphinized rats. Paper presented at the 47th regional meeting of the Japanese Pharmacological Society, November 1972.

33. M. Nozaki and E. Hosoya, Hourly changes of the body weight of rats by the repeated administration of morphine (in Japanese). Paper presented at the 42nd regional meeting of the Japanese Pharmacological Society, June 1970.

34. M. Nozaki and E. Hosoya, Hourly changes of the body weight of morphinized rats after withdrawal. Paper presented at the 43rd regional meeting of the Japanese Pharmacological Society, November 1970.

35. C. Maggiolo and F. Huidobro, Administration of pellet of morphine to mice abstinence syndrome. Acta Physiol. Latinoamer. 11:70-98 (1961).

36. P. G. Goode, An implanted reservoir of morphine solution for rapid induction of physical dependence in rats. Brit. J. Pharmacol. 41: 558-566 (1971).

37. M. Nozaki and E. Hosoya, Studies on the grade of physical dependence caused by the continuous injection of morphine to rats. Paper presented to the 48th regional meeting of the Japanese Pharmacological Society, June 1973.

38. M. Nozaki and E. Hosoya, Measurement of the intensity of physical dependence due to the repeated administration of morphine to rats. Jap. J. Pharmacol. Suppl. 23, 95 (1973).

39. E. L. Way, H. H. Loh, and F. H. Shen, Quantitative assessment of morphine tolerance and physical dependence. Pharmacologist 10:188 (1968).

40. D. L. Francis and C. Schneider, Jumping after naloxone precipitated withdrawal of chronic morphine in the rat. Brit. J. Pharmacol. 41: 4249 (1971).

41. A. Weissman, Jumping in mice elicited by 1-naphthyloxyacetic acid. J. Pharmacol. Exp. Ther. 184:11-17 (1973).

42. M. Nozaki, S. Shimada, and E. Hosoya, Effect of propranolol upon the withdrawal symptoms of morphinized rats (in Japanese). Paper presented to the 49th regional meeting of the Japanese Pharmacological Society, November 1973.

Chapter 13

THE NARCOTIC WITHDRAWAL SYNDROME IN THE RAT

GERALD GIANUTSOS
and MARTIN HYNES

Department of Pharmacology and Toxicology
College of Pharmacy
University of Rhode Island
Kingston, Rhode Island

RICHARD DRAWBAUGH
and HARBANS LAL

Department of Pharmacology and Toxicology
College of Pharmacy
Department of Psychology
University of Rhode Island
Kingston, Rhode Island

I. INTRODUCTION

In order to study the pathophysiology of narcotic dependence, it is necessary to evolve an appropriate animal model. The rat has proven to be a useful subject for the study of the mechanism of narcotic addiction since it is easily made dependent on narcotics by a variety of methods. The most reliable dependence in the rat has been produced by the chronic injection of morphine sulfate [1], subcutaneous implantation of pellets containing insoluble morphine alkaloids [2], or continuous administration of orally acting drugs, such as fentanyl, in the daily drinking water.

It generally takes a period of 2 weeks to produce a reliable dependence. Several short procedures to produce dependence in a few hours or a few days have been reported [3-5]. However, before one accepts these procedures, one must wait until their relevance to clinical dependence is proven. According to the presently accepted definition of narcotic dependence, it must result from repeated administration of a narcotic drug for prolonged periods of time. Therefore, the physiological changes occurring after brief treatment may not be considered as dependence based upon this accepted definition.

In addition to the ease with which dependence can be produced in the laboratory rat, the withdrawal syndrome exhibited by the rat is consistent, reliable, and can be objectively measured. This syndrome may be brought about either by administering a narcotic antagonist or by the abrupt termination of chronic morphine administration. The withdrawal precipitated by an antagonist is immediate, short-lived, and can be easily quantified. However, except for special circumstances, it is never clinically encountered in man. Since an animal model must correspond to the condition encountered clinically, one can rely on nonantagonist-precipitated withdrawal for this information. In addition, for the purpose of pathophysiological research one must contend with a tissue or organism that contains large quantities of two potent drugs in the body if one uses antagonist-precipitated withdrawal for this research. The presence of two drugs would certainly present difficulties in the interpretation of biochemical data, since any results obtained would have equivocal explanations.

Above all, the antagonist-precipitated withdrawal presents a formidable obstacle to the pharmacologist who is looking for a chemotherapeutic approach to the treatment of narcotic dependence or who must use drugs as tools to determine the role of various neurochemical mechanisms involved in the narcotic abstinence syndrome. In contrast to the spontaneous withdrawal syndrome, the withdrawal precipitated by an antagonist is very difficult, if not impossible, to suppress by other drugs, including opiates. Therefore, the usefulness of the antagonist-precipitated withdrawal is limited to the investigation of carefully selected, specific areas of research. In contrast, the spontaneous withdrawal caused by cessation of narcotic drug administration has wider application to research and the screening of antiabstinence drugs. It has a definite course of onset and duration and, like the clinical situation, can be studied over extended periods. Usually, the organism contains only negligible quantities of exogenous chemicals.

The withdrawal syndrome can be divided into two phases: early or primary abstinence and protracted abstinence [6,7]. The early abstinence begins to appear 12-24 hr after discontinuing chronic morphine. It consists of the following symptoms described by Martin et al. [1]: "wet shakes," loss of body weight, decreased metabolic rate, increased urination and defecation, decreased fluid consumption, hypothermia, sleeplessness, irritability on handling, and enhanced norepinephrine and epinephrine excretion. In addition, there is a decline in the voltage output of the EEG [8], writhing [9], social aggression [10], ptosis, and piloerection [11]. This syndrome lasts for approximately 72 hr. After this time, the syndrome changes. During the protracted phase, food and water intake, body weight, temperature, and locomotor activity increase above normal levels and may persist for several months [1]. In addition, there is a continuation of wet shakes [1,12], aggression [13], and EEG abnormalities [14] during the protracted phase. Many of the other symptoms begin to return to normal levels during this time.

In this chapter, we shall describe the method we use in our laboratory to study the withdrawal phenomenon in the rat.

II. METHODS

A. Intraperitoneal Injection of Narcotic Drugs

The method used to addict rats by intraperitoneal injection of morphine sulfate is discussed in Chapter 8. Briefly, male Long-Evans (hooded) rats weighing 250-350 g are injected intraperitoneally (ip) with systematically increasing doses of morphine sulfate three times a day. The starting dose of 15 mg/kg/injection (45 mg/kg/day) is increased daily by 15 mg/kg/

dose until a terminal dose of 135 mg/kg/injection (405 mg/kg/day) is reached. The rats are maintained at this dose level for several days (minimum of 5 days) before withdrawal.

B. Oral Administration of Narcotic Drugs

The oral administration of narcotic drugs may be reliably used to produce narcotic dependence only if the drugs used are orally active. Morphine sulfate, which is usually employed to produce addiction in the rat, is unsuitable for oral administration because of its poor absorption from the GI tract. Although after several weeks of oral consumption of morphine sulfate some symptoms can be observed during withdrawal, they are usually limited to the signs of physiological disturbances in the GI tract [4]. Recently, narcotic dependence of high reliability has been achieved by oral administration of fentanyl in saccharine solution. This drug possesses high analgesic potency when given orally and the rat readily ingests the saccharine solution containing sufficient fentanyl. Fentanyl is added in increasing concentration to the drinking water in saccharine (0.2 mg/ml). A starting concentration 0.03 mg/ml is increased daily (except Saturday and Sunday) by 0.06 mg/ml until a concentration of 0.48 mg/ml is readily tolerated (10-12 days). This concentration is maintained for at least 3 days before withdrawal. Approximate daily intake is 15 mg/kg/day. At day 0 of withdrawal, the rats are injected ip with 16 mg/kg of fentanyl to ensure that all the rats begin the withdrawal period with high concentrations of the drug in the body.

C. Withdrawal

Besides using narcotic antagonists, there are a variety of ways to cause the abrupt cessation of narcotic administration. Regardless of the method used, care must be taken not only so that the administration of narcotic drug is discontinued, but also so that the environment continuously paired with the drug administration is discontinued [12,15]. We have found that ringing of a bell which is repeatedly paired with the injection of morphine can, when presented without morphine, significantly reduce the incidence and intensity of certain withdrawal symptoms in addicted rats [16,17]. Similarly, in the case of orally active narcotics given in saccharine solution, the saccharine must be discontinued in addition to the narcotic. In rats so addicted, the withdrawal syndrome is markedly more severe if the saccharine-fentanyl solution is replaced with water without saccharine during abstinence. The saccharine solution can reduce the intensity and severity of the withdrawal symptoms if it was previously consistently paired with the narcotic drug.

D. Measurement of Symptoms

Symptoms of withdrawal are measured during both primary and protracted abstinence. Although one may begin recording symptoms as early as a few hours after the last administration of a narcotic, to be practical we have come to the conclusion that measurement of symptoms once every 24 hr during primary abstinence and once every fortnight during protracted abstinence is sufficient. The symptoms are measured 30 min after the last morphine injection and 3 hr after the fentanyl injection in order to serve as baselines for subsequent comparisons. The dependent rats are removed from their home cages and placed singly into novel cages for the measurement of the symptoms. The rats are observed for 30 min, during which time the occurrence of abnormal gross behavior is noted. The following behaviors are consistently seen during withdrawal.

1. Wet shakes: These are violent shaking movements of the head and/or body of the rat which resemble the action of an animal that has been drenched with water and are readily distinguishable from tremors or jerky movements. The number of shakes during this 30-min observation is recorded. One will notice that there are two types of wet shakes: one involving the whole body and one involving just the head and forelimbs of the animal. The frequency of occurrence of wet shakes is greatest shortly after handling the rat or after changing its place of residence and decreases with time. As soon as the rats are placed in new cages, the measurement should begin, since the frequency is reduced as time passes and it will be an important source of error.

2. Writhing: This consists of dragging the abdomen along the floor of the cage and drawing in the abdominal wall [9] or arching the back, neither of which is accompanied by yawning. The presence or absence of writhing during the 30-min observation period is noted.

3. Piloerection: This is the state in which the fur stands on end during most of the observation period. The presence or absence of piloerection is noted during the 30 min of observation, except for the period immediately after placing the rat in the observation cage, since this may be the result of handling. Piloerection may also be graded on a 4-point scoring system [18]. Score 0 is given for no piloerection, 1 for doubtful piloerection, 2 for piloerection which is present but which could be more intense, and 3 for highest intensity of piloerection.

4. Ptosis: This is defined as a condition in which the rat's eyelids are drooping so that the eyes appear as slits. To be recorded as

ptosis, the eyes must not be completely closed and the rat must be capable of movement, in order to distinguish this state from normal resting and sleep. Eye closure in ptosis is sometimes reversed when the animal is handled. The amount of time during the observation period that the rat is exhibiting ptosis is measured with the aid of a cumulative timer. Ptosis can also be graded on a 5-point scoring system [18]. A score of 0 is given if the eyes are completely closed and 4 is given when exophthalmia is present. Intermediate scores are given for different levels of eye opening.

5. Agitation and inhibition of habituation: When a control rat is placed in a novel environment, exploratory movements and grooming are seen. These behaviors usually subside after a few minutes. During narcotic withdrawal, initial exploratory activity, grooming, and scratching are exaggerated. Habituation to these activities is markedly reduced. Chewing and stereotypy are also observed occasionally.

6. Spasms: Frequently, spastic muscle twitches are observed along the back or thighs of the dependent rat. The presence of these spasms is noted during the observation.

7. Hypothermia: Body temperature is reduced during morphine withdrawal. The temperature is measured during morphine abstinence with a digital thermister thermometer (Digitec Model 8500-3, United Systems Corp.). The rectal probe is inserted 5 cm into the colon of the rat, which is held as loosely as possible. The probe is kept in place for 1 min before the rectal temperature is recorded. Because no other satisfactory baseline is available, we use the temperature obtained 30 min after the morphine injection in order to calculate the magnitude of hypothermia. The figure thus obtained is inflated, as morphine causes a marked hyperthermia. One must take this into account when interpreting withdrawal data.

8. Loss of body weight: For the purpose of determining the weight loss during withdrawal, the weight of the abstinent rat is compared with the rat's weight immediately before the last injection of morphine.

9. Aggression: Measurement of aggression is described in Chapter 8.

All these observations are made at various time intervals after the final injection of morphine. We have systematically looked at these signs at 30 min and 4, 12, 24, 48, and 72 hr after terminating morphine injection.

III. CHARACTERISTICS OF WITHDRAWAL SYNDROME

There is little difference, qualitatively, between the withdrawal symptoms of the various narcotic drugs that have been studied to date. Therefore, we shall limit our discussion to the details of the symptoms of withdrawal following chronic morphine injections.

A. Onset and Duration

During abstinence from morphine, a rat exhibits a large variety of measurable signs [1]. The parameters which are quantified in our laboratory are listed in Table I. These signs were chosen because they are highly reproducible, easily quantifiable, and objective.

TABLE I

Occurrence of Withdrawal Signs During Abstinence from Morphine

Parameter observed	Peak intensity (hr of abstinence)	Duration	Blockade by morphine	Blockade by methadone
Wet shakes	24-48	Months	Yes	Yes
Writhing	24-48		Yes	Yes
Weight loss	24-72[a]	5-7 days	No[b]	No[c]
Hypothermia	24	4-5 days	Yes	No[d]
Piloerection	24-72		Yes	Yes
Ptosis	24	3-4 days	Yes	No
Aggression	72	30 days or more	Yes	Yes

[a] The largest weight loss for a 24-hr interval occurs in the first 24 hr, but the weight continues to fall, reaching a minimum at 72 hr.

[b] Continuation of morphine prevents the occurrence of weight loss, but administration of morphine during withdrawal does not immediately reverse it.

[c] Initially there is a prevention of weight loss, but a tolerance very rapidly develops to this effect so that after 72 hr there is no difference between rats given methadone or saline.

[d] Temperature reversal is partial, but not complete (see text).

To evaluate the symptoms of withdrawal, we measured them in a manner such that a large number of measurements could be handled by an average-sized research group. However, for the detailed study of the characteristics of the syndrome or the underlying mechanism, one can measure it with still greater precision. Other symptoms that we do not routinely measure include tolerance to analgesics; body injuries, such as self-mutilation of paws and tail; increased locomotor activity; hyperreflexia; changes in sleep characteristics; and decreased food and water consumption.

Initially, we conducted a detailed study of the symptoms every 6 hr for a total of 96 hr during withdrawal. Analysis of these data suggested that observation of the symptoms at 24-hr intervals encompasses all of the important information. Values obtained at 30 min after the last morphine injection are used for comparison. However, when using narcotic drugs other than morphine, we must accordingly modify the interval between observations. The course of the withdrawal syndrome differs depending on the pharmacokinetic properties of the drug used.

Prior to 24 hr, the withdrawal syndrome is relatively mild, with some measureable signs beginning to appear at the 12-hr mark. It should be noted from Table I that, with the exception of aggression, the peak intensity of all the withdrawal signs occurs within 24-48 hr following termination of morphine administration. It is during this period (24-48 hr of withdrawal) that the most severe withdrawal is observed.

B. Weight Loss

Weight loss is the most frequently used criterion of the withdrawal syndrome. It can be reliably recorded and has been observed by numerous investigators. Results from pooling of the data from several runs of experiments in our laboratory are summarized in Table II. The rats begin losing weight approximately 12 hr after their last dose of morphine and continue to lose weight up to the 72 hr mark. The total weight loss is more than 10% of the prewithdrawal body weight. For the first 4-6 hr after receiving an injection of morphine, the rats gain weight, so that the total weight loss during withdrawal may actually be greater. It is not clear whether the weight loss can be attributed primarily to the decrease in food and water consumption during withdrawal or to the loss of bulk and fluids through increased defecation, diarrhea, and urination during withdrawal.

C. Body Shakes

Body shakes constitute a widely used and reliable criterion for narcotic withdrawal. Results from pooling the data from several runs of

TABLE II

The Morphine Withdrawal Syndrome

Hours of withdrawal	N	Symptom (mean ± SE)					
		Body weight loss (g)	Temperature drop (deg)	Shakes	Ptosis (sec)[a]	Pilo-erection[b]	Writhing[b]
24	57	13.0 ± 1.1	2.03 ± 0.05	7 ± 0.8	282 ± 38	57/57	26/57
48	57	26.1 ± 1.4	1.77 ± 0.05	6 ± 0.5	92 ± 18	57/57	47/57
72	7	35.6 ± 2.8	1.53 ± 0.08	6 ± 0.8	384 ± 92	7/7	7/7

[a] Duration of ptosis during 30-min observation.

[b] Number of animals showing positive reaction out of total number observed.

experiments in our laboratory are summarized in Table II. It will be noted that abstinent rats exhibit approximately 7 shakes during the 30-min observation period. We have looked for similar shakes in nondependent drug-free rats and have found that less than 1 rat out of 10 will shake, indicating a marked increase in frequency during withdrawal. Although pooling of the data obscures any differences during the withdrawal period, it has been generally found that during a particular run of the experiment, the greatest frequency of shakes is observed at 24 hr of withdrawal, with a slight decrease in frequency thereafter.

D. Hypothermia

Hypothermia is one of the most consistent and reliable parameters of withdrawal in the rat. Data pooled from several runs of experiments in our laboratory are summarized in Table II. The nadir is observed at 24 hr of withdrawal with a highly reproducible drop of 2° in the body temperature at this time. The temperature slowly begins to rise thereafter. As mentioned earlier, the withdrawal temperature is compared with the temperature of the same animal 30 min after it receives its last morphine injection. Since morphine raises body temperature, the magnitude of the hypothermia may be slightly inflated. In studies conducted in our laboratory, designed to pharmacologically alter the withdrawal syndrome, it has been difficult to completely prevent the hypothermia during withdrawal using drugs. Morphine injected into these rats returns the temperature to its elevated level, where it remains for 8 hr. Methadone, at a dose which blocks other withdrawal signs (20 mg/kg), partially reverses the hypothermia, but is unable to reverse it to the same level as morphine. It is not yet clear whether these results are due to the inflated initial temperature or to some characteristics of the hypothermia. It has been demonstrated that a conditioned stimulus (bell) that has been repeatedly paired with a morphine injection will significantly reverse the withdrawal hypothermia if that stimulus is presented during withdrawal [16,17].

E. Autonomic Symptoms

In addition to the above symptoms, during withdrawal there are autonomic reactions that resemble cholinergic discharge. These symptoms include diarrhea, lacrimation, salivation, and rhinnorhea. It has been our experience that the incidence of these symptoms is low during spontaneous withdrawal, but they are very prevelant after the administration of naloxone.

Another aspect of withdrawal is piloerection, which is observed in virtually all rats during the abstinence period. It is possible that piloerection may be related to the withdrawal hypothermia.

F. Aggression

Aggression is reliably observed as a consequence of spontaneous withdrawal. Unlike the other withdrawal symptoms, aggression appears at a later time during withdrawal and has a peak effect (72 hr) at a time when other symptoms are reversing. A detailed discussion of withdrawal aggression appears in Chapter 8.

G. Miscellaneous

In addition to the above symptoms, there are other reliable signs during narcotic abstinence. The data for some of these other symptoms are summarized in Table II. Writhing is observed in approximately 90% of all rats during abstinence. Because of the wide variability in the frequency of writhing among animals, we generally determine whether or not this symptom appears in a parcitular rat rather than count the number of writhes, although the latter procedure could be followed. Similarly, ptosis is generally observed during withdrawal to various degrees. We have found that measuring the duration of ptosis provides a reliable value.

It should be pointed out that several symptoms observed during naloxone-precipitated withdrawal, such as teeth chattering, lacrimation, and salivation [19], are rarely noted in our laboratory during spontaneous withdrawal.

IV. MECHANISM

A. Specificity

Since the purpose of this chapter is to discuss methodology, theoretical interpretations will not be attempted here. Several recent reports [20-22] adequately describe current theories of addiction. However, it may be relevant to comment on these symptoms from the point of view of their evaluation.

1. Selection of Symptoms

It must be remembered that morphine produces a wide variety of pharmacological effects on numerous sensitive physiological systems. It is assumed that after repeated interference with these systems, compensatory mechanisms take over and the activity of these compensatory mechanisms is reflected during withdrawal. However, it is not yet clear which of the resulting symptoms are specifically due to narcotic withdrawal and which symptoms are nonspecific but possibly related to withdrawal. A convenient rule of thumb would be to limit the symptoms to those which are blocked by morphine or other narcotic drugs. However, this still does not exclude the possibility of focusing on nonspecific effects. For example, morphine reverses the hypothermia observed during withdrawal. However, morphine has a hyperthermic action of its own in naive rats, and it is unclear whether the temperature reversal is a reflection of morphine action on the centers involved with withdrawal or whether the hyperthermic action of morphine is superimposed on some other mechanism. In order to screen an antiabstinence drug, it would be important to know which symptoms are a direct consequence of the withdrawal state.

2. Lack of Specificity

It should also be pointed out that none of the observed symptoms are encountered solely in narcotic withdrawal. For example, hypothermia can be produced by a variety of pharmacological agents. Weight loss can occur after the administration of anorexics. Ptosis occurs after neuroleptic administration. Similarly, it has been shown that wet shakes can be observed in rats after cessation of chronic treatment with the neuroleptic haloperidol [23] or in drug-free rats that have received a lesion of the dopaminergic nigrostriatal bundle [24]. Neither of these groups had any exposure to narcotic drugs. It remains to be seen, therefore, which symptoms are particularly relevant to narcotic withdrawal.

B. Drug Effects

Naturally induced morphine withdrawal in the rat provides a convenient and useful system for the study of drugs that attenuate the severity of the symptoms associated with narcotic abstinence. Alterations of the measured responses by drugs give valuable information about potential chemotherapeutic treatment of narcotic withdrawal in man and also provide a framework for the study of CNS mechanisms that are responsible for the withdrawal phenomenon. Because of the extended length of time of natural withdrawal compared with naloxone-induced withdrawal, it is possible to gain insight into the duration of action of various treatments and the advantages or disadvantages of multiple dosing as well as the potential development of tolerance to these treatments.

The study of the action of drugs on the withdrawal syndrome begins with ascertaining the effect of continued narcotic administration. It was previously noted that both morphine and methadone prevent the occurrence of signs of narcotic abstinence in the rat. The effectiveness of both agents is short-lived, lasting less than 24 hr, after which the syndrome again emerges. In addition, the effectiveness of methadone on certain parameters (e.g., body weight loss, wet shakes) disappears during repeated treatment, indicating the rapid development of tolerance (see Table III).

TABLE III

Effect of Methadone[a] on Morphine Withdrawal Syndrome

Hours of withdrawal	N	Body weight loss (g)	Temperature drop (deg)	Shakes	Ptosis (sec)[b]	Pilo-erection[c]	Writhing[c]
24	18	4.4 ± 1.2	0.64 ± 0.11	0.3 ± 0.2	66 ± 16	4/18	4/18
48	18	24.0 ± 3.0	0.66 ± 0.09	2.1 ± 0.6	230 ± 44	17/18	4/18

[a] Methadone was given at a dose of 20 mg/kg every 12 hr beginning 10 hr after terminal morphine injection. Observations were made at 2 hr after injection.

[b] Duration of ptosis during 30-min observation period.

[c] Number of rats showing positive reaction out of total number observed.

Since haloperidol has been used to treat heroin addicts [25], it became important to see what effects it had on this animal model of narcotic addiction. Given acutely, haloperidol blocked certain symptoms (e.g., wet shakes, writhing, aggression) but aggravated others (e.g., weight loss, hypothermia). Similarly, we have found that p-chloroamphetamine blocks some of the symptoms (e.g., wet shakes, ptosis, hypothermia) but aggrevates the loss of body weight [26]. It is important, therefore, to look at the entire syndrome in order to more accurately assess the effect of a drug. However, it would be of great interest, in subsequent studies, to determine whether one sign has a greater predictive value than others for the treatment of narcotic withdrawal in man. Of course, this could be accomplished only after comparison of treatments that prove to be effective in clinical trials.

Currently, the effect of other compounds having mechanisms of action different from haloperidol are being studied in our laboratory in order to determine the underlying mechanism that produces the abstinence syndrome. Further animal experimentation should provide needed information that will be relevant to the treatment of drug addiction.

V. CLINICAL SIGNIFICANCE

Ideally, the narcotic withdrawal syndrome in the rat should sufficiently mimic the clinical situation so that it may be used as a screening procedure for the development of agents that can be used to treat withdrawal in humans. It is essential to design chemotherapeutic agents that can reduce the severity of the withdrawal syndrome and aid in the rehabilitation of human addicts.

By using this model in the rat, it should be possible to obtain information in order to produce these drugs. It is not necessary, theoretically, to relate a specific symptom in the rat to specific aspects of the clinical picture. That is, it is not necessary, for example, to ascertain the human equivalent of wet shakes. It is necessary, however, to determine whether therapeutic agents which block wet shakes in the rat will be effective in treating withdrawal in human addicts. Wet shakes are, in fact, blocked by methadone or haloperidol, agents that have been used to treat human narcotic addiction.

For this research, spontaneous withdrawal is far superior to withdrawal precipitated by narcotic antagonists, as discussed earlier. Since it is very difficult to reverse the effects of naloxone-induced withdrawal even by administering opiates, it would be futile to attempt to screen chemotherapeutic agents using this approach.

Furthermore, by investigating the role of various neurochemicals in the elaboration of the withdrawal syndrome, it may be possible to determine the mechanisms underlying the phenomenon of addiction. With this information, it would be possible to treat addiction with specific drugs of known activity and bring the addiction under control.

ACKNOWLEDGMENTS

The investigations described in this chapter were partially supported by research grants from McNeil Laboratories, Roche Laboratories, and Searle Laboratories. Drugs were provided free of charge. Mrs. Kathleen McGovern provided secretarial assistance in preparing this manuscript.

REFERENCES

1. W. R. Martin, A. Wikler, C. G. Eades, and F. T. Pescor, Tolerance to and physical dependence on morphine in rats. Psychopharmacologia 4:247-260 (1963).

2. H. O. J. Collier, D. L. Francis, and C. Schneider, Modification of morphine withdrawal by drugs interacting with humoral mechanisms: Some contradictions and their interpretation. Nature (London) 237: 220-223 (1972).

3. H. Kaneto, M. Koida, and H. Nakanishi, Studies on physical dependence inducible by hours exposure of mice to morphine. Jap. J. Pharmacol. 22:755-766 (1972).

4. M. E. Risner and K. A. Khavari, Morphine dependence in rats produced after five days of ingestion. Psychopharmacologia 28:51-62 (1973).

5. E. L. Way, H. H. Loh, and F. H. Shen, Simultaneous quantitative assessment of morphine tolerance and physical dependence. J. Pharmacol. Exp. Ther. 167:1-8 (1969).

6. W. R. Martin and J. W. Sloan, The pathophysiology of morphine dependence and its treatment with opioid antagonists. Pharmakopsychiat. Neuro-Psychopharmakol. 1:260-270 (1971).

7. W. R. Martin, Pathophysiology of narcotic addiction: Possible roles of protracted abstinence in relapse. In Drug Abuse: Proceedings of the International Conference (C. J. D. Zarafonetis, ed.). Philadelphia: Lea and Febiger, 1972, pp. 153-159.

8. N. Khazan, J. R. Weeks, and L. A. Schroeder, Electroencephalographic electromyographic and behavioral correlates during a cycle of self-maintained morphine addiction in the rat. J. Pharmacol. Exp. Ther. 155:521-531 (1967).

9. W. R. Buckett, A new test for morphine-like physical dependence (addiction liability) in rats. Psychopharmacologia 6:410-416 (1964).

10. H. Lal, J. O'Brien, and S. K. Puri, Morphine-withdrawal aggression: sensitization by amphetamines. Psychopharmacologia 22:217-223 (1971).

11. A. Wikler, P. Green, H. Smith, and F. T. Pescor, Use of benzimidazole derivative with potent morphine-like properties orally as a presumptive reinforcer in conditioning of drug seeking behavior in rats. Fed. Proc. Fed. Amer. Soc. Exp. Biol. 19:22 (1960).

12. A. Wikler, W. R. Martin, F. T. Pescor, and C. G. Eades, Factors regulating oral consumption of an opioid (etonitazene) by morphine-addicted rats. Psychopharmacologia 5:55-76 (1963).

13. G. Gianutsos, M. D. Hynes, S. K. Puri, R. B. Drawbaugh, and H. Lal, Effect of apomorphine and nigrostriatal lesions on aggression and striatal dopamine turnover during morphine withdrawal: Evidence for dopaminergic supersensitivity in protracted abstinence. Psychopharmacologia 34:37-44 (1974).

14. N. Khazan and B. Colasanti, EEG correlates of morphine challenge in post-addict rats. Psychopharmacologia 22:56-63 (1971).

15. A. Wikler and F. T. Pescor, Classical conditioning of a morphine abstinence phenomenon, reinforcement of opioid drinking behavior and "relapse" in morphine addicted rats. Psychopharmacologia 10:255-284 (1967).

16. M. Roffman, C. Reddy, and H. Lal, Control of morphine-withdrawal hypothermia by conditioned stimuli. Psychopharmacologia 29:197-201 (1973).

17. R. B. Drawbaugh and H. Lal, Reversal by narcotic antagonist of a narcotic action elicited by a conditional stimulus. Nature (London) 247: 46-47 (1974).

18. P. A. J. Janssen, C. J. E. Niemegeers, and K. H. Schellekens, Is it possible to predict the clinical effects of neuroleptic drugs from animal data? I. The neuroleptic activity spectra of rats. Arzneimittal-Forsch. 15:104-117 (1965).

19. E. Wei, H. H. Loh, and E. L. Way, Quantitative aspects of precipitated abstinence in morphine-dependent rats. J. Pharmacol. Exp. Ther. 184:398-403 (1973).

20. W. R. Martin, Pharmacological redundancy as an adaptive mechanism in the central nervous system. Fed. Proc. Fed. Amer. Soc. Exp. Biol. 29:13-27 (1970).

21. J. H. Jaffe and S. K. Sharpless, Pharmacological denervation supersensitivity in the central nervous system. A theory of physical dependence. Ass. Nerv. Ment. Dis. 46:226-246 (1968).

22. A. Goldstein and D. B. Goldstein, Enzyme expansion theory of drug tolerance and physical dependence. Ass. Nerv. Ment. Dis. 46:265-278 (1968).

23. G. Gianutsos, R. B. Drawbaugh, M. D. Hynes, and H. Lal, Behavioral evidence for dopaminergic supersensitivity after chronic haloperidol. Life Sci. 14:887-898 (1974).

24. M. D. Hynes, R. B. Drawbaugh, G. Gianutsos, and H. Lal, Simulation of narcotic withdrawal symptoms by brain lesions in non-dependent rats. In preparation.

25. Y. Karkalas and H. Lal, A comparison of haloperidol with methadone in blocking heroin-withdrawal symptoms: A pilot study. Int. Pharmacopsychiat. 8:248-251 (1973).

26. H. Lal, S. K. Puri, R. B. Drawbaugh, and C. Reddy, Morphine withdrawal syndrome in mice and rats: Partial blockade by p-chloroamphetamine. Fed. Proc. Fed. Amer. Soc. Exp. Biol. 33:487 (1974).

Chapter 14

METHODS TO INDUCE METHADONE ADDICTION IN RATS*

JASBIR M. SINGH

Alcoholism Services Unit
Department of Psychiatry
Charity Hospital of Louisiana
New Orleans, Louisiana[+]

*Presented in part at the New York meeting of the Society of Toxicology, 1973, and the fall meeting of the Society of Pharmacology and Experimental Therapeutics, East Lansing, Michigan 1974.

+Present address: Alcoholism Out-Patient Treatment Clinic, Singh Behavior Therapy Clinic, Metairie, Louisiana.

I. INTRODUCTION

The degree of tolerance and withdrawal symptoms depend on (a) the nature of the compound, (b) doses used, routes and duration of administration, and (c) miscellaneous factors, i.e., liver, adrenals, and thyroid involvement [1]. Withdrawal symptoms with some of the over-the-counter drugs (alcohol, caffeine, tobacco, and others) may be very mild and at the same time can be controlled easily with compounds because they are easily available without prescription. However, compounds that are not easily available over the counter pose a problem. Many times tolerance and withdrawal symptoms are produced in a patient because not enough is known about the addiction liabilities of the compound in question; methadone is a good example [2]. Methadone was synthesized by a German chemist in 1941 and came into clinical use at the end of World War II. Because of certain characteristics of methadone, (a) effective analgesic activity, (b) efficacy by the oral route, (c) extended duration of action, and (d) less sedation or euphoria than morphine, Dole et al. introduced it for the treatment of narcotic withdrawal symptoms [2,12]. At that time, dependence and change in behavioral characteristics with methadone were not completely known. The question raised is how long can a patient be maintained on methadone without developing addiction, tolerance, and change in behavioral characteristics? The answer to this question was to come from either animal or human studies. It was observed that patients maintained on methadone, in methadone maintenance programs, do develop tolerance and addiction. In addition to this, they also develop a change in behavior [13,14]. No models for studying development of tolerance, change in behavior, and addiction has been reported in the literature previously. This chapter describes models for the study of development of addiction with methadone.

II. METHOD

A. Production of Methadone Addiction by Oral Route

Male rats weighing 150-200 g were fed 0.1% methadone in drinking water for 180 days. Methadone solution was made with distilled water. To test for methadone addiction, the animals were injected with nalline, 2.5 mg/kg, 24, 48, and 72 hr after methadone withdrawal.

Methadone-withdrawal-induced aggression (tremors, irritability, vocalization on handling) in animals was intensified by treating methadone-treated animals with reserpine, 2.5 mg/kg (24 hr after withdrawal), and amphetamine (72 hr after withdrawal). These animals were observed at regular intervals for 14 days.

B. Production of Methadone Addiction by Parenteral Route

Rats weighing 150-220 g were injected ip with methadone twice daily at intervals of approximately 12 hr for 30 days. Induction of methadone addiction was divided into three stages:

1. Methadone doses up to 20 mg/kg were given twice daily in increasing doses (2 mg) for up to 10 days.
2. The animals were maintained on 20 mg/kg methadone for the next 10 days.
3. Methadone doses of up to 60 mg/kg were given twice daily in increasing doses (4 mg) for the next 10 days.

C. Clinical Symptoms

Before methadone was withdrawn, body weight was recorded, rectal body temperature was taken with a Telethermometer, and any tremors, vocalization on handling, and any actual fighting that was initially present were noted.

D. Experimental Design

Two series of experiments were performed with these methadone-addicted animals (parenteral route).

In the first series, the animals were divided into five groups: (1) control, (2) methadone-addicted (MA), (3) methadone-withdrawn (MW), (4) MW plus apomorphine, and (5) MW plus amphetamine plus apomorphine. Behavioral changes (sniffing, licking, gnawing, and stereotyped posture) and signs of aggression (irritability and actual fighting) were graded on a scale of 0 to 3 (0, no change; 3, maximum change).

A similar experimental design was followed with animals that were addicted by an oral route. In these animals, reserpine was used instead of apomorphine.

III. RESULTS: EVIDENCE OF METHADONE ADDICTION

A. Oral Route

When methadone was withdrawn after 180 days from the addicted animals, mild to severe tremors and irritability (vocalization on handling) were present. Body weight decreased (8-10%) and body temperature decreased (1-2°) 72 hr after drug withdrawal in 70% of the animals.

1. Treatment with Nalline

The symptoms of withdrawal syndrome were intensified (tremors, "wet shakes," and piloerection) when nalline, 1 mg/kg, was injected into methadone-withdrawn animals 24-72 hr (days 181-183) after withdrawal.

2. Treatment with Reserpine and d-Amphetamine Sulfate

Methadone withdrawal symptoms were aggravated when reserpine-treated animals were given d-amphetamine sulfate, 2.5 mg/kg, 72 hr after methadone withdrawal. Delayed fighting was induced in 70% of the animals, and this lasted for 2 weeks. All the drug-treated animals were placed in one cage. The rectal body temperature increased (1.5-3°) after amphetamine treatment.

B. Parenteral Route

The withdrawal findings, similar to those observed after oral administration, were recorded in animals that were addicted by the parenteral route. The withdrawal symptoms were also precipitated by nalline administration.

1. Treatment with Apomorphine and d-Amphetamine Sulfate

The animals were treated with 1 mg/kg nalline 24-74 hr after the methadone withdrawal for methadone withdrawal symptoms. The symptoms of a withdrawal syndrome appeared (tremors, wet shakes, and piloerection). The results of the effects of apomorphine, 1 mg/kg, and d-amphetamine sulfate, 2.5 mg/kg, are shown in Table I. Separately, the apomorphine and d-amphetamine sulfate produced mild behavioral changes and symptoms of aggression, but when they were given together, the behavioral changes and symptoms of aggression were intensified. Actual fighting was induced 2 or 3 min after the administration of apomorphine and amphetamine together. The rectal body temperature increased significantly ($p < 0.05$) at 15 and 60 min after the administration of both drugs. Body temperature also increased in the control animals, but not to such a significant degree as in those receiving both drugs.

The comparison between methadone-addicted and methadone-withdrawn animals is shown in Table II. When amphetamine and apomorphine were injected into control and methadone-addicted animals, irritability was induced, but no actual fighting was present, whereas the identical treatment in methadone-withdrawn animals did induce irritability to the point of actual fighting.

TABLE I

Effect of Apomorphine (1 mg/kg) and d-Amphetamine Sulfate (2.5 mg/kg) on Methadone-Withdrawn Animals

Animal[a]	Behavioral changes[b]			
	Sniffing, licking, and gnawing	Stereotype posture	Aggression	
			Irritability	Actual fighting
Control, NT	0	0	0	0
MW	0	1	1	0
MW + A	1	1	1	1
MW + AS	1	1	1	1
MW + AS + A	3	3	3	3

[a] NT, no treatment; MW, methadone-withdrawn, 48 hr; A, apomorphine; AS, amphetamine sulfate.

[b] Grading scale: 0, no change; 3, maximum change.

TABLE II

Comparison between Methadone-Addicted and Methadone-Withdrawn Animals

Animal[a]	Behavioral changes[b]			
	Sniffing, licking, and gnawing	Stereotype posture	Aggression	
			Irritability	Actual fighting
Control + A + AS	1	1	1	0
MA + A + AS	1	1	1	0
MW + A + AS	3	3	3	3

[a] MW, methadone-withdrawn, 48 hr; MA, methadone-addicted; AS, amphetamine sulfate, 2.5 mg/kg; A, apomorphine 1 mg/kg.

[b] Grading scale: 0, no change; 3, maximum change.

2. Development of Tolerance

The slow development of tolerance to lethal effects of methadone is shown in Fig. 1.

IV. DISCUSSION

The following question should be raised: Is methadone addiction actually produced in our suggested models? Yes; these animals were addicted to methadone because, upon withdrawal, the animals did exhibit such symptoms of addiction as mild to severe tremors, mild aggression as indicated by irritability (vocalization on handling), loss of body weight, and a decrease in body temperature in 70% of the animals. These are the clinical signs on which the index of morphine addiction is based [3]. Singh and Singh [4] have shown that if a colony of animals is maintained on 0.1% methadone in the drinking water for 180 days, all animals exhibit clinical signs of withdrawal (drug addiction) and the injection of nalline, 1 mg/kg, also intensifies the withdrawal syndrome. In our model, nalline administration produces a methadone withdrawal syndrome. Miller and Singh [5,15]

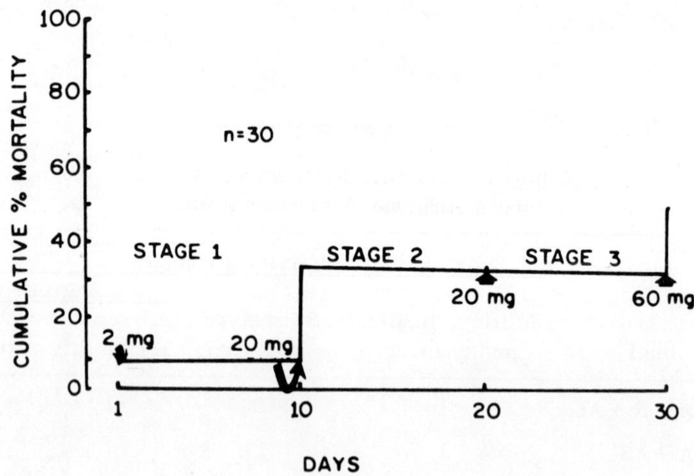

FIGURE 1. Development of tolerance to the lethal effects of methadone. Stage 1: Methadone doses up to 10 mg/kg increasing by milligram twice daily up to 10 days. Stage 2: The animals were maintained on 20 mg/kg for 10 days. Stage 3: The doses up to 60 mg methadone, with 4 mg daily, increased for the next 10 days.

have reported that the administration of nalline induces the withdrawal syndrome (piloerection, body shakes) without affecting the electrophysiological activity of the central nervous system. Therefore, it is suggested from our findings that treatment (with methadone) does produce drug dependence or addiction in the treated animals. When methadone is withdrawn from the addicted animals, mild aggression, indicated by irritability, is present and this mild aggression can then be intensified by treatment with apomorphine plus amphetamine. This treatment produces spontaneous fighting. Singh and Singh [4] have also reported that the mild aggression present in animals that have been withdrawn from methadone after 180 days of treatment can be intensified by reserpine and amphetamine treatment. Such treatment induces delayed aggression. Again, such treatment with apomorphine plus amphetamine or reserpine plus amphetamine does not produce aggression in normal animals.

Why is it necessary to pharmacologically manipulate methadone animals in order to produce spontaneous or delayed aggression? The answer is to implicate the involvement of cerebral biogenic amines. It is now a well-established fact that brain neurons store dopamine, norepinephrine, and serotonin [6]. Apomorphine is known for its dopaminergic stimulating effects. Neurochemically, this action of apomorphine is manifested in the reduced turnover of dopamine [7]. Reserpine treatment is known to cause release of norepinephrine, dopamine, and serotonin from the brain [8]. Large doses of reserpine cause an almost complete depletion of brain norepinephrine and dopamine. It has also become increasingly clear that d-amphetamine sulfate acts on central neurons. A single injection of amphetamine was found to persist for 6-7 days [8]. Amphetamine blocks the uptake and release of norepinephrine from sympathetic nerves [9]. Taylor and Snyder have proposed that amphetamine stimulates dopaminergic receptors [10]. Therefore, in order to induce spontaneous or delayed aggression, the cerebral biogenic amines, norepinephrine and dopamine, must first undergo a change in the cerebral neurons that at this time is not completely understood.

Addiction or physical dependence is also contingent on the development of tolerance to the drug in question. The animals are able to tolerate more of the drug; therefore, tolerance to the lethal effects is developed more slowly. Alvares [11] has shown that methadone does stimulate drug-metabolizing enzymes. In spite of the fact that tolerance to methadone is developed, lethal effects do appear at some point in treatment. Methadone, 60 mg/kg, was found to produce over 50% mortality on the 30th day of treatment. This is a strong indication that, had we exceeded the dose of 60 mg/kg, all the animals would have been killed. Thus, this is the most important reason for testing our model for drug addiction on the 30th day.

Methadone addiction or dependence is produced by oral and parenteral routes [4,13,14]. The production of addiction via the oral route is less tedious than that via the parenteral route. However, it takes longer to produce addiction via the oral route. The withdrawal symptoms produced by either the oral or the parenteral route should be examined very carefully because the animals may be passive or aggressive. The passive animals show mild withdrawal symptoms upon drug withdrawal, and these symptoms may not be changed to severe fighting as seen in aggressive animals. Decrease in body temperature is not one of the best indexes for determining withdrawal. Handling of animals can give a false index because it elevates the body temperature, and for this reason the animals should be handled with great care. Also, the body weight does not decrease uniformly in all the animals. In order that these pitfalls be avoided, the withdrawal symptoms should not be based on decrease in body temperature and weight only, but also on the production of wet shakes after nalline administration and on the production of aggressive episodes after apomorphine plus amphetamine injection. It is possible to obtain a correct drug addiction index if drug addiction or dependence is based on temperature, body weight, wet shakes, and induction of aggression with apomorphine plus amphetamine.

REFERENCES

1. J. M. Singh, Factors affecting the development of tolerance to pentobarbital and thiopental. In Drug Addiction: Experimental Pharmacology (J. M. Singh, L. H. Miller, and H. Lal, eds.). Mt. Kisco, N. Y.: Futura, 1972, pp. 235-246.

2. L. S. Goodman and A. Gilman, The Pharmacological Basis of Therapeutics. New York: Macmillan, 1971, pp. 260-262.

3. H. Lal and S. K. Puri, Morphine-withdrawal aggression: Role of dopaminergic stimulation. In Drug Addiction: Experimental Pharmacology (J. M. Singh, L. H. Miller, and H. Lal, eds.). Mt. Kisco, N.Y.: Futura, 1972, pp. 301-310.

4. M. D. Singh and J. M. Singh, Methadone-induced aggressive behavior. Toxicol. Appl. Pharmacol. 25:452 (1973).

5. L. H. Miller and J. M. Singh, Electrophysiological correlates of methadone tolerance abstinence and blockade in cortex and deep brain centers. In Drug Addiction: Neurobiology and Influences on Behavior (J. M. Singh and H. Lal, eds.), Vol. 3. New York: Intercontinental Book Corp., 1974, pp. 287-296.

6. V. Th. F. Brauck, O. Hornykiewiez, and E. B. Sigg, The Pharmacology of Psychotherapeutic Drugs. New York: Springer-Verlag, 1969, p. 53.

7. N. E. Anden, A. Rubenson, and K. Fuxe, Evidence for dopamine receptor stimulation by apomorphine. J. Pharm. Pharmacol. 18: 627-629 (1967).

8. K. Fuxe and U. Ungerstedt, Histochemical, biochemical, and functional studies on central monamine neurons after chronic and acute amphetamine administration. In Amphetamines and Related Compounds (E. Costa and S. Garattini, eds.). New York: Raven Press, 1970, pp. 317-329.

9. J. Axelrod, Amphetamines: Metabolism, physiological disposition, and its effects on catecholamine storage. In Amphetamines and Related Compounds (E. Costa and S. Garattini, eds.). New York: Raven Press, 1970, pp. 201-216.

10. K. M. Taylor and S. H. Snyder, Amphetamine: Differentiation by d and l isomers of behavior involving brain norepinephrine or dopamine. Science 168:1487-1489 (1970).

11. A. P. Alvares and A. Kappas, The influence of phenobarbital on the in vitro and in vivo metabolism of methadone in rats. In Drug Addiction: Experimental Pharmacology (J. M. Singh, L. H. Miller, and H. Lal, eds.). Mt. Kisco, N. Y.: Futura, 1972, pp. 191-198.

12. V. P. Dole, M. E. Nyswander, and M. G. Kreek, Narcotic blockade. Arch. Intern. Med. 206:2708-2711 (1966).

13. J. M. Singh, P. C. Madere, and M. P. Thomas, Methadone-induced behavioral changes. Clin. Toxicol. 7:300 (1974).

14. J. M. Singh, A model study of methadone-induced aggression in rats. In Drug Addiction: Neurobiology and Influences on Behavior (J. M. Singh and H. Lal, eds.). New York: Stratton Intercontinental Medical Book Corp., 1974, pp. 13-18.

15. L. M. Miller and J. M. Singh, Different neurophysiological or neurochemical mechanisms of nalline and apomorphine during methadone withdrawal. Pharmacologist 16:194 (1974).

Part V

EVALUATION OF NARCOTIC ANTAGONISTS

Chapter 15

RESPONDING MAINTAINED BY TERMINATION OR POSTPONEMENT OF NARCOTIC ANTAGONIST INJECTIONS IN THE RHESUS MONKEY*

STEVEN R. GOLDBERG

Laboratory of Psychobiology
Department of Psychiatry
Harvard Medical School
Boston, Massachusetts
New England Regional Primate Research Center
Southborough, Massachusetts

*Preparation of this chapter was supported by USPHS Research Grants DA-00499, MH-02094, MH-07658 and with facilities and services furnished by the New England Regional Primate Research Center, Harvard Medical School, Southborough, Massachusetts (USPHS Grant RR-00168, Division of Research Resources, National Institutes of Health).

I. INTRODUCTION

The behavioral aspects of drug dependence have been increasingly studied in recent years using operant techniques developed by B. F. Skinner and his colleagues [1]. Operant behavior may be simply defined as behavior controlled by its consequences. Consequences are termed reinforcers when they immediately follow the occurrence of a designated response and subsequent occurrences of similar responses increase in frequency. The conditioning of operant behavior usually involves an experimental subject performing some easily repeatable, identifiable response that is intermittently followed by a reinforcer. The parameters of the temporal and sequential relations between stimuli presented to the animal, responses of the animal, and reinforcing events consequent on these responses are called the schedule of reinforcement.

An event that functions as a reinforcer by maintaining behavior leading to its presentation is often called a positive reinforcer. As an example, key-press responses of a food-deprived monkey increase in frequency if responses are followed by delivery of food pellets to the monkey; delivery of a food pellet serves as a reinforcer in this situation. The injection of certain centrally active drugs can also function as a positive reinforcer. For example, key-press responses of a rhesus monkey increase in frequency if responses are followed by intravenous injection of morphine; if the dose per injection is large enough and the opportunity for responding is frequent enough, the monkey will receive sufficient morphine to develop a high degree of physiological dependence [2,3]. A wide variety of drugs from many pharmacological classes (psychomotor stimulants, barbiturates, alcohol, narcotics, narcotic antagonists) have been shown to maintain behavior as positive reinforcers [2,4-8].

An event can also function as a reinforcer by maintaining behavior leading to its termination or postponement. For example, key-press responses by squirrel monkeys increase in frequency if the responses are followed by termination of a stimulus associated with periodic delivery of electric shock [9,10]. When an event maintains behavior leading to its termination it is often called a negative reinforcer. Drugs from only one pharmacological class, the narcotic antagonists, have been shown to function as negative reinforcers and maintain behavior that leads to termination or postponement of their injection [3,11,12].

A critical factor in studying the reinforcing effects of narcotic antagonists is the presence or absence of physiological dependence on morphine [11]. In the absence of physiological dependence on morphine, reinforcing effects are not consistent among different members of the narcotic antagonist class of drug. Narcotic antagonists such as pentazocine and propiram, which have only weak antagonistic properties, have been repeatedly shown to maintain behavior leading to their injection [8,11,13], whereas narcotic antagonists such as nalorphine and cyclazocine, which have strong antagonistic properties, generally fail to maintain behavior leading to their injection [2,8]. In the presence of physiological dependence on morphine, the reinforcing effects of narcotic antagonists have been more consistent. Both narcotic antagonists with weak antagonistic properties and narcotic antagonists with strong antagonistic properties have been reported to maintain behavior leading to termination or postponement of their injection. Goldberg et al. [11] found that key-press responding by morphine-dependent rhesus monkeys was maintained when it resulted in termination of a stimulus associated with periodic injections of either nalorphine, naloxone, pentazocine, or propiram, but was not maintained when it resulted in termination of a stimulus associated with periodic injections of saline.

The behavioral techniques that have been used to study responding maintained by termination or postponement of drug injections are modifications of operant scheduling techniques that were originally developed to study responding maintained by termination or postponement of electric shock [9,10]. This chapter describes in detail a type of schedule that has been successfully employed in morphine-dependent rhesus monkeys for studying responding maintained by termination of a stimulus associated with periodic injections of a narcotic antagonist [3,11]. Representative data obtained with this schedule and recent results obtained with interesting variations of this schedule are also briefly described.

II. METHOD

A. Subjects and Apparatus

Subjects were male and female rhesus monkeys (*Macaca mulatta*) weighing approximately 4 kg. Under pentobarbital anesthesia (30 mg/kg, iv), silicone rubber (Vivosil) catheters (1.0 mm i.d., 2.2 mm o.d.) were passed through the internal jugular vein to the level of the right atrium. Each monkey was then placed in a metal harness that protected the catheter. The harness was attached to a jointed metal restraining arm. The arm attached to the rear wall of a cubicle and allowed almost complete freedom of movement within the cubicle. The surgically implanted catheter led subcutaneously to the monkey's back, where it exited through a stab wound in the skin. An extension of the intravenous catheter was passed from the harness through the restraining arm to the back of the cubicle, where it connected to an automatic injection pump (Cole-Parmer Masterflex). Figure 1 shows the experimental situation. The front of each cubicle was open for observation

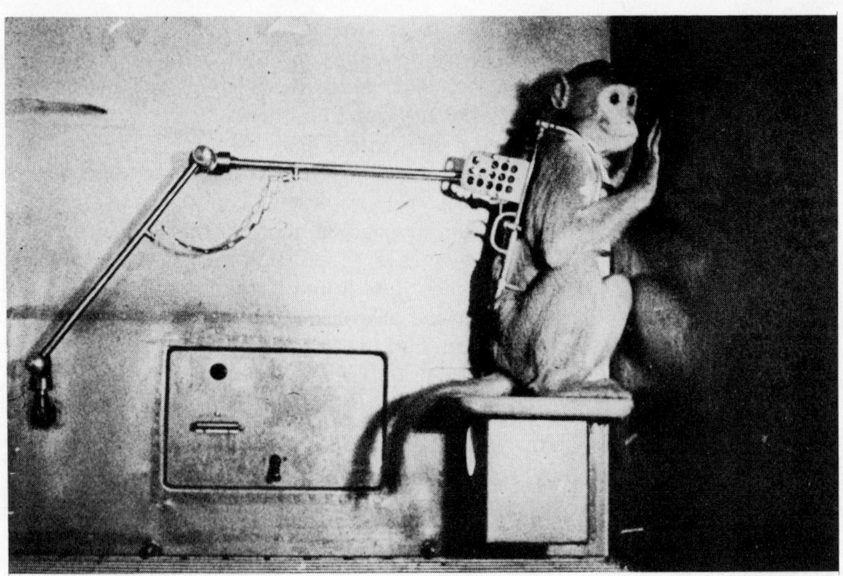

FIGURE 1. A rhesus monkey in the experimental situation. The monkey is restrained by a metal harness and a jointed metal restraining arm which attaches to the rear wall of the cubicle. A response key and a 12-W bulb are mounted on the rear wall of the cubicle. A water spout, located below the response key and the bulb, delivers water when pressure is applied to the end of the spout.

and maintenance of the monkey. A key (Lehigh Valley Electronics no. 1380) and a 12-W bulb (red, white, or green) were mounted in the back wall of the cubicle. When illuminated, the bulb served as a stimulus light. Intravenous injections could be automatically delivered or injections could be programmed to occur when the monkeys pressed the key (response). Injections consisted of 0.2 ml/kg of solution. Activation of the pump was clearly audible to the monkeys. Injection duration (approximately 10 sec) was regulated according to the monkeys' weights. Monkeys remained in their individual cubicles throughout the experiments, with food and water freely available.

Descriptions of the preceding catheterization procedure and the restraint arm and harness have been reported in more detail by Deneau et al. [2]. It should be noted that many modifications of the catheterization procedure and apparatus are possible and, in some instances, desirable. There are many examples. Halothane-oxygen anesthesia, when available, allows a finer control of the level and duration of anesthesia than is possible with pentobarbital anesthesia. Polyvinyl chloride catheters may be used in place of silicone rubber catheters. Light-tight, sound-attenuating cubicles (e.g., model AC-5, Industrial Acoustics Co., Bronx, N.Y.), when available, allow better control of environmental variables than the open-front cubicles described above and still allow the observation of the animals during experimental sessions. Finally, there are numerous possible alternatives to the restraint arm and harness arrangement described above and numerous alternatives to the Cole-Parmer injection pump [14-16].

B. Procedure

In order to develop morphine dependence in the monkeys, morphine was initially made available 24 hr a day so that each key-press response by a monkey produced an intravenous injection of 0.1 mg/kg of morphine. During periods of morphine availability, a white stimulus light was continuously present, except during the injections. Under these conditions, responding of the rhesus monkeys increased and then stabilized within 1-2 months, at a level of 100-210 morphine injections per day [3]. This resulted in a total daily intake of 10-21 mg/kg of morphine, which is sufficient to develop near maximal physiological dependence on morphine, as assessed by intensity of abstinence signs precipitated by abrupt termination of morphine treatment [17].

One month after response rate and daily morphine intake stabilized, the schedule of morphine injections was changed. The white stimulus light was no longer present, key-press responses had no specified consequences, and 3.0 mg/kg of morphine was injected automatically once every 4 hr. Automatic morphine injections were continued throughout the following experiment to maintain the subjects physiologically dependent on morphine.

After five or more days, during which responses had no consequences, monkeys were studied under a schedule in which responses terminated a condition associated with drug injections. Under this schedule, a green stimulus light was continuously present and a 10-sec injection of 10 μg/kg of nalorphine was delivered every 30 sec in the presence of the green light. Each key-press response by the monkey terminated the green light and the associated injections of drug for 60 sec (time-out). Responses during the 60-sec time-out periods had no specified consequences. Each session was 2 hr in duration and was started 1 hr after an automatic morphine injection. Behavior in this situation is maintained by a schedule complex which includes the association of the green light with nalorphine injections, the termination of the green light, the nalorphine dose, and the degree of morphine dependence.

C. Representative Data

After responding was initiated and had increased to a rate that was stable from session to session, pharmacological studies could be conducted. For example, other drugs could be tested by substitution to assess their reinforcing effects in morphine-dependent monkeys. In one series of experiments [3], either saline injections or injections of naloxone were substituted for the nalorphine injections. The sequence employed and the results obtained in these substitution studies are shown in Fig. 2. Responding by the monkeys in the presence of the green light was initially maintained by nalorphine at a rate of approximately 105 responses per 2-hr session. In the presence of the green light, the majority of responses occurred either in the 30-sec periods between injections or within a second of the onset of injection. Since each response terminated the green light and the associated injections and produced a 60-sec time-out period, monkeys spent very little time in the presence of the green light and received fewer than five complete injections per session. When saline injections were substituted for nalorphine injections, behavior changed dramatically. Within three sessions, rate of responding sharply decreased to less than 40 responses per 2-hr session; consequently, monkeys spent long periods of time in the presence of the green light and received over 100 complete injections per session. Responding, which decreased to low rates during saline substitution, could be immediately restored to previous high rates by replacing injections of saline with injections of either nalorphine or naloxone. These findings demonstrate that nalorphine and naloxone can function as reinforcers in rhesus monkeys physiologically dependent on morphine by maintaining behavior leading to termination or postponement of their injection.

In a more extensive series of experiments, Goldberg et al. [11] studied substitution of saline and different doses of nalorphine, naloxone, pentazocine, and propiram. Figure 3 shows the mean number of responses in the presence of the green light and the mean number of complete injections during sessions with either saline, nalorphine, naloxone, pentazocine, or propiram injections. During sessions with injections of higher doses of nalorphine, naloxone, pentazocine, or propiram, over 100 responses per session occurred in the presence of the green light and, consequently, there were very few complete injections. During sessions with injections of saline, however, very few responses occurred in the presence of the green light and, consequently, the number of complete injections was very high. Thus, pentazocine and propiram, as well as nalorphine and naloxone, can function as reinforcers in rhesus monkeys physiologically dependent on morphine by maintaining behavior leading to termination or postponement of their injection. It seems likely that maintenance of behavior leading to termination or postponement of drug injection in morphine-dependent rhesus monkeys will prove to be an effect common to narcotic antagonists as a drug class.

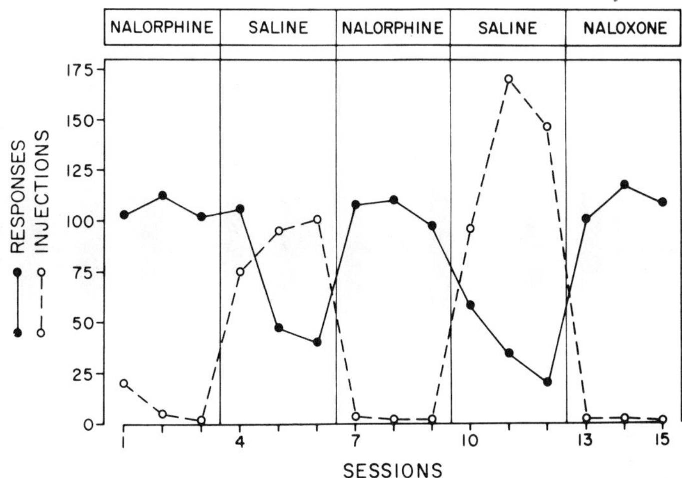

FIGURE 2. Effects of substituting saline injections or naloxone injections for nalorphine injections under a schedule in which each response terminated a stimulus (green light) associated with periodic injections. Abscissa: successive 2-hr sessions. Ordinate: number of key-press responses per session in the presence of the green light (closed symbols, solid lines) and number of injections per session that were not terminated by a response (complete injections; open symbols, broken lines). Nalorphine injection dose was 10 μg/kg and naloxone injection dose was 1 μg/kg. Each point represents the mean of results with two monkeys. Note that responding is well maintained by both nalorphine and naloxone injections but not by saline injections. (Modified from Goldberg et al. [3], p. 273.)

III. MODIFICATIONS OF THE METHOD

A. Intermittently Reinforced Responding

Under the preceding schedule, every response terminated the green light and the associated narcotic antagonist injections. Although this schedule is useful for evaluating the presence or absence of reinforcing effects with different drugs, more information about how narcotic antagonists function as reinforcers and control behavior can be obtained under schedules where responses are only intermittently reinforced. There are many possible schedules of intermittent reinforcement [1], but two simple types have been frequently employed to study the behavioral effects of drugs.

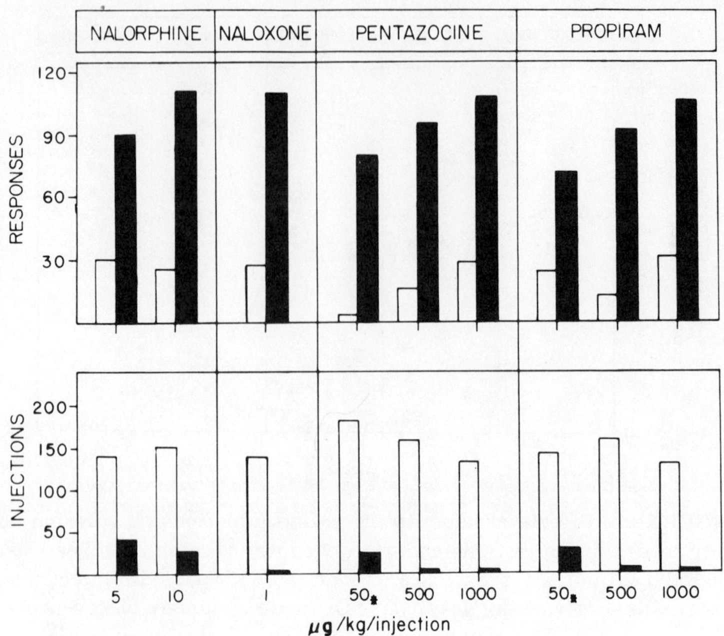

FIGURE 3. Responding maintained by saline and by different doses of nalorphine, naloxone, pentazocine, and propiram under a schedule in which each response terminated a stimulus (green light) associated with periodic injections. Abscissa: injection dose. Ordinate of upper panel: number of key-press responses per session during nalorphine, naloxone, pentazocine, or propiram sessions (solid bars) compared to intervening saline sessions (open bars). Ordinate of lower panel: number of injections per session that were not terminated by a response (complete injections) during nalorphine, naloxone, pentazocine, or propiram sessions (solid bars) compared to intervening saline sessions (open bars). Each dose of drug was studied for three sessions and was followed by three saline sessions. Each point represents the mean of results of the last two sessions at each condition for two monkeys. Asterisks indicate that results of only one monkey are shown. Note that responding is well maintained over a range of doses by narcotic antagonist injections but not by saline injections. (Modified from Goldberg et al. [11], p. 39.)

One type of schedule, termed a fixed-interval schedule (FI), is based on time. Under a fixed-interval schedule, reinforcement follows the first response that occurs after a constant minimum interval of time has elapsed; responses during this interval have no specified consequences.

Responding under this schedule is characterized by a period of no responding at the beginning of each interval, followed by progressively increasing responding up to the point at which the interval ends. This type of schedule has been of particular interest because, under diverse conditions and in different species, the characteristic pattern of positively accelerated responding can be maintained by a variety of events, including presentation of food or water [18,19], intravenous injection of cocaine [20,21], and termination of a stimulus associated with periodic electric shocks [10,22]. Unfortunately, there have been no studies of fixed-interval responding maintained by termination of a stimulus associated with periodic injections of a drug. Whether characteristic fixed-interval rates and patterns of responding can be maintained by termination of a stimulus associated with periodic injections of a narcotic antagonist is an interesting question that remains to be explored.

A second type of frequently studied schedule, termed a fixed-ratio schedule (FR), is based on number of responses. Under a fixed-ratio schedule, reinforcement follows the occurrence of a constant number of responses. Responding under this schedule is characterized by a pause before the initial response in each ratio, followed by a sustained high rate of responding until the ratio is completed. Characteristic fixed-ratio rates and patterns of responding can be maintained by a variety of events, including presentation of food [1,16], intravenous injection of certain drugs such as cocaine or codeine [8,16], and termination of a stimulus associated with periodic electric shocks [9,22].

Characteristic fixed-ratio rates and patterns of responding can also be maintained by termination of a stimulus associated with periodic injections of a narcotic antagonist in morphine-dependent rhesus monkeys [3,23]. For example, once responding by morphine-dependent monkeys was consistently maintained by nalorphine or naloxone injections under the schedule described in Sec. II,B, Goldberg et al. [3] changed the schedule to a fixed-ratio schedule. Under the fixed-ratio schedule, injection time was only 5 sec, responses during 5-sec injections had no programmed consequences, and the number of responses required to terminate the green light and the associated injections was raised gradually until responding was maintained under a 10-response fixed-ratio schedule (FR 10; every tenth response terminated the green light and the associated injections for 60 sec).

Figure 4 shows a cumulative-response record of responding maintained by termination of a green light associated with periodic injection of 0.5 μg/kg naloxone injections under the 10-response fixed-ratio schedule. The green light and the associated injections of naloxone exerted powerful control over behavior. In the presence of the green light, characteristic fixed-ratio patterns of responding were maintained. A pause in responding

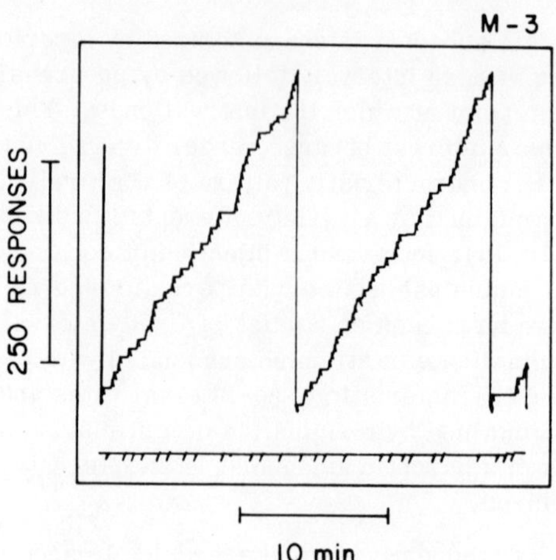

FIGURE 4. A representative cumulative-response record from one monkey (M-3) under a fixed-ratio schedule in which 10 key-press responses were required to terminate a green light associated with periodic injections of 0.5 μg/kg naloxone. On a cumulative-response record the recording pen moves vertically with each response and moves horizontally with time. Abscissa: time. Ordinate: cumulative number of responses. The short diagonal strokes on the cumulative record indicate completion of the fixed-ratio requirement and termination of the green light for 60 sec (time-out). Similar strokes on the lower event line indicate 5-sec injections of naloxone. During 5-sec injections and during 60-sec time-out periods, the recording pen did not move and responses had no specified consequences. The recording pen reset to the bottom of the record whenever 420 responses had accumulated and at the end of the session. At any point on the cumulative record, the positive slope of the record is directly related to the rate of responding. The steep slope of the record indicates that this schedule engendered high rates of responding. (Modified from Goldberg et al. [3], p. 274.)

at the onset of the green light was followed by a steady high rate of responding until the ratio was completed and the green light was terminated. In contrast, when the green light was not present (time-out periods), responding occurred at a very low rate. Almost identical results were obtained with nalorphine at an injection dose of 5 μg/kg. When saline injections were substituted for narcotic antagonist injections, however, responding decreased dramatically. Thus, intermittent scheduling techniques provide powerful control over large amounts of behavior occurring at high rates. The strong control of behavior possible under the present schedules in which responses intermittently terminate a stimulus associated with periodic narcotic antagonist injections is comparable to the strong control of behavior possible under similar schedules in which responses intermittently lead to the injection of drugs such as cocaine (see, e.g., Goldberg [16]).

An interesting modification of the fixed-ratio schedule described above has been reported by Downs and Woods [23]. Subjects and apparatus were similar in all respects to those previously described (Secs. II,A and II,B). Schedules of drug injection, however, were quite different. In the presence of one color stimulus light, monkeys responded under a fixed-ratio schedule to produce intravenous injections of morphine. In the presence of a different color stimulus light, monkeys received a continuous infusion of the narcotic antagonist naloxone at a dose of 1-3 μg/kg/minute. Completion of a fixed number of responses by the monkeys (e.g., 30 responses; FR 30) terminated the infusion of naloxone and the light for 60 sec (time-out). Responses during the time-out periods had no programmed consequences. Under this schedule, stable high rates of responding (over one response per second) were maintained by termination of naloxone infusion. When saline infusion was substituted for naloxone infusion, responding markedly decreased within a few sessions; fixed-ratio responding was immediately reinstated with naloxone infusion. Under this fixed-ratio termination of drug infusion schedule, monkeys are repeatedly exposed to small amounts of the drug each session and this appears to facilitate extinction of responding when saline is substituted for the narcotic antagonist [23]. It is likely that repeated exposure to small amounts of drug each session would also allow a more rapid comparison of the reinforcing effects of different drugs.

B. Responding Maintained in Nondependent Monkeys

A common feature of the experiments described so far was that subjects were physiologically dependent on morphine. Physiological dependence on morphine was maintained either by automatically injecting morphine [3,11], or by allowing animals frequent opportunities to response and produce morphine injections [23]. Although the presence of physiological dependence on morphine is important, an experiment by Hoffmeister and Wuttke [12] indicates that, at least with certain narcotic antagonists, responding can be maintained by termination of a stimulus associated with periodic injections in the absence of any history of physiological dependence on morphine. Initial training of the subjects was different, but the final schedule employed in this experiment by Hoffmeister and Wuttke was identical in all respects to the schedule described in Sec. II,C.

Monkeys were first trained to press a key to terminate a stimulus associated with periodic electric shocks. Shocks could be delivered through gold plate electrodes placed subcutaneously under the skin of the head, below the major occipital nerve. Monkeys were tested under a stimulus-shock termination schedule for 2 hr each day. A 10-sec electric shock was delivered every 30 sec in the presence of a white light. Each response terminated the white light and the associated electric shocks for 60 sec (time-out). Responses during the time-out period had no programmed consequences.

After monkeys initiated responding, 10-sec shock deliveries were discontinued and replaced by 10-sec injections of saline solution. Responding decreased to very low levels within 1-2 weeks and monkeys received large numbers of saline injections each session. Saline injections were then replaced by injections of a test drug. Each dose of a test drug was studied for six consecutive sessions, followed by additional saline sessions. The narcotic antagonists nalorphine (500-10 μg/kg/injection) and cyclazocine (10-2.5 μg/kg/injection) maintained high rates of responding. In contrast, the narcotic antagonists naloxone (100-5 μg/kg/injection), pentazocine (50 μg/kg/injection), and propiram (50 μg/kg/injection) failed to maintain responding at rates above saline levels, and monkeys received large numbers of injections. These findings suggest that, in the absence of physiological dependence on morphine, maintenance of behavior leading to termination or postponement of drug injection in rhesus monkeys may not be an effect common to the narcotic antagonists as a drug class.

IV. SUMMARY AND CONCLUSIONS

A drug can function as a reinforcer either by maintaining behavior leading to its injection or by maintaining behavior leading to termination or postponement of its injection. A wide variety of methods for studying behavior leading to drug injection are already available and there have been repeated demonstrations that drugs from many different pharmacological classes can maintain behavior leading to their injection. The present chapter describes recently developed methods for studying behavior maintained by termination or postponement of drug injections. Experiments that have employed these methods are reviewed which demonstrate that, in rhesus monkeys physiologically dependent on morphine, the narcotic antagonists nalorphine, naloxone, pentazocine, and propiram can maintain behavior leading to termination of a stimulus associated with their periodic injection. The maintenance of behavior leading to termination or postponement of drug injections in morphine-dependent rhesus monkeys may prove to be an effect common to narcotic antagonists as a drug class. Methods for studying behavior maintained by termination or postponement of drug injections provide a new and already fruitful approach for the experimental analysis of the reinforcing effects of narcotic antagonist drugs in morphine-dependent animals.

The methods described in this chapter have also been used to study behavior maintained in the absence of physiological dependence on morphine. Experiments are reviewed which demonstrate that, in the absence of physiological dependence on morphine, nalorphine and cyclazocine can maintain behavior leading to termination of a stimulus associated with their periodic injection. These findings suggest that these methods may have a more general use in the analysis of the reinforcing effects of drugs from a variety of pharmacological classes.

ACKNOWLEDGMENT

I am indebted to Dr. W. H. Morse and Dr. R. T. Kelleher for helpful comments about the manuscript.

REFERENCES

1. C. B. Ferster and B. F. Skinner, Schedules of Reinforcement. New York: Appleton-Century-Crofts, 1957.
2. G. A. Deneau, T. Yanagita, and M. H. Seevers, Psychopharmacologia 16:30 (1969).
3. S. R. Goldberg, F. Hoffmeister, U. Schlichting, and W. Wuttke, J. Pharmacol. Exp. Ther. 179:268 (1971).
4. S. R. Goldberg, F. Hoffmeister, U. U. Schlichting, and W. Wuttke, J. Pharmacol. Exp. Ther. 179:277 (1971).
5. U. U. Schlichting, S. R. Goldberg, W. Wuttke, and F. Hoffmeister, Excerpta Med. Int. Congr. Ser. 220:62 (1971).
6. G. D. Winger and J. H. Woods, Ann. N.Y. Acad. Sci. 215:162 (1973).
7. M. C. Wilson, M. Hitomi, and C. R. Schuster, Psychopharmacologia 22:271 (1971).
8. F. Hoffmeister and U. U. Schlichting, Psychopharmacologia 23:55 (1972).
9. N. H. Azrin, W. C. Holz, D. G. Hake, and T. Ayllon, J. Exp. Anal. Behav. 6:449 (1963).
10. W. H. Morse and R. T. Kelleher, J. Exp. Anal. Behav. 9:267 (1966).

11. S. R. Goldberg, F. Hoffmeister, and U. U. Schlichting, in Drug Addiction: I. Experimental Pharmacology (J. M. Singh, L. Miller, and H. Lal, eds.). Mt. Kisco, N. Y.: Futura, 1972.

12. F. Hoffmeister and W. Wuttke, Psychopharmacologia 33:247 (1973).

13. J. H. Woods and J. E. Villarreal, Pharmacologist 12:230 (1970).

14. T. Thompson and C. R. Schuster, Psychopharmacologia 5:87 (1964).

15. C. R. Schuster and R. L. Balster, in Agonist and Antagonist Actions of Narcotic Analgesic Drugs (H. W. Kosterlitz, H. O. J. Collier, and J. E. Villarreal, eds.). Baltimore: University Park Press, 1973.

16. S. R. Goldberg, J. Pharmacol. Exp. Ther. 186:18 (1973).

17. G. A. Deneau and M. H. Seevers, Advan. Pharmacol. 3:267 (1964).

18. P. B. Dews, Fed. Proc. Fed. Amer. Soc. Exp. Biol. 17:1024 (1958).

19. R. T. Kelleher and W. H. Morse, Ergebn. Physiol. 60:1 (1968).

20. R. L. Balster and C. R. Schuster, J. Exp. Anal. Behav. 20:119 (1973).

21. J. Dougherty and R. Pickens, J. Exp. Anal. Behav. 20:111 (1973).

22. R. T. Kelleher and W. H. Morse, Fed. Proc. Fed. Amer. Soc. Exp. Biol. 23:808 (1964).

23. D. A. Downs and J. H. Woods, Pharmacologist 15:237 (1973).

Chapter 16

CLINICAL EVALUATION OF NARCOTIC ANTAGONISM IN MAN

MAX FINK

Health Sciences Center
State University of New York at Stony Brook
Stony Brook, New York

I. INTRODUCTION

The narcotic antagonists are a diverse group of substances that prevent or reverse the expression of the agonistic effects of the opioids, analgesic substances that have pharmacological effects similar to those of morphine. Clinical interest in these substances comes from two directions: (a) the relief of narcotic overdose, as in analgesia and anesthesia, or in accidental overdose, and (b) the treatment of opiate dependence. These two uses of the narcotic antagonists require drugs with different characteristics. For overdose, one needs a substance with a rapid onset of activity, a duration measured in hours, and high antagonist potency. For treatment of opiate dependence, compounds must be effective for periods measured in days or longer, without stimulating tolerance to antagonistic activity, with low toxicity on chronic usage, and very high potency, for a likely application is the use of an implant releasing such a substance over many weeks or even months.

Since their first elaboration in 1915, the principal use of the narcotic antagonists has been in the treatment of narcotic overdose. Early in the 1960s, however, Wikler and Martin at the Narcotic Addiction Research Center in Lexington, Kentucky, viewing opiate dependence as a conditioned response to environmental and pharmacological factors, suggested that a long-acting narcotic antagonist might serve to extinguish learned drug-seeking behavior [1,2]. This suggestion was tested in studies of cyclazocine and naloxone, two novel experimental narcotic antagonists. The studies demonstrated extinction of drug-seeking behavior in opioid-dependent persons, despite some drawbacks for each compound (naloxone, its short duration of action, and cyclazocine, its persistent agonistic activity). The studies not only demonstrated the feasibility of a therapy designed to extinguish drug-seeking behavior, but also defined the characteristics of the ideal antagonist. A number of substances have been assayed, the latest in clinical testing being naltrexone [3].

The methods of evaluation of narcotic antagonists are designed to assay many characteristics, such as the degree of narcotic antagonism, duration of action, concurrent agonistic effects, tolerance development, effects on drug-seeking behavior, euphoria and other subjective feelings, in addition to toxicity, bioavailability, and CNS activity. The specific action of narcotic antagonists used in their evaluation is their ability to precipitate abstinence symptoms in opioid-dependent animals and man. They elicit the withdrawal symptoms of pupillary dilation, lacrimation, hyperthermia, tachycardia, salivation, and insomnia in such subjects. Pupillary dilatation and hyperthermia are sufficiently reliable responses to be used as quantitative indices.

Many known antagonists retain some opioid activity, which is measured by their ability to suppress the abstinence syndrome following withdrawal of an opioid. The degree to which the compound has morphine-like activity is defined by the suppression of withdrawal symptoms. Some narcotic antagonists, notably cyclazocine and pentazocine, do retain a significant degree of abstinence suppression and to that extent are "impure" antagonists.

II. METHODS

It is difficult to specify a single flow chart for evaluation, since the characteristics of a compound may be developed differently in different laboratories, but the following are some essential measures. We assume that the accepted methods of evaluation of toxicity to single and multiple doses in animals, and the initial human acute and subacute toxicology in suitable volunteers, have been done. For the measurement of specific antagonist and opioid activities, many tests are used including rising dose tolerance, precipitated abstinence, blockade (antagonism) to injected opiate, and cross-tolerance studies.

A. Subjects

Opioid substances are subject to particular governmental regulations and social attitudes that preclude studies in normal or prisoner volunteers. Most, if not all, investigations are done either with experienced, opiate-using subjects, dependent and tolerant to administered opiates (usually methadone, morphine, or Dilaudid), or with postwithdrawal ("postaddicts"), drug-free subjects after detoxification with rapidly decreasing doses of methadone. In subjects who have recently been detoxified, it is preferable to have a 10- to 14-day drug-free period before testing putative narcotic antagonists. Administration of an active antagonist earlier than 10 days after the last dose of methadone may elicit abstinence symptoms, which may be difficult to separate from direct effects of the study compound.

Thus, two populations are necessary for testing: drug-free postaddicts and maintained drug-dependent addicts. Screening studies are usually done in males, not only because of their higher incidence of opiate usage, but to preclude the risk of teratogenicity and interference of menstrual cycles in physiological measures.

Volunteers must be capable of giving consent without duress, and the accepted standards of informed consent must be met. Volunteers, prior to participation, should have a medical and psychiatric history and examination and laboratory tests including electrocardiogram, hemogram, serology, and urinalysis. Subjects with recent medical or psychiatric disability are usually excluded from study.

B. Clinical Measures

1. Measures of Opioid Activity

a. Single-dose tolerance study. If the usual single-dose toxicology studies in normal volunteers are definitive, the following single-dose studies designed to test for opioid effects may be abbreviated.

In a sufficient number of postaddicts, usually 10-15, single doses of the compound under study are administered, starting with a dose found safe in the initial testing and increasing by doubling for each two observations to the highest single dose given. Observations made before, at 30 min, and hourly include observed behavior, blood pressure, temperature, pulse rate, respiratory rate, and pupillary diameter. In addition, an electrocardiogram and electroencephalogram are done prior to, and 2-4 hr after, drug intake.

Conventional methods are used for blood pressure, pulse rate, and respiratory rate. Temperature is measured by skin thermistor or orally using a thermometer. Pupillary size is recorded photographically using a Polaroid camera assembly and measured using calipers or a plastic card consisting of graduated circles used by commercial artists.

Behavior is rated by an observer and by the subject. Various symptom scales have been published, but the best known are those developed by the Addiction Research Center in Lexington, Kentucky. One set of scales for evaluating drug effects on chronic dosage is shown in Figs. 1 and 2 [4]. These should be modified for single-dose as well as multiple-dose studies.

b. Subacute rising-dose tolerance study. To measure opioid effects, beginning with median doses and rising to the maximum single dose, four to six postaddicts receive single daily doses of the compound for periods of up to 4 weeks. Observations are the same as in Sec. II,B,1,a. In this study, such opioid effects as elevated blood pressure, temperature, and heart rate, and miosis, bradypnea, behavioral euphoria, and sedation are assessed.

This study should be controlled by the random assignment of from half the number to an equal number of subjects, treated by a placebo under the same laboratory conditions.

At the end of 2-4 weeks of observation, the active medication should be replaced by an equivalent placebo, without the prior knowledge of the subject or observers. This transfer should be done on a Monday or Tuesday, and subjects should be observed during the succeeding 48 hr for symptoms of withdrawal. In addition to the measures described in Sec. II,B,1,a, changes in the subjective check list, sleep patterns, food intake, and interpersonal interactions with other subjects should be observed. (For comparison, similar observations should be made on the same days during the buildup week while subjects are receiving an active compound.)

From these studies, safely tolerated dosages, both single and multiple, will be defined, as will the degree to which opioid effects are elicited, both as direct effects and on withdrawal. If active opioid effects are observed, further testing for antagonist activity may be deferred until specific tests for analgesic activity and tolerance development are done.

Date________________

Name____________________No.__________Drug____________Study______

ANSWER ALL QUESTIONS ACCORDING TO HOW THIS DRUG IS AFFECTING PATIENT TODAY.

1. Has the patient shown a drug effect today? Yes______ No_____

2. Does its effect resemble any of the following drugs? Check one or more.

a. Dope (heroin)	______	e. Marihuana (pot)	______
b. Barbiturate (goofball)	______	f. LSD	______
c. Cocaine	______	g. Thorazine	______
d. Amphetamines (speed, benny, Methedrine)	______	h. Miltown and Librium	______

3. Does the patient like its effects? (Check one)

a. Dislikes	______	d. Moderately	______
b. Doesn't care one way or the other	______	e. A lot	______
c. Slightly	______		

4. Is the patient hooked? Yes __ No__

5. Have you observed any of the following signs in the patient today?

a. Relaxed	______	m. Driving	______
b. Tired	______	n. Coasting	______
c. Anxious	______	o. Nodding	______
d. Nervous	______	p. Sleepy	______
e. Drunk	______	q. Scratching	______
f. Depressed	______	r. Uncooperative	______
g. Disheveled	______	s. Rides the bed	______
h. Unfriendly	______	t. Complaining	______
i. Primping	______	u. Can't sleep	______
j. Vomiting	______	v. Irritable	______
k. Soapboxing or rapping	______	w. Moody	______
l. Stays to himself		x. Stays close to ward	______
		y. Room disorderly	______

6. Is the patient kicking? Yes___ No___

7. How do you think the patient feels?

a. Very good	______	e. Moderately bad	______
b. Good	______	f. Bad	______
c. Average	______	g. Very bad	______
d. Slightly bad	______		

FIGURE 1. Chronic dosage attitude questionnaire (aide's rating). (Taken from Martin et al. [4] by permission of the American Medical Association.)

Date________________

Name______________________No.__________Drug__________Study_____

ANSWER ALL QUESTIONS ACCORDING TO HOW THIS DRUG IS AFFECTING YOU TODAY.

1. Have you felt a drug effect during the last 24 hours? Yes____No____

2. Does its effects resemble any of the following drugs? Check one or more.
   - a. Dope (heroin) ______
   - b. Barbiturate (goofball) or alcohol ______
   - c. Cocaine ______
   - d. Amphetamines (speed, benny, Methedrine) ______
   - e. Marihuana (pot) ______
   - f. LSD ______
   - g. Thorazine ______
   - h. Miltown and Librium ______

3. Do you like the effects? Check one
   - a. Dislike ______
   - b. Don't care one way or the other ______
   - c. Slightly ______
   - d. Moderately ______
   - e. A lot ______

4. Are you hooked? Yes___ No___

5. Have you had any of the following feelings or symptoms during the last 24 hours? Check the ones you have had.
   - a. Relaxed ______
   - b. Tired ______
   - c. Anxious ______
   - d. Nervous ______
   - e. Drunk ______
   - f. Pins and needles ______
   - g. Rush or flush ______
   - h. Cold or chills ______
   - i. Joint, bone, muscle or back pains ______
   - j. Soapboxing or rapping ______
   - k. Nausea or vomiting ______
   - l. Feel hot
   - m. Driving ______
   - n. Coasting ______
   - o. Nodding ______
   - p. Sleepy ______
   - q. Skin itchy ______
   - r. Stomach cramps ______
   - s. Diarrhea ______
   - t. Gooseflesh ______
   - u. Can't sleep ______
   - v. Irritable ______
   - w. Weak ______
   - x. Nervous or jumping stomach ______

6. Are you kicking? Yes___ No___

7. How do you feel?
   - a. Very good ______
   - b. Good ______
   - c. Average ______
   - d. Slightly bad ______
   - e. Moderately bad ______
   - f. Bad ______
   - g. Very bad ______

FIGURE 2. Chronic dosage attitude questionnaire (patient's rating). (Taken from Martin et al. [4] by permission of the American Medical Association.)

2. Measures of Antagonist Activity

a. Precipitated abstinence. Volunteers are made opiate dependent on fixed doses of morphine, usually to 15 mg subcutaneously four times daily [5]. Using a crossover design, subjects receive increasing single doses of the experimental compound or a reference compound, and symptoms of abstinence are measured using both behavioral and physiological measures. The doses of the experimental compound are usually calculated on a milligram per kilogram basis beginning with doses that were without symptoms in single or multiple administrations and increasing to the maximum single dose given earlier. Reference drugs are usually nalorphine, 1.0-3.0 mg/70 kg, or naloxone, 0.4-1.0 mg/70 kg. One way to assess the antagonist activity of the experimental compound is to calculate the relative potency and 95% confidence limits according to Finney [6].

b. Duration of antagonist activity (single doses). In drug-free postaddicts, acute experiments are used to define the short-term intensity of antagonist activity. Using appropriate random selection of subjects and randomized treatments at weekly intervals, subjects receive single doses of the experimental compound with morphine, or at 3, 6, or 12 hr before morphine. For comparison, the same regimen is done with naloxone (0.4-1.0 mg).

Three measures are used: pupillary diameter, subjective symptoms, and an observer rating scale.

Should the experimental compound be available in an oral as well as parenteral form, the tests should be repeated for the oral form. If the duration and potency of the experimental compound compare favorably to those of naloxone or naltrexone, further testing may be warranted.

c. Duration and potency of antagonist activity (chronic dosage). Drug-free postaddicts are given appropriate single daily doses of the experimental compound, usually for 2-3 weeks until tolerance has been established to any opioid effects. At these levels, subjects receive in an appropriate double-blind, randomized fashion single doses of subcutaneous morphine, intravenous heroin, or saline. One variable under study is opiate dosage, usually 15-45 mg morphine or 25-75 mg heroin, the latter in 2 ml saline given in 60-120 sec intravenously. Another is the time since the last dose of experimental compound to assess duration of antagonist activity. The criteria of antagonism are subjective effects, pupillary size, breathing rate, and heart rate. Temperature is also occasionally measured, and some authors have added index of how much the subject is willing to pay for this dose of opiate [7].

The data developed for the experimental compound should be compared to data from similar studies using an established narcotic antagonist, either naloxone or naltrexone.

3. Measures of Tolerance and Withdrawal

Substances that demonstrate active narcotic antagonism with minimal or no opioid activity may be considered candidates for long-term treatment of opiate dependence. In such instances, two additional measures may be considered: the development of tolerance to antagonist activity and withdrawal symptoms after prolonged use. In subjects receiving the experimental compound for 6 months, tests of antagonism using subcutaneous morphine or intravenous heroin may be repeated, as in Sec. II,B,2,c, and the active drug may be replaced by an identical placebo and withdrawal symptoms evaluated, as in Sec. II,B,1,b.

III. DISCUSSION

These methods of evaluation are undergoing development, as new drugs are developed and as new uses for antagonists are formulated. A special challenge to evaluation methods results from the search for compounds or formulations that are active for extended periods, measured in weeks and months, after single administration.

For the most part, the methods described here have been developed at the Addiction Research Center in Lexington, Kentucky, and modified at the New York Medical College. Particular examples of studies that describe the methods of the Addiction Research Center in detail are found in Martin et al. [4,8] and Jasinski et al. [5,9].

For the New York Medical College studies, reference may be made to Freedman et al. [10], Fink et al. [11], and Zaks et al. [7,12,13]. For recent reviews of the clinical uses, methods of evaluation, and description of narcotic antagonists, see Martin [14], Fraser and Harris [15], or Fink [3].

A special aspect of the evaluation of narcotic antagonists in man is the measure of their electrophysiology. These compounds affect brain function and, to the extent that these effects are generalized in brain functions, they do alter cerebral electrophysiological measures, particularly the resting electroencephalogram, the contingent negative variation, and the sleep electroencephalogram. These specialized measures have been used to define aspects of drug activity in addition to the behavioral and physiological measures described here, such as the thymoleptic, antidepressant activity of cyclazocine [16,17].

IV. SUMMARY

Narcotic antagonists have two principal uses today, the reversal of opiate overdose and the extinction treatment of opiate dependence. Methods for clinical evaluation of experimental compounds for narcotic antagonism have been described, and references to established studies have been given.

REFERENCES

1. W. R. Martin, Pharmacological factors in relapse and the possible use of the narcotic antagonists in treatment. Ill. Med. J. 130:489-494 (1966).

2. A. Wikler, Opiates and opiate antagonists. A review of their mechanisms of action in relation to clinical problems, Public Health Monograph 52. Washington, D. C.: U. S. Govt. Printing Office, 1958.

3. M. Fink, Narcotic antagonists. In National Commission of Marijuana and Drug Abuse, Drug Use in America: Problem in Perspective, Appendix IV. Washington, D. C.: U. S. Govt. Printing Office, 1973, pp. 143-157.

4. W. R. Martin, D. R. Jasinski, and P. A. Mansky, Naltrexone, an antagonist for the treatment of heroin dependence. Arch. Gen. Psychiat. 28:784-791 (1973).

5. D. R. Jasinski, W. R. Martin, and C. A. Haertzen, The human pharmacology and abuse potential of N-allynoroxymorphone (naloxone). J. Pharmacol. Exp. Ther. 157:420-426 (1967).

6. D. J. Finney, Experimental Design and its Statistical Basis. Chicago: Univ. of Chicago Press, 1955.

7. A. Zaks, A. Bruner, M. Fink, and A. M. Freedman, Intravenous diacetylmorphine (heroin) in studies of opiate dependence. Dis. Nerv. Syst. (Suppl.) 30:89-92 (1969).

8. W. R. Martin, C. W. Gorodetzky, and T. K. McClane, An experimental study in the treatment of narcotic addicts with cyclazocine. Clin. Pharmacol. Ther. 7:455-465 (1966).

9. D. R. Jasinski, W. R. Martin, and J. D. Sapira, Antagonism of the subjective, behavioral, pupillary, and respiratory depressant effects of cyclazocine by naloxone. Clin. Pharmacol. Ther. 9:215-222 (1968).

10. A. Freedman, M. Fink, R. Sharoff, and A. Zaks, Clinical studies of cyclazocine in the treatment of narcotic addiction. Amer. J. Psychiat. 124:1499-1504 (1968).

11. M. Fink, A. Zaks, R. Sharoff, A. Mora, A. Bruner, S. Levitt, and A. M. Freedman, Naloxone in heroin dependence. Clin. Pharmacol. Ther. 9:568-577 (1968).

12. A. Zaks, T. Jones, M. Fink, and A. M. Freedman, Naloxone treatment of opiate dependence: A progress report. J. Amer. Med. Ass. 215:2108-2110 (1971).

13. A. Zaks, M. Fink, and A. M. Freedman, Duration of methadone induced cross-tolerance to heroin. Brit. J. Addict. 66:226-229 (1971).

14. W. R. Martin, Opioid antagonists. Pharmacol. Rev. 19:463-521 (1967).

15. H. F. Fraser and L. H. Harris, Narcotic and narcotic-antagonist analgesics. Annu. Rev. Pharmacol. 7:277-300 (1967).

16. M. Fink, Electrophysiology of drugs of dependence. In Chemical and Biological Aspects of Drug Dependence (S. J. Mule and H. Brill, eds.). Cleveland, Ohio: Chemical Rubber Co., 1972, pp. 379-387.

17. M. Fink, J. Simeon, T. M. Itil, and A. M. Freedman, Clinical antidepressant activity of cyclazocine, a narcotic antagonist. Clin. Pharmacol. Ther. 11:41-48 (1970).

Part VI

CHEMICAL AND BIOCHEMICAL TECHNIQUES FOR STUDYING NARCOTIC DRUG ACTION

Chapter 17

METHODS USED IN THE STUDY OF OPIATE RECEPTORS

ERIC J. SIMON

Department of Medicine
New York University Medical Center
New York, New York

I. INTRODUCTION

Less than two years ago, the existence of stereospecific binding sites for opiates in animal brain was reported independently by three laboratories [1-3]. Such binding sites have also been demonstrated in human brain obtained at autopsy [4]. There is now a considerable body of evidence consistent with the view that these sites represent recognition sites for opiates of pharmacological importance. Some authors have referred to these binding sites as opiate receptors. However, the correct definition of a receptor requires that it contain a recognition site for a given drug or hormone as well as a transducing element that permits binding to trigger biochemical reactions leading to the pharmacological effect. The latter has not yet been demonstrated for any of the opiate binding sites studied. We will, nevertheless, occasionally refer to the stereospecific binding sites as receptors for the sake of brevity.

Goldstein and his collaborators [5] have reported the existence of stereospecific binding sites that can be extracted into lipid solvents. They differ from the above-mentioned binding sites in localization, affinity for opiates, and sensitivity to enzymes and reagents.

This chapter describes the methods that have been utilized to date in the study of opiate receptors and mentions some techniques that have proved useful in the study of other receptors and may eventually prove equally useful for opiate receptors.

II. PREPARATION OF LABELED LIGANDS

A number of opiates and opiate antagonists, labeled with tritium at high specific activity (2-30 Ci/mmole), are now available commercially or can be readily obtained by custom labeling from one of the radioisotope supply houses. The preparations are carried out by standard methods of catalytic exchange or reduction of double bonds and are therefore not described here. For descriptions of exchange procedures see Simon et al. [1] and Pert and Snyder [2]. [^{3}H]Etorphine is not yet available commercially but can be prepared as described by Simon et al. [1]. A better preparation involves the reduction with tritium of the double bond in 15,16-dehydroetorphine. Amersham-Searle & Co. is planning to make available [15,16-^{3}H]etorphine in the near future. [^{3}H]Naltrexone (15.3 Ci/mmole) is now available upon request from Dr. Robert Willette, Biomedical Research Branch, National Institute on Drug Abuse, Washington, D. C.

III. PURIFICATION

The radio purity of labeled ligands is assayed by thin-layer chromatography (tlc). Purification is generally done by preparative tlc on silicic acid plates. Table I lists a number of solvent systems used in our laboratory and the R_f values for a number of opiates and opiate antagonists.

I will illustrate purification procedures by the manner in which [^{3}H]-etorphine is purified in our laboratory. Labeled etorphine (10-100 μCi) is spotted on silica gel plates containing fluorescent indicator (E. Merck 60 F 254) under a stream of nitrogen. Unlabeled etorphine (10-30 μg) is spotted in lanes on both sides of the lane containing the radioactive material. The unlabeled etorphine is readily visualized under ultraviolet (uv) light by the quenching of the fluorescence of the indicator. The plates are developed in a suitable solvent system, usually system 1 (Table I), which requires 4-5 hr (solvent front moves 12-15 cm from origin). Plates are removed from the tank and dried in a stream of nitrogen. When barely dry, the etorphine zones are visualized and marked. The silica in the corresponding zone on the [^{3}H]etorphine lane is scraped off the plate and placed overnight in the dark in 5 ml of chloroform-ethanol (3:1). The extract is counted, and purity is checked by chromatography in at least two solvent systems. The solvent is removed from the silica gel by decantation or filtration and evaporated to dryness in a stream of nitrogen. The residue is dissolved in water and diluted to appropriate concentration. The specific activity can be estimated by measuring uv absorption of a suitable solution at 285 nm.

IV. TISSUE PREPARATIONS FOR BINDING STUDIES

Initially, all binding studies were carried out with whole brain homogenates. These were prepared from a variety of animals but most commonly from rats. Male Sprague-Dawley rats (200-300 g) were decapitated by guillotine. The brain was dissected and, once it was established that the cerebellum was devoid of binding capacity, the cerebella were removed. The brain was homogenized at 2 °C in 6-10 volumes per gram wet weight of brain of 0.32 M sucrose in a motor-driven tissue homogenizer (Teflon pestle). These homogenates are readily stored at -20 °C for 1-2 weeks with little loss in binding activity. For binding experiments, the homogenates are thawed and diluted to suitable tissue concentrations (usually 10-40 mg wet weight per milliliter) with 0.05 M tris-HCl buffer, pH 7.4. The hypotonicity breaks the synaptosomes, but the binding sites remain sedimentable and are presumed to be tightly bound to membranes.

TABLE I

Thin-Layer Chromatographic Solvent Systems[a] for Opiates

Opiate	1	2	3	4	5
	R_f values				
Etorphine	0.53	0.73	0.90	0.84	0.85
Naltrexone	0.38	0.75	0.48	0.72	0.56
Naloxone	0.30		0.80	0.86	0.07
Levorphanol	0.53		0.34		0.85
Morphine	0.37	0.54		0.22	0.21

[a] 1, Butanol:acetic acid:water (60:15:25); courtesy of Reckitt and Coleman, Ltd., Hull, England. 2, Ethanol:acetic acid:water (60:30:10); from Cochin and Daly [6]. 3, Methanol:benzene:butanol:water (60:10:15:15); courtesy of New England Nuclear Corp., Boston, Massachusetts. 4, Ethanol:pyridine:dioxane:water (50:20:25:15); from Cochin and Daly [6]. 5, Methanol:chloroform:ammonium hydroxide (25:75:3 drops); courtesy of Research Triangle Institute, Research Triangle Park, North Carolina.

More recently, in our laboratory most binding studies have been performed using rat brain synaptosomal-mitochrondrial fractions (P_2), prepared essentially as described by Gray and Whittaker [7]. A rat brain homogenate (1:10, w/v) in 0.32 M sucrose is centrifuged at 1000 x g for 10 min. The supernatant fluid is removed and the pellet washed once with 0.32 M sucrose at the same centrifugal force. The wash is added to the supernatant and the combined supernatant (S_1) is centrifuged at 17,000 x g for 15 min. The supernatant is discarded and the pellet (P_2) is resuspended in the original volume of sucrose. Upon dilution with tris buffer it is ready for use. This fraction contains over 90% of the binding capacity of the whole homogenate and is equally stable at -20°C.

Pert et al. [8] use a washed homogenate prepared as follows: Rat brains, after removal of cerebella, are homogenized in ice-cold 0.05 M tris-HCl buffer, pH 7.4 (100 ml per gram wet weight), for 20 sec in a Polytron PT-10 homogenizer, 3000 rpm. After centrifugation at 10,000 x g for 10 min, the supernatant fluid is discarded and the pellets are reconstituted in the original volume of tris buffer.

Goldstein and his collaborators [5] perform their binding studies in lipid extracts of mouse brain prepared as follows: Each mouse brain (~500 mg wet weight) is homogenized at room temperature in 9.5 ml of chloroform-methanol (2:1, v/v). After centrifugation, the extract is washed once with 0.2 volume of distilled water and then precipitated with 4 volumes of cold ether. The precipitate is sedimented by centrifugation at 8000 x g for 5 min and redissolved in chloroform-methanol.

V. ASSAYS

A. Assay of Stereospecific Binding on Membranes

1. Centrifugation Techniques

The first use of stereospecific binding as an assay for putative opiate receptors was reported by Goldstein et al. [9] in 1971. These authors incubated mouse brain homogenate with labeled levorphanol in the presence of a 100-fold excess of either unlabeled levorphanol or its inactive enantiomorph, dextrorphan. Since levorphanol blocks both specific and nonspecific binding of [^{3}H]levorphanol, whereas dextrorphan would be expected to block only nonspecific binding, the difference in bonding observed should be a measure of stereospecific binding. The binding assay was carried out as follows: A mouse brain homogenate (10%, w/v) in 0.32 M sucrose in 0.01 M tris-HCl, pH 7.0, was prepared and diluted to give concentrations of 50-150 μg protein/ml. Five-milliliter aliquots were incubated at 25°C in 10-ml polypropylene tubes with 50 μg/ml of unlabeled dextrorphan or levorphanol. Tritiated levorphanol (37.6 μCi/mg, 0.5 μg/ml) was added to the tubes 5 min later and incubation continued for 15 min. Tubes were centrifuged for 1 hr at 105,000 x g. The supernatant fluid was discarded and adhering moisture was removed with absorbent cotton. Pellets were dissolved in 0.1 M NaOH or in Hyamine hydroxide and counted by liquid scintillation. By this technique only about 2% of total radioactivity adhering to the tissue pellet represented stereospecific binding.

Modifications of this technique, which resulted in 50-80% of total binding being stereospecific, were adopted independently in three laboratories [1-3]. These consist of (a) the use of labeled opiates or antagonists with very high specific activities (2-30 Ci/mmole) which permit use of very low drug concentrations (10^{-10}-10^{-8} M) and (b) washing of the homogenates after incubation with cold buffer to remove contaminating unbound and loosely bound radioactivity. The modified sedimentation technique is done as follows: Brain homogenate, 2 ml containing 1-2 mg protein/ml, is incubated at 37°C for 5 min with either unlabeled dextrorphan or levorphanol (10^{-7} or 10^{-6} M). Labeled opiate or antagonist (10^{-10}-10^{-8} M) is added and incubation is continued for 15 min. The homogenate is then sedimented at 20,000 x g for 15 min. The supernatant is removed and the pellets are washed twice with cold 0.05 M tris-HCl buffer, pH 7.4, by resuspension and centrifugation at the same centrifugal force. The washed pellets are transferred to counting vials provided with Teflon-lined screw caps, using 0.3 ml of water in two portions. Protosol (1 ml) is added and digestion is allowed to proceed at 55°C for at least 3 hr. Samples are allowed to cool and 10 ml of Aquasol counting fluid and 3 drops of glacial acetic acid (to minimize chemoluminescence) are added. Samples are counted by liquid scintillation, preferably in a refrigerated counter.

2. Filtration Technique

A rapid filtration technique was introduced by Pert and Snyder [2] which has been found useful for a variety of brain homogenates and fractions. For a given tissue it is necessary to compare the results of filtration with those of sedimentation. Thus, in our studies of opiate receptors in the brain of dog fish (*Mustelus canis*), the filtration technique gave low and erratic results and sedimentation had to be used.*

Brain homogenates or P_2 fractions are diluted with 0.05 M tris buffer to give protein concentrations of 0.5-2 mg/ml. Two-milliliter aliquots are incubated as described for the sedimentation assay. Samples are then filtered through Whatman GF/B glass fiber filters, 24 cm in diameter, and washed twice with 4-ml volumes of ice-cold tris buffer. Filters are dried under an infrared lamp and counted in toluene scintillation cocktail (10 ml) in a liquid scintillation counter. Proteins are determined by the method of Lowry et al. [10]. Results are reported as picomoles drug bound stereospecifically per milligram brain protein.

B. Assay of Stereospecific Binding in Lipid Extracts

The technique used by Lowney et al. [5] for studying stereospecific opiate binding in liquid extracts was adapted from the method used in the laboratory of De Robertis [11]. To tissue extract in chloroform-methanol (50-100 μl), or an equivalent volume of the solvent, is added 1 ml of n-heptane and 1 ml of 0.1 M tris-HCl, pH 7.4. [^{14}C]Levorphanol or [^{3}H]-dextrorphan (aqueous phase concentration 10^{-7}-10^{-6} M) is added to separate samples and allowed to equilibrate between the two phases by three treatments, for 10 sec each, on a Vortex mixer. The tubes are centrifuged for 1 min at 1000 x *g* at room temperature to separate the phases before sampling each phase for radioactivity. The increase in the apparent partition coefficient (organic/aqueous) caused by the tissue extract is the measure of binding. The binding of [^{3}H]dextrorphan is subtracted from the binding of [^{14}C]levorphanol to obtain the amount of stereospecific binding.

*Simon, Sher, and Meilman, unpublished results.

C. Suggested Assays of Stereospecific Binding in Aqueous Solution

When the solubilization of opiate receptors in aqueous media is achieved, special techniques will be required to determine stereospecific binding. A number of techniques have been successfully utilized for other soluble receptors. Because of their potential, but not immediate, application to the opiate receptor field, we shall merely enumerate a number of these techniques with illustrative literature citations.

Equilibrium dialysis has frequently been used for studies of binding of small ligands to soluble proteins. Changeux et al. [12] used it for studies of solubilized acetylcholine receptor. Precipitation with polyethylene glycol followed by Millipore filtration was found useful by Cuatrecasas [13] for solubilized insulin receptor. Filtration through DEAE cellulose discs has been used by several investigators, including Klett et al. [14] studying solubilized acetylcholine receptor. Another frequently used method is gel filtration through a column of Sephadex G-25, which was employed by Lefkowitz et al. [15] for assaying a solubilized catecholamine-binding protein. Finally, ultrafiltration using the recently developed Diaflo membranes (Amicon Corp.) has been reported to be a rapid, sensitive assay for ligand-soluble protein interactions [16,17].

D. Assay for Agonist and Antagonist Properties of Opiates

We reported profound inhibition of stereospecific etorphine binding by increasing concentrations of salt [1], whereas no such effect was observed by Pert and Snyder [2] on naloxone binding. On the basis of these observations, we suggested that this may represent a general difference in the manner in which opiate agonists and antagonists are bound. Pert et al. [8] subsequently showed that, indeed, all agonists tested exhibit reduced binding in the presence of salt, whereas the binding of antagonists is significantly enhanced. They also found that this discriminatory effect is specifically exerted by sodium ions.

When competition of opiate drugs is studied using a labeled "pure" antagonist as the ligand ([^{3}H]naloxone or [^{3}H]naltrexone) the ED_{50} concentration of the competing opiate is increased only slightly or not at all in the presence of 0.1 M NaCl if the latter is also an antagonist. If the competing drug is an agonist, its ED_{50} concentration increases from 10- to 60-fold in 0.1 M sodium chloride, whereas drugs that exhibit mixed agonist-antagonist properties show an intermediate (3- to 7-fold) increase [8,18].

It is therefore possible to obtain an idea of the pharmacology of a new drug with respect to its opiate agonist and/or antagonist potencies by assaying its stereospecific binding to rat brain homogenate in the absence and presence of salt. If the new drug is not available in labeled form, this is done by measuring its competition for binding with a known labeled antagonist, such as [^{3}H]naloxone or [^{3}H]naltrexone. Binding assays are carried out as described previously, in both the presence and absence of 0.1 M NaCl, using 5-6 concentrations of the unknown drug. Percentage of control binding of labeled antagonist is plotted on probit paper against the log of the drug concentration. The concentration of the unknown (ED_{50}), which reduces the binding of the labeled antagonist by 50%, is determined from the plot.

E. Preparation of Affinity Chromatography Beads for Receptor Purification

Purification of receptors is most readily accomplished once the receptor molecules are solubilized in aqueous medium. This has not been achieved at the time this chapter is being written. We have, however, some preliminary results suggesting that membranes containing opiate receptors may be purified by affinity chromatography. Moreover, once opiate-binding molecules are obtained in water solution, affinity beads will be of considerable usefulness for purification. We shall therefore describe several preparations of opiates linked covalently to solid beads, suitable for affinity chromatography.

1. Preparation of Morphine-Sepharose Beads [19]

It is best to couple a drug to its support via a functional group known not to be required for pharmacological activity. The hydroxyl group in position 6 of morphine is such a group. The specific esterification of the 6 position with a succinyl group is readily achieved by refluxing morphine (free base) with excess succinic anhydride for 3 hr in a solvent (20 ml/g) such as benzene (pyridine was used in earlier experiments, but yields and purity of product are better in benzene). After decantation of benzene, the residue is dissolved in water. Unreacted morphine is removed by filtration at pH 9, where succinylmorphine remains in solution. The pH is then adjusted to 5, where 6-succinylmorphine crystallizes at 4°C overnight. The yield is 60-70% of theoretical.

The 6-succinylmorphine is coupled via the free carboxyl group to agarose beads containing side arms ending in free amino groups. Sepharose 4B with hexylamine side arms is now available from Pharmacia (AH-Sepharose 4B). The coupling is done by a procedure similar to that described by Cuatrecases [20] for coupling succinylestradiol to agarose, except that the reaction is carried out in aqueous medium. Fifty milligrams of 6-succinylmorphine (usually tritium labeled to facilitate determination of bound residues) is dissolved in 20 ml of H_2O. The solution is added to 12 ml of AH-Sepharose 4B beads. The pH is adjusted to 5 and 250 mg of 1-ethyl-3-(3-dimethylaminopropyl)carbodiimide is added slowly over 5 min. The pH is monitored frequently and readjusted to 5 with 0.1 N HCl. The reaction is allowed to proceed at room temperature for 20 hr. The beads are washed in a column successively with 1 liter of 0.1 N NaCl/0.01 N tris-HCl, pH 7; 100 ml of 1 N NaCl; and again with 1 liter of NaCl-tris buffer. The yield of morphine bound is 0.1-0.3 μmole/ml of settled beads. The beads are stored with sodium azide (0.025%) and washed extensively immediately before use to remove the azide and small amounts of released morphine.

Morphine-glass beads have been made in an identical manner by using glass beads with alkylamino side arms (GAO-3940, Pierce Chemical Co.).

2. Preparation of Opiates Covalently Attached to Glass Beads by Diazotization

The use of glass beads with side arms that terminate in aromatic amine groups allows the coupling by diazotization of a variety of morphine derivatives. The drugs can be used directly without previous derivatization. The method used is essentially that described by Venter et al. [21] for immobilizing catecholamines.

Glass beads containing alkylamine side chains are obtained from Pierce Chemical Co. (GAO-3940). Arylamino groups are added by the introduction of nitrobenzene groups and subsequent reduction with sodium dithionite as follows: To 1 g of the GAO glass, add 10 ml of a chloroform solution containing 100 mg of p-nitrobenzoyl chloride and 50 mg of triethylamine. The reaction mixture is refluxed for 1 hr; the solution is then decanted and the glass washed three times with chloroform. The glass can be air dried or heated for 30 min at 80°C to remove the chloroform.

The nitrated glass is reduced by adding 10 ml of a 1% aqueous sodium dithionite solution and refluxing for 30-60 min. The reaction solution is decanted and the aromatic amine product is washed three times with water.

The resulting arylamine glass is diazotized and coupled to a drug in the following manner: 10 ml of 2 N HCl are added to 1 g of glass beads in an ice bath followed by 0.25 g of sodium nitrite. The nitrous oxide gas evolved is evacuated by placing the reaction mixture in a vacuum dessicator attached to a water pump for 30 min. The solution is decanted and the beads are washed on a coarse sintered glass filter with large quantities of cold distilled water, followed by cold 1% sulfamic acid and again by cold water.

The diazotized beads are coupled to a drug by adding 5 ml of a solution of the drug (10 mg/ml) to the beads and incubating in ice for 60 min, by which time the beads assume a deep yellow to red color. The color frequently intensifies upon overnight incubation in the refrigerator. The beads are washed on a coarse glass filter with 1 liter of HCl (pH 1) and 1 liter of water. Under these conditions approximately 50 μmoles of drug are bound per gram of beads. The beads are stored at 4°C in 0.1 N HCl as a slurry. This procedure has been used to attach morphine, levorphanol, dextrorphan, and etorphine to the glass beads.

F. Affinity Labeling

One method, which has proved powerful in the isolation of a variety of biological macromolecules and may eventually be exceedingly useful in the isolation and purification of opiate receptors, is affinity labeling. This technique involves the synthesis of molecules closely related to the ligands, in our case opiates, but containing an active chemical group able to form a covalent bond with functional groups at the active binding sites of the receptors. An even more elegant technique is photoaffinity labeling, developed by Westheimer and his collaborators [22], in which molecules are constructed which react with the active site in the usual reversible manner, but which form a covalent bond when irradiated with ultraviolet light.

A photoaffinity labeling derivative of levorphanol has been synthesized by Winter and Goldstein [23]. The structure of this compound, [^{3}H]N-β-(p-azidophenyl)ethylnorlevorphanol, is as follows:

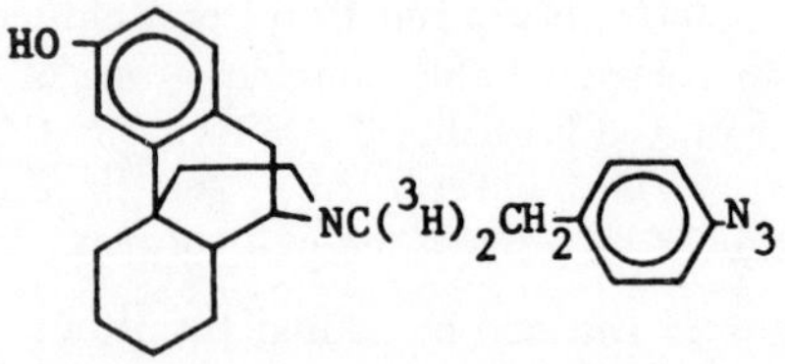

This drug has potent opiate-like pharmacological activity in mice and in the isolated guinea pig ileum. Upon photolysis for 10-15 min in the presence of brain homogenate, using a Hanovia medium-pressure mercury arc lamp, radioactivity was irreversibly incorporated into the particulate matter of the homogenate. To date, no stereospecific blocking of this incorporation has been reported. However, compounds of this kind should be exceedingly useful once suitable conditions for their use have been worked out.

VI. CONCLUDING REMARKS

It is the object of this brief chapter to summarize the more important methods used to date in the study of stereospecific opiate binding sites (receptors). This survey is clearly not exhaustive but presents the investigator who wishes to enter this interesting area of research with enough methods and literature references to get him or her launched in this direction. The field is very active so that new techniques will be introduced or adapted for these studies, even as this chapter is being written and published. A number of techniques expected to be useful in future investigations of opiate receptors have also been enumerated or discussed.

REFERENCES

1. E. J. Simon, J. M. Hiller, and I. Edelman, Proc. Nat. Acad. Sci. U. S. 70:1947 (1973).
2. C. B. Pert and S. H. Snyder, Science 197:1011 (1973).
3. L. Terenius, Acta Pharmacol. Toxicol. 32:317 (1973).
4. J. M. Hiller, J. Pearson, and E. J. Simon, Res. Commun. Chem. Pathol. Pharmacol. 6:1052 (1973).
5. L. I. Lowney, K. Schulz, P. J. Lowery, and A. Goldstein, Science 183:749 (1974).
6. J. Cochin and J. W. Daly, Experientia 18:294 (1961).
7. E. G. Gray and V. P. Whittaker, J. Anat. (London) 96:79 (1962).
8. C. B. Pert, G. Pasternak, and S. H. Snyder, Science 182:1359 (1973).
9. A. Goldstein, L. I. Lowney, and B. K. Pal, Proc. Nat. Acad. Sci. U. S. 68:1742 (1971).
10. O. H. Lowry, N. J. Rosebrough, A. L. Farr, and R. J. Randall, J. Biol. Chem. 193:265 (1951).
11. G. Weber, D. P. Borris, E. De Robertis, F. J. Barrantes, J. L. LaTorre, and M. deCarlin, Mol. Pharmacol. 7:530 (1971).
12. J. P. Changeux, J. C. Meunier, and M. Huchet, Mol. Pharmacol. 7: 538 (1971).
13. P. Cuatrecasas, Proc. Nat. Acad. Sci. U. S. 69:318 (1972).
14. R. P. Klett, B. W. Fulpius, D. Cooper, M. Smith, E. Reich, and L. D. Possani, J. Biol. Chem. 248:6841 (1973).
15. R. J. Lefkowitz, E. Haber, and D. O'Hara, Proc. Nat. Acad. Sci. U. S. 69:2828 (1972).
16. H. Paulus, Anal. Biochem. 32:91 (1969).

17. M. T. Ryan and N. S. Hanna, Anal. Biochem. 40:364 (1971).

18. E. J. Simon, J. M. Hiller, J. Groth, and I. Edelman, J. Pharmacol. Exp. Ther. 192:531 (1975).

19. E. J. Simon, W. P. Dole, and J. M. Hiller, Proc. Nat. Acad. Sci. U. S. 69:1835 (1972).

20. P. Cuatrecasas, J. Biol. Chem. 245:3059 (1970).

21. J. C. Venter, J. E. Dixon, P. R. Maroko, and N. O. Kaplan, Proc. Nat. Acad. Sci. U. S. 69:1141 (1972).

22. A. Singh, E. R. Thornton, and F. H. Westheimer, J. Biol. Chem. 237:PC3006 (1962).

23. B. A. Winter and A. Goldstein, Mol. Pharmacol. 6:601 (1972).

Chapter 18

RADIOIMMUNOASSAY FOR MORPHINE

SYDNEY SPECTOR

Roche Institute of Molecular Biology
Nutley, New Jersey

I. INTRODUCTION

A number of chemical methods have been described for the determination of morphine in biological fluids and tissues. The chemical techniques are photometric procedures involving reactions to detect either a phenolic group or an alkaloid substance [1]. Also available are fluorometric methods [2,3], as well as gas chromatographic procedures [4]. The latter procedures afford far greater sensitivity and specificity for morphine determinations than the photometric methods. However, these methods require extraction procedures or derivatization in order to quantify morphine from biological materials. The pioneering work of Berson and Yalow introduced into the field of endocrinology the radioimmunoassay technique for the measurement of protein and polypeptide hormones. This concept has applicability for smaller molecules; thus, radioimmunoassay principles have been applied for steroid hormones [5-10], cyclic AMP [11,12], digoxin [13-15], and barbiturates [16], to cite a few. These low molecular weight compounds are not antigenic, but it had been demonstrated by Landsteiner [17] that when low molecular weight substances are chemically conjugated to an antigenic substance, the antibodies produced will recognize not only the conjugated molecule, but also the small molecular moiety that is referred to as a haptenic group. There are a number of chemical procedures to covalently link a haptenic group to a large molecular weight carrier substance, and any treatise on organic chemistry affords the reader details for conjugating reactive groups of one molecular with reactive groups of another molecule.

Morphine has a number of sites, C-3, C-6, and the phenol ring, which lend themselves for conjugation to a protein carrier. Morphine was coupled to protein by a carbamido linkage at the C-3 position by first preparing 3-O-carboxymethylmorphine, which was then coupled to bovine serum albumin in the presence of a water-soluble carbodiimide [18]. The alcoholic group of the cyclohexane ring of morphine, C-6, can be, and was, used as a site for conjugating the drug to bovine serum albumin. Succinic anhydride was reacted with morphine in a pyridine solvent and then the succinic acid derivative of morphine in C-6 was conjugated to bovine serum albumin in the presence of a water-soluble carbodiimide. Another immunogen of morphine was prepared by utilizing the phenolic hydroxyl. Morphine was initially diazotized to form 2-(p-aminophenylazo)morphine, which in turn was coupled to the protein carrier. The rationale for preparing these various immunogens of morphine was based on investigations on the preparation of antibodies to steroids. It was found that the specificity of the antibody to the haptenic group is influenced by determinant groups on the haptenic moiety of the immunogen farthest from attachment to the protein carrier. Thus, the morphine molecule was coupled at various sites to a carrier protein with the thought that the various immunogens would stimulate the production of antibodies having different specificities. Figure 1 shows the structures of the three derivatives of morphine used to couple to a protein carrier.

II. PRINCIPLES

The radioimmunoassay technique is based on the principle of a competition between a labeled and unlabeled antigen for a limited number of binding sites on their specific antibodies. The concentration of the antibody is made limiting by appropriate dilution of the antiserum.

Antigen + antibody = antigen-antibody

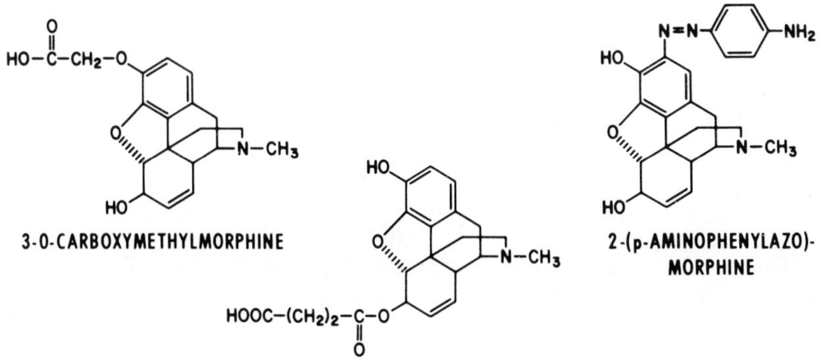

3-O-CARBOXYMETHYLMORPHINE

6-MORPHENYL HEMISUCCINATE

2-(p-AMINOPHENYLAZO)-MORPHINE

FIGURE 1. Morphine derivatives used for preparation of morphine-protein conjugates.

If the antigen is labeled and incubated with antibody, the antigen-antibody complex formed will be labeled. If unlabeled antigen is added to the incubation medium, a competition is established between the labeled and unlabeled antigen for the limited available sites on the antibody, so that the addition of the unlabeled antigen diminishes the radioactivity of the antigen-antibody complex. The degree of competitive inhibition observed in unknown samples is compared with that obtained in known standard solutions. The concentration of morphine in an unknown sample is determined from the observed reduction in binding of labeled morphine by reference to a standard curve.

Antibodies to the various morphine-conjugated protein immunogens were stimulated by injecting an emulsion of the immunogen in complete Freund's adjuvant into the footpads of rabbits. It should be pointed out that goats, guinea pigs, and chickens can also be used to produce antibodies. The rabbits were boosted every few weeks. Serum is then obtained either by a cardiac puncture or from the central ear artery.

The requirements for the antibody depend on the substance to be measured by the assay. If the drug to be measured is administered in high concentrations, then sensitivity may not be that critical a factor; rather, specificity is the attribute sought in assay. However, when low concentrations of the drug may be present in biological fluids because of rapid metabolism, distribution, or excretion of the drug, then one seeks an antibody possessing great sensitivity. Sensitivity is assessed on the basis of (a) the rate of change of the ratio between the labeled drug bound to the antibody and unbound labeled drug and (b) the concentration of the unlabeled drug.

With a sensitive antiserum at hand and a labeled drug with high specific activity, one can consider the development of a radioimmunoassay. The radioimmunoassay can provide information regarding plasma and tissue concentrations of the drug for pharmacokinetic and toxicological studies.

III. METHODS

Since a commercial kit* is available, a protocol is described for measuring morphine in biological fluid (urine or plasma) using the radioimmunoassay kit. To a number of culture tubes (10 mm x 75 mm) one adds 0.1 ml of morphine-positive urine, and to other tubes one adds 0.1 ml of unknown urine. Then, 0.2 ml morphine antibody reagent is added to these tubes and vortexed. The labeled morphine (0.2 ml) is next included in the incubation medium. The tubes are permitted to incubate for a period of 10 min at room temperature. Following the incubation period, 0.5 ml of saturated ammonium sulfate is added to precipitate globulins. Each tube's content is mixed well on a Vortex mixer and then allowed to stand at room temperature for about 10 min. The tubes are centrifuged at about 2000 x g, and 0.5 ml of the supernatant fluid is added to 12 ml of Bray's scintillation counting fluid and counted in a scintillation spectrometer. A standard curve for known concentrations of morphine is concommitantly determined by the same procedure, so that one can plot concentrations of unknown from the standard curve.

The antibody present in the commercial kit is diluted to a concentration so that the labeled hapten saturates all the available binding sites of the antibody. If one effectively elicits morphine antibodies following immunization with the morphine-containing antigen, then the protocol is essentially the same as described above, except that one has to determine the concentrations of antiserum to add to the incubation medium. Various dilutions of antiserum in a 0.1 ml volume are incubated with the labeled morphine so as to give a 50-80% binding of the labeled hapten.

In any consideration of a method, the specificity of the method is of prime importance. The antibodies for the various morphine immunogens will recognize codeine and heroin to the same extent as they do morphine. Thus, substitution on C-3 or C-6 with a methyl group or acetyl groups does not impair the binding to the antibody sites. However, the insertion of a bulky hydrophilic group such as a glucuronide at C-3 markedly diminishes binding to all of the antibodies but to a much lesser extent to the antibodies stimulated by the 6-morphenyl hemisuccinate. The other metabolite of morphine metabolism, normorphine, is recognized by the antibodies generated by the three immunogens to different extents. Antibodies produced by

*Abuscreen-Roche Diagnostics, Division of Hoffman-La Roche Inc., Nutley, New Jersey 07110.

3-O-carboxymethylmorphine recognize the demethylated product of morphine as well as they do morphine; whereas the 6-morphenyl hemisuccinate and 2-(p-aminophenylazo)morphine antibodies require a little over 10 times and 100 times, respectively, the concentration of normorphine to be bound to the same extent.

Antibodies generated by all three immunogens of morphine failed to bind synthetic surrogates of morphine to any extent. In order to determine concentrations of naloxone in biological fluids, we formed an immunogen with naloxone as the haptenic group [19].

The principle of radioimmunoassay has afforded us a technique to measure with great sensitivity and accuracy small molecular weight substances such as morphine.

REFERENCES

1. E. L. Way and T. K. Adler, The Biological Disposition of Morphine and its Surrogates. Geneva, Switzerland: World Health Organization, 1962.

2. H. J. Kupferberg, A. Burkhalter, and E. L. Way, A sensitive flurometric assay for morphine in plasma and brain. J. Pharmacol. Exp. Ther. 145:247 (1964).

3. A. E. Takemori, An ultrasensitive method for the determination of morphine and its application in experiments in vitro and in vivo. Biochem. Pharmacol. 17:1627 (1968).

4. G. R. Wilkensen and E. L. Way, Submicrogram estimation of morphine in biological fluids by gas-liquid chromatography. Biochem. Pharmacol. 18:1435 (1969).

5. S. M. Beiser, B. F. Erlanger, F. J. Agate, and S. Lieberman, Antigenicity of steroid-protein conjugates. Science 129:654 (1959).

6. S. M. Beiser and B. F. Erlanger, Estimation of steroid hormones by an immunochemical technique. Nature (London) 214:1044 (1967).

7. B. F. Erlanger, F. Borek, S. M. Beiser, and S. Lieberman, Steroid protein conjugates: Preparation and characterization of conjugates of bovine serum albumin with progesterone, deoxycorticosterone, and estrone. J. Biol. Chem. 234:1090 (1957).

8. L. Goodfriend and A. H. Sehon, Antigenicity of estrone-protein conjugates. Nature (London) 185:764 (1960).

9. L. Goodfriend and A. H. Sehon, Antibodies to estrone-protein conjugates. Immunochemical studies. Can. J. Biochem. Physiol. 39:941 (1961).

10. S. J. Gross, D. H. Campbell, and H. H. Weetall, Production of antisera to steroids coupled to proteins directly through the phenolic a ring. Immunochemistry 5:55 (1969).

11. A. L. Steiner, D. M. Kipnis, R. Utiger, and C. W. Parker, Radioimmunoassay for the measurement of adenosine 3'5' cyclic phosphate. Proc. Nat. Acad. Sci. U. S. 64:367 (1969).

12. A. L. Steiner, C. W. Parker, and D. M. Kipnis, The measurement of cyclic nucleotide by radioimmunoassay. In Role of Cyclic AMP in Cell Function (P. Greengard and E. Costa, eds.), Vol. 3 of Advances in Biochemistry and Psychopharmacology. New York: Raven Press, 1969.

13. T. W. Smith, V. P. Butler, and E. Haber, Determination of therapeutic and toxic serum digoxin concentrations by radioimmunoassay. N. Engl. J. Med. 281:1212 (1969).

14. T. W. Smith, V. P. Butler, and E. Haber, Characterization of antibodies of high affinity and specificity for the digitalis glycoside digoxin. Biochemistry 9:331 (1970).

15. V. P. Butler, Digoxin radioimmunoassay. Lancet 1:186 (1971).

16. E. J. Flynn and S. Spector, Determination of barbiturate derivatives by radioimmunoassay. J. Pharmacol. Exp. Ther. 181:547 (1972).

17. K. Landsteiner, Specificity of Serological Reactions. Cambridge, Mass.: Harvard Univ. Press, 1946.

18. H. G. Khorana, The chemistry of carbodiimides. Chem. Rev. 53:145 (1953).

19. B. A. Berkowitz, S. H. Ngai, J. Hempstead, and S. Spector, J. Pharmacol. Exp. Ther., in press.

Chapter 19

THE DETERMINATION OF OPIATES IN URINE BY HOMOGENEOUS ENZYME IMMUNOASSAY*

KENNETH E. RUBENSTEIN
RICHARD S. SCHNEIDER
and EDWIN F. ULLMAN

Syva Research Institute
Palo Alto, California

*Contribution no. 56 from the Syva Research Institute.

I. INTRODUCTION

There has been a recent upsurge of interest in determining the presence and amounts of abused drugs, particularly morphine, in biological fluids. Many researchers, toxicologists, and clinical chemists find themselves faced with the task of assaying large numbers of samples, usually urine, with limited funds, limited time, and limited numbers of skilled assistants. Classical techniques involving extraction of the drug followed by spectroscopic or chromatographic identification and quantitation have been found wanting on several grounds (Sec. IV) and are currently giving ground to immunochemical methods, generally known as immunoassay techniques.

These techniques require antibodies that bind tightly to the drug of interest and weakly or not at all to other substances. Any drug can be made to function as a hapten, i.e., a substance that may not be antigenic per se, but becomes so when bound covalently to an appropriate immunogen. Thus, it becomes possible to obtain antibodies to morphine and other drugs such as methadone and phenobarbital. These antibodies are not monospecific and bind with varying strengths to closely related substances. A complete knowledge of the specificity of an antibody preparation is an important prerequisite for its effective utilization in an immunoassay.

A second requirement for an immunoassay is a labeled analog of the drug. The label must be detectable by some means and must be placed so as not to interfere seriously with the binding of the antibody to the drug. In performing an immunoassay one combines a solution suspected of containing the target drug with a limited quantity of the antibody. If some drug is present, it will occupy some fraction of the antibody sites. A measured quantity of the labeled drug must also be present. The more drug present in the sample, the less labeled drug will bind to the antibody. By comparing the amount of label left unbound to the antibody (or conversely the amount bound) with a calibration curve obtained with standards, the amount of drug present in the sample may be estimated.

In the technique known as radioimmunoassay (RIA), described in Chapter 18, the label is a radioactive atom, usually tritium or one of the radioactive isotopes of iodine. In order to distinguish bound labeled drug from free labeled drug, the two must be separated. This may be done, for example, by precipitating the antibody along with bound label or by selective adsorption of unbound low molecular weight compounds. Because of this separation requirement, RIA and related techniques have been termed "heterogeneous" immunoassays [1]. Techniques that feature an intrinsic discrimination between bound and free label, and hence do not require a separation step, called "homogeneous" techniques, have recently been devised. One of these, spin immunoassay [2], uses a stable nitroxide free radical as the label and electron spin resonance (esr) spectrometry as the detection method. The shape of the esr signal produced by a nitroxide radical depends on its mobility. When the labeled drug is bound to an antibody, the label is relatively immobile and the esr signal is broad and weak; when it is free and mobile, the signal is sharp and intense.

Homogeneous enzyme immunoassay utilizes an enzyme as the label. In this method the drug is bound covalently to an enzyme, e.g., lysozyme, amylase, or malate dehydrogenase. The enzyme activity of the enzyme-drug conjugate is inhibited upon complexation with an antibody against the drug (Fig. 1). The mechanism of this inhibition has not yet been fully elucidated, but it is believed in the case of lysozyme that the binding of an antibody to a hapten located near the enzyme active site provides a steric blockade to admission of the enzyme substrate [1]. This is particularly likely in the case of lysozyme, where the substrate is contained on the surface of a bacterium and is thus very large.

The method consists simply of (a) mixing a solution suspected of containing the target drug with a limited quantity of antibody and (b) adding a measured quantity of the enzyme-drug conjugate. A portion of the latter binds to any unoccupied antibody and is rendered inactive. The portion of conjugate left unbound is determined by measuring the enzyme activity of the solution. One then relates that activity to the amount of drug present in the sample by means of standards.

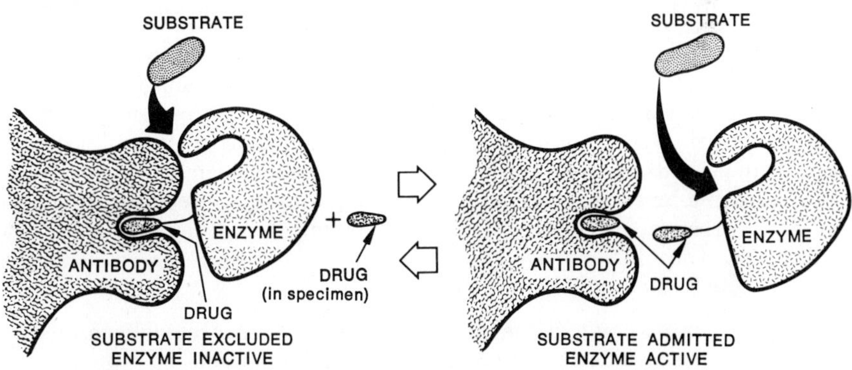

FIGURE 1. Principle of homogeneous enzyme immunoassay.

The method to be described is for the semiautomated assay of opiates in urine and utilizes the enzyme lysozyme. A completely automated assay and an assay applicable to serum and saliva have been developed and will be described in the near future.

II. DESCRIPTION OF THE METHOD

A. Instrumentation

The assay consists of combining measured volumes of sample and reagents, and determining the lysozyme activity. Lysozyme catalyzes the hydrolytic cleavage of the mucopeptide layer of bacterial cell walls, a process that leads to lysis of the bacteria. Lysis results in clearing of an initially turbid bacterial suspension. The rate of clearing, which is traditionally measured with a spectrophotometer at 436 nm, is proportional to the enzyme activity and, in the present case, to the amount of drug present in the sample. Since plots of turbidity against time for such a lysozyme assay are not linear, timing becomes important. The intervals between starting the reaction, introducing the sample into the instrument, attainment of assay temperature, initial measurement, and final measurement must be held constant.

The following instrument package has proved adequate to satisfy these requirements.

Spectrophotometer. A Gilford Model 300-N is employed with a Model 3017 ThermoCuvette, an electrically heated 0.5-ml cuvet that is operated at 37°C. Alternatively, a Bausch and Lomb Spectronic 100 or a Beckman 24/25 may be used.

Printer. An automatic printer (Model 5B069, Syva Company) is used which provides direct digital readout in optical density difference (ΔOD) units and permits entry of sample identification numbers. Upon introduction of the sample into the spectrophotometer, the printer begins a sequence that includes a brief delay for temperature equilibration, recording of an initial absorbance, recording of absorbance after 40 sec, and automatic calculation of the difference. The latter number may be compared directly with the standard curve (see below).

Diluter/pipet. An instrument is employed that can precisely sample 50 μl of solution and deliver it along with 250 μl of buffer.

B. Reagents*

Lysozyme-morphine conjugate. The conjugate is prepared from O^3-carboxymethylmorphine and lysozyme [1], and contains 4-5 morphines per enzyme molecule. A solution of this conjugate is prepared that contains sufficient enzyme in 50 μl for one assay (reagent B).

Antibody. The opiate antibody is prepared by injection of a bovine serum albumin conjugate of morphine into any of a variety of animals, usually sheep. Both the enzyme conjugate and the antibody are stable for at least 1 year if kept at 4°C. The concentration of the antibody solution (reagent A) is likewise adjusted to provide sufficient antibody in 50 μl for one assay.

Buffer. A tris-maleate buffer, pH 6.0, is employed.

Substrate. Nonpathogenic bacteria, *Micrococcus luteus*, are employed. A suspension is prepared by adding 100 ml of the buffer to 75 mg of the lyophilized powder in a clean plastic bottle and shaking the mixture vigorously for at least 30 sec. The suspension should be stored in the refrigerator for at least 12 hr prior to use and remains usable for 7 days if kept refrigerated.

Calibration standards. Stable lyophilized powders are prepared from solutions of drugs in pooled human urine collected from healthy drug-free adults. Four calibrators are employed which, when reconstituted, contain, respectively, 0, 0.5, 5.0, and 50.0 μg/ml of morphine as well as quantities of other drugs including methadone, amphetamine, secobarbital, and benzoyl ecgonine. The other drugs permit use of the same calibrators for other assays and do not interfere with the morphine assay. After reconstitution, the calibrators are stable for 14 days with refrigeration.

Urine specimen. Untreated urine is employed in the assay. Addition of preservatives is not recommended since their effect on the assay has not been established. For optimal results the pH of the urine should fall between 5.5 and 8.0. Samples that are aged more than 7 days at ambient temperature or 20 days in the refrigerator may become more alkaline than pH 8. If necessary, samples may be neutralized with 1 M HCl.

C. Procedure

The procedure will be given in general form only. In principle, the assay can be performed with a wide variety of instrumentation, but in

*These are proprietary reagents supplied by Syva Company under the trademark EMIT.

practice users have encountered various difficulties in attempting to adapt their own instrumentation for use with the assay system. Therefore, the following procedure is intended only to acquaint the reader with the types of manipulations required.

Step 1. The wavelength of the spectrophotometer is set at 436 nm, the cuvet temperature at 37°C, and the diluter/pipet is primed with buffer.

Step 2. Disposable 1-ml plastic beakers (not all brands are satisfactory) are filled with 0.2 ml each of bacteria suspension.

Step 3. Fifty microliters of negative calibrator and 250 μl of buffer are transferred into a sample cup by means of the diluter/pipet. The force of the stream on discharge is sufficient to mix the solutions.

Step 4. In the same way, 50 μl of the antibody solution (reagent A) is transferred to the same beaker.

Step 5. Then 50 μl of the enzyme solution (reagent B) is transferred.

Step 6. Within 5 sec after completing step 5, the sample must be aspirated into the spectrophotometer flowcell. After a brief delay (preferably less than 10 sec) for temperature equilibration, the initial absorbance is recorded. After another 40 sec, the final absorbance is taken and the difference (ΔOD) between the two numbers is determined.

Step 7. A standard curve is obtained by repeating the above procedure with the 0.5, 5.0, and 50.0 μg/ml calibrators. It is convenient to plot the ΔOD readings vs the log of the drug concentration.

Step 8. The procedure is repeated with the urine sample to be assayed. The drug concentration corresponding to the observed ΔOD reading is read from the standard curve.

D. Assay Performance

A typical standard curve (Fig. 2) suggests that the morphine assay could detect as little as 0.1 μg/ml morphine. In practice, however, sensitivity is limited by urine-to-urine background variation. A histogram showing the results from a study in which 100 drug-free urine samples were assayed before and after spiking with morphine to a concentration of 0.5 μg/ml illustrates this point (Fig. 3). All of the normal urines give readings corresponding to 0.25 μg/ml or less of morphine. The morphine-spiked urines give values ranging from 0.3 to 0.7 μg/ml with a mean of 0.49 μg morphine/ml. Thus, readings in excess of 0.3 μg/ml morphine can safely

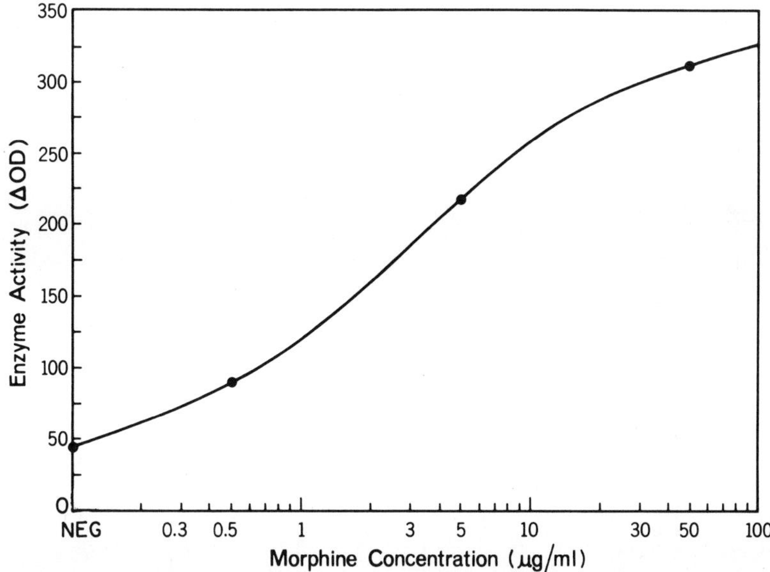

FIGURE 2. Typical standard curve for the assay of opiates in urine.

be assumed to indicate the presence of morphine and readings below this value indicate that less than 0.5 μg/ml morphine is present, each with greater than 95% certainty. We refer to 0.3 μg/ml as the "cutoff" value, below which samples should be considered negative. In practice 0.5 μg/ml is frequently used as the cutoff. At this value more than 95% of the samples containing greater than 0.7 μg/ml morphine are detected. Depending on the user's needs, the cutoff may be raised or lowered as long as he is cognizant that the lower the cutoff, the greater will be the incidence of false positive results.

A possible source of error arises from the presence of abnormally high concentrations of lysozyme in a small percentage of urine samples. Endogenous lysozyme will add to the observed enzyme activity and can give a false positive result. With 0.5 μg/ml as the cutoff the incidence of false positives is only about 1%. If this is unacceptable, the user can run blanks on samples giving values in excess of the cutoff level. A blank is run just like an assay except that the antibody and enzyme solutions are replaced by buffer. The blank ΔOD reading is then subtracted from the assay reading. Data relating to the reliability of the assay have been published [3].

The specificity of any immunoassay depends much more on the antibody than on the nature of the label. All antibodies exhibit some degree of

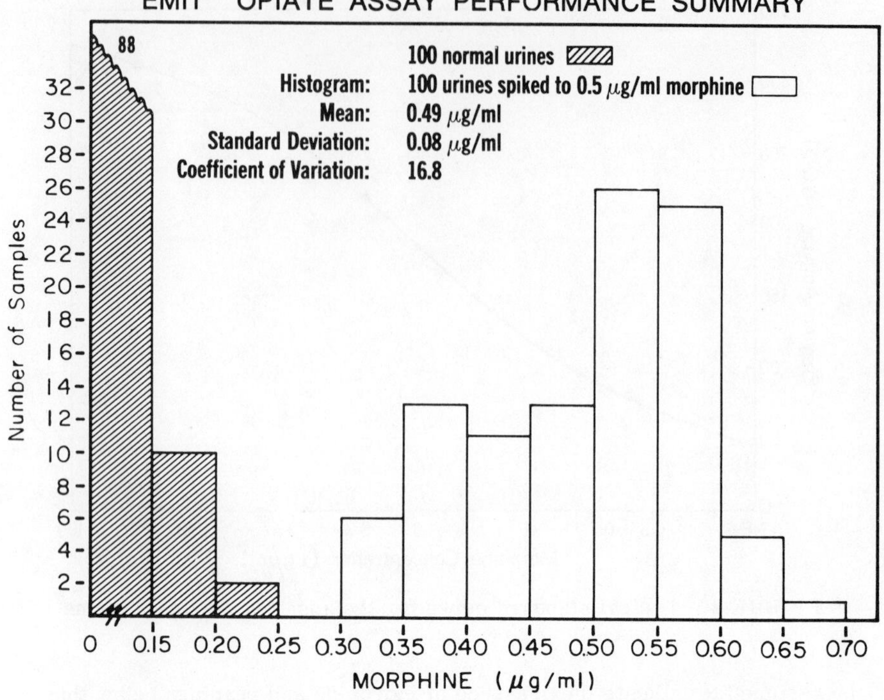

FIGURE 3. Performance summary for the assay of opiates in urine.

cross-reactivity. For example, the present morphine assay is highly sensitive to morphine, morphine glucuronide, and codeine (Table I). Heroin and nalorphine are moderately cross-reactive, and other opiate-like substances and nonrelated drugs do not interfere significantly. The high sensitivity to morphine glucuronide can be considered a plus factor in detecting morphine usage since the major part of metabolized morphine is excreted in this form. Experiments performed with urine samples from subjects taking usual doses of the slightly cross-reacting drugs chlorpromazine and dextromethorphan showed no interference at the 0.5 μg/ml cutoff level [3].

E. Pitfalls and Precautions

As mentioned earlier, the user must be cognizant of the occasional incidence of elevated lysozyme levels in urine samples. The user should also be aware that certain surfaces may absorb the enzyme. This is particularly true of the plastic tips supplied with some diluters. Control of pH

TABLE I

Reactivity of Some Drugs in the Opiate Assay

Drug	Concentration[a] (μg/ml)
Codeine	0.35
Morphine	0.5
Nalorphine	5.5
Heroin	5.5
Meperidine	55
Dextromethorphan	150
Diphenoxylate	>1000
Chlorpromazine	200
Naloxone	200
Methadone	>1000
Dextropropoxyphene	>1000
α-Acetylmethadol	>1000

[a]Concentration of the drug in aqueous solution that gives a response equivalent to 0.5 μg morphine/ml.

within narrow limits is essential for obtaining valid results. Since, as mentioned, aged urine samples often become rather alkaline, due care must be taken to see that the buffer strength is not overrun. The use of buffers with higher ionic strength is not recommended since lysozyme activity decreases with increasing ionic strength. Also, it is well to remember that the optical density of the bacterial suspension during lysis is a nonlinear function of time. Consequently, it is important to control rather strictly the time intervals between adding the enzyme to the assay mixture, introducing the sample into the cuvette, taking the initial measurement, and taking the final measurement.

III. TYPES OF DATA OBTAINABLE

The assay for opiates in urine that has been described is designed to establish whether the subject has recently taken an opiate. It is usually capable of detecting opiates from 24 to 48 hr following injection. It does not distinguish among the several opiates that bind strongly to the antibody nor between morphine and its major metabolite, the glucuronide. Consequently, the assay has proved highly useful in drug rehabilitation programs where it is desirable to know whether the subject has been using opiates in any form. It can be considered only a semiquantitative assay, since the magnitude of the assay response depends not only on the amount of drug present but on the ratios of the various metabolites. Good quantitative results may be obtained if the technique is applied to urine samples or extracts containing morphine as the only opiate.

IV. COMPARISON WITH OTHER TECHNIQUES

The techniques available for assaying opiates in urine fall into the categories of immunological and nonimmunological. In general, the former are more sensitive than the latter. They require no prior extraction or concentration of the drug and hence are less costly in terms of manpower. They detect morphine glucuronide as well as morphine, a distinct advantage since some samples contain virtually no free morphine. Although other opiates are weakly detected, the cross-reactivity problem has been well defined and provides no serious impediment to obtaining results that are reliable within clearly defined limits.

The spin immunoassay technique [2], known commercially by the trade name FRAT, is a homogeneous technique requiring no sample manipulation beyond combining reagents. It found intensive and successful application in urine screening by the U. S. military starting in 1971 in Vietnam. The sensitivity and other performance parameters are quite similar to those of the enzyme system and, like the enzyme system, it can be used to assay for barbiturates, methadone, amphetamine, and cocaine metabolite. The relatively high cost and lack of general utility of electron spin resonance spectrometers have so far limited the application of spin immunoassay to large volume users.

Radioimmunoassay [4] is a heterogeneous technique. After combining sample and reagents it is necessary to precipitate proteins to centrifuge out the precipitate, and remove the supernatant without disturbing the pellet. When large numbers of samples are assayed batchwise, the time per assay becomes quite reasonable; however, a single sample along with standards takes about 1 hr as compared to 5 min for the enzyme method. Of the two methods, RIA is currently the more sensitive; however, modified enzyme immunoassays using different enzymes have been found to offer sensitivity comparable to that of the RIA assay. Additionally, the known hazards associated with radioactive materials require special controls to comply with government regulations and ensure safety.

The last of the immunological methods to be discussed is hemagglutination inhibition (HI) [5]. Hemagglutination inhibition relies on the ability of antibodies to agglutinate (clump) red blood cells labeled with the substance of interest. Agglutination, or lack of it, is determined by visual examination and, hence, in borderline cases requires that a subjective decision be made. A single determination gives a yes or no answer to the question of whether the drug is present in excess of a particular cutoff level. Like RIA, over an hour is required for a single assay. The method is subject to interference from other substances present in biological fluids that can agglutinate red blood cells. Hemagglutination inhibition has so far failed to gain widespread acceptance due, presumably, to the erratic performance of commercial products.

The rapid nonimmunological techniques are generally characterized by low reagent costs coupled with low reliability or long assay times requiring inefficient utilization of expensive equipment. The chromatographic methods, while qualitative, have the potential advantage of identifying several substances in a single operation.

Thin-layer chromatography (tlc) is the most widely used of these methods [6]. Whereas equipment and reagent costs are quite low, the time and degree of skill required are rather high. Posttreatment of the plates with various reagents can increase the objectivity of identification. However, the morphine spot is sometimes obscured by other substances and the reliability and sensitivity of the assay are far less than those of immunochemical techniques.

Gas chromatography (gc) is similar in many respects to tlc, although it is much more reliable. Equipment costs are in the moderate range. The major serious disadvantage is the time required for a single assay (10-20 min), which remains constant no matter how many samples are to be analyzed. Despite this fact, gc has proved useful as a confirmatory technique for immunoassays.

Fluorescence methods comprising extraction of morphine and conversion to fluorescent materials have also been used. Both semiautomated [7] and fully automated [8] versions are available, with instrumentation costs being quite high ($20,000) for the latter. Major problems of these assays include their insensitivity to morphine glucuronide and interference by fluorogenic materials in urine.

A combination of gas chromatography and mass spectrometry [9] has been applied to the analysis of morphine in urine with excellent results in terms of both sensitivity and reliability. Major disadvantages are high cost (around $100,000), low throughput (around 15 min per sample), and high level of operator skill required.

V. CONCLUSION

Homogeneous enzyme immunoassay is a powerful tool for assaying haptens in biological fluids. In addition to opiates, assays for methadone, barbiturates, amphetamines, and benzoyl ecgonine (cocaine metabolite) in urine are available.

The technique is not limited to urine. Assays for opiates in both serum and saliva have been devised and data will be published shortly. The latter assay utilizes malate dehydrogenase as the enzyme and can detect as little as 5 ng/ml morphine in saliva with a high level of confidence. This 100-fold increase in sensitivity over the lysozyme system, which is by no means a limit, opens new vistas for the enzyme technique. A great many drugs and hormones of interest both to clinicians and researchers will someday be assayed with this convenient and accurate method.

REFERENCES

1. K. E. Rubenstein, R. S. Schneider, and E. F. Ullman, Biochem. Biophys. Res. Commun. 47:846 (1972).
2. R. K. Leute, E. F. Ullman, and A. Goldstein, J. Amer. Med. Ass. 221:1231 (1972).
3. R. S. Schneider, P. Lindquist, E. T. Wong, K. E. Rubenstein, and E. F. Ullman, Clin. Chem. 19:821 (1973).
4. D. H. Catlin, R. Cleeland, and E. A. Grunberg, Clin. Chem. 19:216 (1973).
5. F. L. Adler, C. T. Lin, and D. H. Catlin, Clin. Immunol. Immunopathol. 1:53 (1972).
6. B. Davidow, N. KiPetri, and B. Quame, Amer. J. Clin. Pathol. 50:714 (1968).
7. S. Mulé and P. L. Hushin, Anal. Chem. 43:708 (1971).
8. D. J. Blackmore, A. S. Curry, T. S. Hayes, and E. R. Rutter, Clin. Chem. 17:896 (1971).
9. R. Foltz and P. Clark, Clin. Chem., in press.

AUTHOR INDEX

Numbers in brackets are reference numbers and indicate that an author's work is referred to although his name is not cited in the text. Underlined numbers give the page on which the complete reference is listed.

C

H

SUBJECT INDEX

L

M

S